Healing the Inner City Child

Healing the Inner City Child
Creative Arts Therapies with At-risk Youth

Edited by Vanessa A. Camilleri

1/08

Jessica Kingsley Publishers
London and Philadelphia

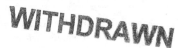

First published in 2007
by Jessica Kingsley Publishers
116 Pentonville Road
London N1 9JB, UK
and
400 Market Street, Suite 400
Philadelphia, PA 19106, USA

www.jkp.com

Library of Congress Cataloging in Publication Data
A CIP catalog record for this book is available from the Library of Congress

British Library Cataloguing in Publication Data
A CIP catalogue record for this book is available from the British Library

ISBN 978 1 84310 824 5

Printed and bound in the United States by Thomson-Shore, Inc.

To the children we serve.
With thanks for the gifts they offer.

"Perhaps there is more understanding and beauty in life when the glaring sunlight is softened by the patterns of shadows. Perhaps there is more depth in a relationship that has weathered some storms. Experience that never disappoints or saddens or stirs up feeling is a bland experience with little challenge or variation in color. Perhaps when we experience confidence and faith and hope…this builds up within us a feeling of inner strength, courage, and security."

Virginia M. Axline, *Dibs In Search of Self*

Acknowledgements

I would like to personally thank all the authors who have contributed their unique perspectives to this book. They each added personal, professional and creative experiences to this compilation which have combined to create a diverse and highly inspiring publication.

I would like to thank the many people who have guided and advised me personally through this process – specifically the following people who read portions of the manuscript and provided invaluable feedback: Barbara Hesser, MCT, Director of Music Therapy at New York University; Ken Aigen, DA, MT-BC, NRMT, Co-Director of the Nordoff-Robbins Center for Music Therapy at New York University; James Garbarino, PhD and Macude C. Clarke, Chair in Humanistic Psychology at Loyola University; and Lisa Edwards, PhD, Assistant Professor in the Department of Counseling and Educational Psychology at Marquette University. I would also like to thank George Murer and Barrie Trimmingham for their guidance.

I would like to thank Dr Flaum Cruz, PhD, ADTR, Editor-in-Chief of the international journal *The Arts in Psychotherapy* for reading and endorsing this manuscript. Dr Flaum Cruz is Vice-President of the American Dance Therapy Association and Associate Professor and Coordinator of Dance Therapy in the Expressive Therapies Division at Lesley University in Cambridge, Massachusetts. Her voice is respected and well recognized in the creative arts therapies community.

I would like to thank Jessica Kingsley Publishers for their attention and responsiveness during the editing process. I thank them for providing me with the opportunity to give voice to these inspiring accounts.

I would like to thank my husband, Steve, and my family and friends for their patience and encouragement during this process.

Lastly, I would like to thank all the children, named and unnamed, who have allowed us the privilege of helping them heal.

Vanessa A. Camilleri

Contents

Figures and tables

Preface

This book emerged out of a desire to highlight an often under-served population and a mission to promote a thriving profession. After working with inner city, at-risk children as a music therapist for ten years in New York City and Washington DC, I have a clear understanding of their needs and a clear vision of how the creative arts therapies are uniquely suited to address them. The complexities faced by inner city children are overwhelming when taken as larger societal issues, but are extremely basic when broken down into the individual needs of each child: to be fed, loved, and heard.

This book describes the lives of children growing up in some of the most dazzling, yet notorious cities in the world: New York, Chicago, San Francisco, Washington DC, New Orleans, Philadelphia, Calcutta, and Melbourne. This international compilation crystalizes the fact that common challenges, needs and outcomes exist, no matter which city a child grows up in. As we will see, the creative arts therapies can address and positively impact on children no matter what their location or their specific situation.

Part I gives detailed information about the context in which these children live. While the research and statistics used are specific to the United States, the issues outlined can be recognized internationally. Describing life in the inner city proved challenging as so many of the processes are cyclical in nature. Specific societal, environmental, and domestic stressors are described with an emphasis on community and family deterioration as an inevitable fact of daily life. Behavioral and emotional outcomes for at-risk children living in the inner city are described, as well as moderating factors that counteract the ills. Part I ends with a description of specific therapeutic interventions that are relevant to this population as well as a description of the goals and processes that are common to the creative arts therapies.

Complex global trends have created a mounting mental health crisis, placing thousands of inner city children at risk of negative consequences. Part II compiles a diverse and practical selection of creative arts therapies approaches that meet the ever-increasing needs of inner city children. With attention to pervasive stressors faced by this population, the authors address deficits in important developmental indicators that dispose children to crippling social, emotional, and behavioral outcomes. Through the disciplined use of music, art, drama, and dance therapy, with attention to relevant research and an awareness of current psychoeducational trends, this book builds a compelling case for the use of creative arts therapies with inner city, at-risk children.

Despite the necessary description of a generalized context, it is essential to view each child as a unique individual. It becomes clear that the children described here are so much more than the sum of the obstacles they face and the negative outcomes they present. These at once challenging and inspiring accounts highlight the resilience of children and the perseverance of creative arts therapists, social workers, and educators who truly believe in the human ability to heal.

Ideal for creative arts therapists, psychologists, social workers, and educators, this book offers a range of detailed information for those interested in improving the lives of children growing up in inner cities, using relevant research, case studies, intervention descriptions, and theoretical discussions. It is my hope that this publication will go forth into the world of the helping professions to serve as a tool for professionals who will touch the lives of countless children in need.

Vanessa A. Camilleri

PART 1

Setting the Scene

CHAPTER I

The Inner City

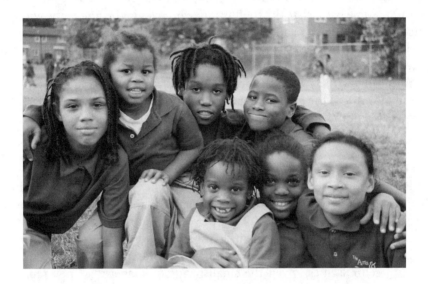

In the United States, large cities such as New York, Chicago, Washington DC, and Los Angeles are known as Metropolitan Areas (MA). An MA is defined by the US Census Bureau (July 2001) as being "a core area containing a large population nucleus, together with adjacent communities having a high degree of economic and social integration with that core". Most are based around primary central cities containing 50,000 or more inhabitants, with a population density of at least 1,000 people per square mile.

For the purpose of this book, the term "inner city" will be used interchangeably to describe central cities. As we shall see through the course of this book, inner cities are at times plagued with seemingly insurmountable conditions such as violence and racism, which create layers of obstacles preventing people from leading happy, safe, and successful lives. Ironically, many families migrate from rural areas within the United States, or immigrate from overseas to over-crowded inner cities with the hope of finding work, community and prosperity. What they often find instead is unemployment and poverty.

Not only do some inner city families lack basic material resources such as food, shelter, and healthcare, they also have inadequate access to community resources such as good schools, safe neighborhoods, and government services. In these resource-poor environments, seemingly mild physical or psychological vulnerabilities may escalate into more serious disorders for lack of treatment.

As described by Garbarino (1997), many children today are growing up in "socially toxic environments" (p.13) that are plagued with violence, poverty, trauma, depression, and alienation. These environments threaten human well-being, survival, and development, and demoralize families and communities. Below are some basic statistics to illustrate who lives in the inner city, with particular emphasis on the children who reside there. In the following chapters, the specific challenges that they face, as well as the outcomes that they demonstrate, will be described in detail.

According to the year 2000 Census of Population and Housing (US Census Bureau May 2001) the total population of the United States was 281,421,906. Thirty per cent of the total population lived in central cities. Of those people living in central cities, 51 per cent were white, 21 per cent were African-American, 19 per cent were Hispanic, and five per cent were Asian. Thirty per cent of inner city residents were under the age of 19.

Furthermore, according to Proctor and Dalaker of the US Census Bureau (September 2003) of the 12.1 per cent of people living at or below the poverty level in the United States in 2002, 40 per cent lived in inner cities – bringing the percentage of inner city residents living in poverty to 16.7 per cent. There is a disproportionately large concentration of poor families, especially children, living in central cities, given the small geographic area that they represent. Using poverty as one of the many risk-factors faced by children, it is clear that many at-risk children live in inner cities.

References

Garbarino, J. (1997) 'Educating children in a socially toxic environment.' *Educational Leadership* 54, 7, 12–16.

Proctor, B. D. and Dalaker, J. (September 2003) Poverty in the United States: 2002. Current Population Reports: Consumer Income, pp.60–222. Washington, DC: US Census Bureau.

US Census Bureau (May 2001) *Profiles of General Demographic Characteristics: 2000 Census of Population and Housing.* Washington DC.

US Census Bureau (July 2001) *Metropolitan Areas: Cartographic Boundary Files Descriptions, and Metadata.* Cartographic Boundary Files. Washington, DC.

CHAPTER 2

At-risk Children

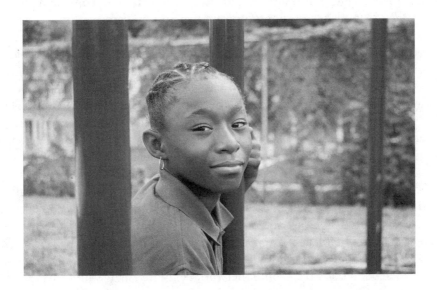

The term "at risk" is defined in different ways, depending on which field you approach it from. For the purpose of this book, "at risk" will be defined as being "in danger of negative future events" (McWhirter *et al.* 1998, p.7). These events, or their outcomes, can include depression, educational failure, addiction, unemployment, incarceration, poverty, or death, and are a result of a complex and often correlated set of risk factors. The children described here are at risk of enduring potentially damaging consequences should intervention not take place. Children become at risk as a result of exposure to risk factors. With information about risk factors and their outcomes, counselors and educators can work to prevent children from becoming victims of their circumstances.

Risk factors or stressors have been described by Attar, Guerra, and Tolan (1994), as being classified into two types, chronic and discrete. Chronic stressors are pervasive within entire communities and affect all inhabitants in that area. Examples in urban areas include poverty, unemployment, limited community resources, weak social support networks, substandard housing, and high crime rates. Discrete stressors occur within particular families and affect the people in that household alone. Examples include the death of a family member, divorce, or relocation.

As described by McWhirter *et al.* (1998), as stressors accumulate in a child's life, he becomes more at risk of negative outcomes. Often, risk factors are bundled, one leading to another in a vicious cycle. This "accumulation of risk model" (Garbarino 2001, p.362), hypothesizes that most children are able to cope with low levels of risk, but once a certain number of risk factors are prevalent in a child's life, there must be structured interventions or consistent moderating factors in place in order to prevent negative outcomes.

McWhirter *et al.* (1998) describe these risk factors or stressors as being a "series of steps along a continuum" (p.7). The first step he identifies is that of having specific demographics, such as living in an impoverished neighborhood, having a low socio-economic status, or being a member of a minority ethnic group. Children are not at risk because of their personal circumstances, but because children with this background often have reduced access to adequate services (school, insurance, housing), and may be victims of personal or material racism. This causes trauma that can affect their quality of life.

The next stressor involves family and school environments. Families and schools that provide caring, nurturing, predictable and safe environments allow children to develop a sense of security and confidence. Families and schools that are chaotic, dangerous, and unpredictable (for example, where there is substance abuse and violence) can provoke feelings of fear and hopelessness. The lack of stable home and school environments reduces access to positive adult role models and potential support networks. Children may want to avoid these situations by skipping school, or to replace them with alternative environments like gangs, which provide a sense of belonging and identity (Garbarino 2001; Batmanghelidjh 1999).

The third stressor is experiencing negative psychosocial or environmental events such as divorce, death, suicide, teenage pregnancy, abuse, incarceration, loss of a job and insurance, and eviction. These can cause psychological trauma and can create physical circumstances such as homelessness, foster care, hunger, poverty, or illness that increase the potential for a child being at risk.

The fourth important factor in determining whether children are at risk, is psychological make-up. Personal characteristics determine how children deal with their circumstances and how they will be affected by them. The more negative their attitudes, the more at risk they will be. Further, if their outlook is hopeless, this can lead to symptoms of depression, anxiety, and aggression, often recognizable as deficits in social skills and coping mechanisms. Negative psychological states can, in addition, lead to dangerous activities and behaviors. These may be self-destructive, or destructive to others. Children may start to skip school, smoke, drink, use drugs, fight, or engage in criminal activity such as theft, mugging, or vandalism. These maladaptive behaviors may result in incarceration, hospitalization, or death.

Each of these circumstances taken alone can lead to children being at risk, but the risk increases as stressors accumulate in a child's life without adequate moderating effects. The more risk factors that the child faces, the more adverse the outcomes will be. These circumstances are not necessarily predictive of children becoming at risk, but make them more vulnerable to negative outcomes, and are factors to look for during evaluation and treatment.

Bryson (September 1997), for the US Census Bureau, has identified six risk factors that can severely impact on outcomes for children. Children living in poverty, in welfare-dependent families, with both parents absent, in single-parent households, with an unmarried mother, or with a parent who has not graduated from high school are considered at high risk for developing problems such as hyperactivity, dropping out of school, becoming pregnant, being unemployed, and becoming involved in criminal activity.

Sawhill and Chadwick (1999) examined four risk factors faced by pre-school age children and determined geographic prevalence. The four risk factors were: having an unmarried mother, having a teen mother, having a mother with educational attainment lower than a high school degree, and living in a family at or below the poverty level. They associated these risk factors with poor adult outcomes such as poverty, unemployment, and dependence on social agencies. They defined children with exposure to at least three of the risk factors as being "high risk" for poor adult outcomes. They found that 50 per cent of high-risk children lived in central cities, as compared with 30 per cent who lived in the suburbs, and 20 per cent who lived in rural areas. When comparing exposure to risk factors of children in cities versus children in the suburbs, it became obvious that children in cities experienced risk factors at about double the rate of children in the suburbs. For example, in 1996 32 per cent of urban children were born to unmarried mothers, as compared with 17 per cent of suburban children. They also found that high-risk inner city children were predominantly of minority backgrounds. Fifty per cent were found to be African-American, 34 per cent were other minorities, and 16 per cent were white.

Kominsky, Jamieson, and Martinez (June 2001) at the US Census Bureau examined the prevalence of risk factors in school-age children in the United States. They identified three personal risk factors – presence of a disability, retention in school (repeating a grade-level for failing to complete all grade-level benchmarks), and not speaking English well. They also identified four familial risk factors – either or both parents being absent from home, at least one foreign-born parent or recent immigration, low family income, and unemployed parents. They found that most school-age children (54 per cent) had no significant risk factors. They also found that 36 per cent of all children had one familial risk factor, and 18 per cent had a personal one. The most common familial risk factor was not living with both parents, and the most common personal risk factor was being retained in school. Taken together, 46 per cent of all children had at least one of the seven risk factors examined here. Of these, 11 per cent were white, 18 per cent were Asian, 27 per cent were Hispanic, and 34 per cent were African-American. Eighteen per cent of all children had more than one risk factor. It was further determined that a higher proportion of children living in central cities had at least one risk factor (59 per cent) as compared with those living in non-metropolitan areas (43 per cent).

Taken together, the above research paints a clear demographic picture of the children described in this book: children often of minority descent, under the age of 18, living in the inner city, faced with significant environmental and domestic stressors, causing them to exhibit serious and often debilitating outcomes.

References

Attar, B. K., Guerra, N.G. and Tolan, P.H. (1994) 'Neighborhood disadvantage, stressful life events, and adjustment in urban elementary school children.' *Journal of Clinical Child Psychiatry 23*, 391–400.

Batmanghelidjh, C. (1999) 'Whose political correction? The challenge of therapeutic work with inner city children experiencing deprivation.' *Psychodynamic Counseling 5*, 2, 231–244.

Bryson, K. (September 1997) *America's Children at Risk.* Census Brief, CENBR/97–2. Washington DC: US Census Bureau.

Garbarino, J. (2001) 'An ecological perspective on the effects of violence on children.' *Journal of Community Psychology 29*, 3, 361–378.

Kominski, R., Jamieson, A., and Martinez, G. (June 2001) *At-risk Conditions of US School-age Children.* Working Paper Series No. 52. Washington, DC: US Census Bureau.

McWhirter, J.J., McWhirter, B.T., McWhirter, A.M., and McWhirter, E.H. (1998) *At-Risk Youth: A Comprehensive Response.* Pacific Grove, California: Brooks/Cole Publishing Company.

Sawhill, I. and Chadwick, L. (1999) *Children in Cities: Uncertain Futures.* Survey Series. Washington DC: The Brookings Institution, Center on Urban & Metropolitan Policy.

CHAPTER 3

Challenges Faced by At-risk Children in the Inner City

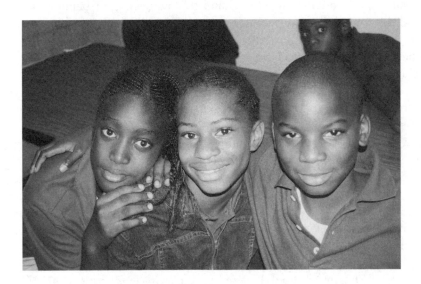

The complex challenges faced by inner city children cause many children to become at risk. Despite the discrete headings below, most stressors are bundled and occur simultaneously. Many of the stressors described here occur in conjunction with associated outcomes and vice versa, making causality difficult to determine. None of the challenges and outcomes present in the lives of inner city children happen in a vacuum, and all are intricately related, often occurring in cycles.

3.1 Societal stressors

a. Racism

In the United States, institutionalized racism continues to exist in domains such as housing, education, and employment. Overt and intentional discriminatory acts are less common than they were historically; however, covert racism is still rampant in schools which lack funding, companies which lack a diverse workforce, and segregated neighborhoods with few resources. Living in a society where advantages are more accessible to the dominant white majority creates a demoralizing situation which takes a toll on some minority groups who are trying to compete in such an environment. Some children see the larger society and the opportunities it presents as unattainable. The lack of role models and successful adults in their own lives leads them to believe that society has largely abandoned them (Halpern 1992). Lacking positive reflections of the self causes some children to internalize feelings of self-hate, which prevents success and achievement.

Simons *et al.* (2002) studied the causes of depressive symptoms among African-American children. They found that witnessing or being a victim of racial discrimination was positively correlated with depressive symptoms in this population. They showed that experiences such as hearing racial slurs, police harassment, physical threats, disrespectful treatment by retail employees, exclusion from social activities, or false accusations by authority figures had a negative impact on the mental health of children. Children tended to internalize these negative experiences, which had detrimental effects on self-worth and self-concept.

When minority authors are omitted from college curricula, racial slurs are used in every day conversations, or people cross the street when they see an African-American male approaching, very clear messages are sent about the status of minorities in our society. Such an atmosphere creates tension, fear, and alienation, which are based on stereotypes and assumptions. Owing to a system of advantages that exists in the United States (Wellman 1977), minorities are at a constant disadvantage when it comes to housing, education, healthcare, and employment. As described by Tatum (1997), "institutionalized racism results in the loss of human potential, lowered productivity (and) stifles…growth and development" (p.200). Racism is a societal stressor that many inner city children have to contend with and will continue to battle as they attempt to complete their education, find employment, and become home owners.

b. Poverty

Living in poverty is stigmatizing and demoralizing. It leaves individuals vulnerable and often unable to adequately cope with additional stressors that arise owing to poverty. This vulnerability often leads to severe psychological distress, creating a cycle of despair. Poverty often comes with visible and humiliating external indicators such as living in a housing project or homeless shelter, using food stamps, or not having adequate material possessions. For children living in poverty, these experiences can have devastating emotional and behavioral consequences.

According to the US Census Bureau (Proctor and Dalaker 2003), the total poverty rate in 2002 was 12.1 per cent, and the poverty rate for children under the age of 17 was 16.7 per cent. According to the US Department of Education (2003), 24 per cent of all school-age children living in poverty resided in inner cities. However, poverty rates for young children in many large cities exceeded this percentage. According to the National Center for Children in Poverty (NCCP) (August 2003) 64 per cent of Hispanic children lived in poverty, 57 per cent of African-American children lived in poverty and 34 per cent of white children lived in poverty. A child living in poverty is defined as lacking basic items considered essential to human well-being such as food, clothing, and shelter and is poor by virtue of her family's economic situation.

As described by the National Center for Children in Poverty (1996), there are clear predictors that a child will grow up in poverty. Poverty is most likely in homes headed by single or teenage mothers, where parents have achieved a low educational level, where parents are unemployed, and in families of minority status. Slow economic growth, widening economic inequality, an increase in families headed by females, an increase in family size, and increasing unemployment rates are pushing more and more families into poverty.

The risk of poverty is highest among those who are unemployed and second highest among the working poor, especially in single-parent families where the parent is earning the minimum wage. The number of children growing up in working but poor families is increasing, indicating that wages are not keeping up with the cost of living (Kamerman *et al.* 2003).

Families in poverty have shown disproportionately high levels of domestic violence, substance abuse, and mental health problems (Knitzer 2000). As a result, children living in poverty often live in less than adequate environments, lacking basic necessities such as food, clothing, housing, medical care, and insurance. The daily struggle for survival often depletes precious energy and resources, leaving little for families to rely upon when in need. Living in constant fear of eviction, hunger, or violence takes a toll on families and children, leaving them in a state of perpetual turmoil and uncertainty. As described by Brooks-Gunn and Duncan (1997), poverty affects children through a number of "pathways" (p.64) such as health and nutrition, home environment, parental interactions with children, parental mental health, and neighborhood conditions. Children living in these conditions often develop physical, cognitive, academic, social, emotional, and behavioral difficulties.

Households in poverty can be chaotic and unpredictable. Paschall and Hubbard (1998) showed a direct relationship between poverty and increased family stress and conflict in a sample of African-American adolescent males. Children in these circumstances may be victims of poor parenting, psychological distress, malnutrition, and exposure to violence stemming from marital conflict, lack of education and poor support systems. Garrett, Ng'andu and Ferron (1994) found that families stressed by poverty provided a home environment that was less supportive of child development than families that were financially secure. As a result, children were often ill prepared for school, showed low test scores, were retained, or dropped out of school (Duncan *et al.* 1998; Guo 1998).

Many children are trapped in a cycle of poverty which is transmitted from generation to generation owing to a lack of alternatives. Children in poor families not only lack in very basic material resources, but are also less likely to have access to community resources such as good schools, safe neighborhoods, and adequate governmental services.

c. Violence

Despite the fact that over the past ten years the rate of violent crime has declined in the United States, there continue to be disparities according to geographic location, victim characteristics and perpetrator characteristics. Based on data from the US Department of Justice (2002a), urban area residents are more likely than suburban and rural residents to be victims of homicide, aggravated assault, robbery, and property crime. Over half of all homicides occur in central cities and are more commonly drug-related and gang-related than family- or work-related, as they are in suburban and rural areas. In 1998, the homicide rate for males living in central cities was about seven times as high as for males living elsewhere (Eberhardt, Ingram and Makuc 2001). African-American residents in urban areas had a higher victimization rate for violent crime than whites in similar geographic areas, and homicide ranked sixth as the cause of death for the African-American population (Anderson and Smith 2003). Homicide continues to be the leading cause of death for young African-American males between the ages of 15 and 24, and the second leading cause of death for young Hispanic males (Eberhardt *et al.* 2001).

Children growing up in the inner city are daily witnesses to, and victims of, acts of violence such as theft, assault, murder, rape, or abuse. Consistent exposure to guns, knives, and drugs add to the breadth of violent events that children describe. As reported by Farrell and Bruce (1997), 31 per cent of a sample of urban sixth-grade boys and 14 per cent of girls had their lives threatened, 42 per cent of boys and 30 per cent of girls had seen someone shot, and nearly all had seen someone beaten up, had witnessed arrests, or had heard a gunshot. Fitzpatrick and Boldizar (1993) stated that among a sample of urban youth aged 7 to 18, 66 per cent had witnessed an assault, and 43 per cent had witnessed a murder. The inner city has often been described as an urban war zone in that children experience similar events and consequences to children living in war-torn nations (Garbarino, Kostelny, and Dubrow 1991).

Osofsky *et al.* (1993) describe how families exposed to violence in their neighborhoods often discuss events in a matter-of-fact manner, indicating that violence occurs routinely and is part of normal, everyday life. Some mothers describe teaching their children to sit with their heads below the window sills when in the house watching television, in order to avoid random bullets. At a very young age children are taught to dive to the ground or to run away when they hear gunshots.

Violence occurs not only in the community, but in homes and schools, leaving children with little access to safe locations. Children who demonstrate aggression and violence at a young age are often victims of inappropriate disciplining methods and witnesses to domestic and community violence. The use of violence becomes a learned and ingrained response that young children pick up owing to their impressionable nature and their lack of alternative reactions. When these behaviors are demonstrated by close family members or peers, they become validated as acceptable forms of interacting.

According to the US Department of Justice (2002b), in 2001, nine per cent of high school age children reported being threatened or injured with a weapon such as a gun, knife, or club on school property, 6 per cent of students carried such a weapon, and 20 per cent of students reported the presence of gang activity (often associated with violence) in their school. During the same year there were 161,000 serious violent crimes reported involving students aged 12 to 18 on school property, and there were 16 school-associated homicides. The quality of the educational environment affects a student's ability to learn. An unsafe school environment may prevent a child from reaching her fullest academic potential, as she is forced to concentrate on her own personal safety rather than on learning.

As reported by Sheley, McGee, and Wright (1992) in their study of gun-related violence in and around inner city schools, children in these neighborhoods had a far higher victimization rate than the national average. They found that 23 per cent of their sample had been victims of gun-related violence, most of them being male. Furthermore, they found that a major predictor of gun-related perpetration or victimization was the extent of exposure to firearms, including whether family members carried guns, or whether children had access to guns. In addition, involvement in behaviors such as drug trafficking and gang activity, which are known to breed violence, increased the risk of gun-related victimization.

Weist, Acosta and Youngstrom (2001) showed that as life stress increased, the risk of exposure to violence increased. They defined life stress as encountering daily stressors such as living in unsafe and unpredictable environments, being exposed to chronic social problems, and being referred for mental health services to address cognitive and social functioning. Life stress was the most consistent predictor of violence exposure as compared with demographic variables, parental substance abuse, number of people in the home, failing grades, and arrest history.

According to a study conducted by the US Department of the Treasury and the US Department of Justice (June 1999), in 1997 18 to 20-year-olds comprised 22 per cent of all those arrested for murder, and 18-, 19-, and

20-year-olds ranked first, second, and third in the number of gun homicides committed. Seventy-five per cent of all homicides committed by children under the age of 17 involved firearms, as well as 75 per cent of all homicides committed by people in the 18–20 age range. Guns were also used most frequently by those in the 18–20 age range in non-lethal crimes such as assault, rape, and robbery. Despite the fact that it is unlawful to sell handguns to persons under the age of 21, guns are readily available to young children through illegal trafficking, and in homes where parents own guns.

Families living in violent neighborhoods often react to their environments by attempting to isolate themselves from their communities as a way of protecting their children. Children are often prevented from playing outside or attending community events. While this may increase a sense of safety, it also cuts off relationships with potential social supports such as community centers or churches. Constant vigilance for safety of self and loved ones takes a toll on inner city families. Exposure to chronic violence is a leading environmental stressor causing children to experience negative social/emotional and behavioral consequences (Farrell and Bruce, 1997; Fitzpatrick and Boldizar 1993). A higher prevalence of serious psychological impairments such as depression, separation anxiety and post-traumatic stress disorder has been found in children living in violent urban areas as compared with children living in suburban areas (Campbell and Schwarz 1996; Cooley-Quille *et al.* 2001).

Exposure to violence often prevents children from believing in the future, as they are more concerned with surviving from day to day. Too often these children are not aware of alternative ways of living and are forced to develop unsafe and self-injurious coping mechanisms.

3.2 Environmental stressors

a. Housing

The concentration of people living in poverty in inner cities creates a housing crisis. Low-income housing in the form of subsidized housing projects often provides the only alternative for families living at or below the poverty level, and apartments are often overcrowded and in disrepair. As stated by journalist Karl Zinsmeister (1990) "Traditional public-housing complexes tend to be giant conglomerations of the troubled-isolated reservations where dysfunction is not the exception but the norm. Housing projects are petri dishes for family disintegration" (p.57).

Living in disadvantaged neighborhoods negatively affects child outcomes by reducing access to positive role models and exposing children to severe stressors. These neighborhoods tend to be burnt-out residential areas that are devoid of any infrastructure, or highly commercial or industrial. Both are chaotic, offer few opportunities for social exchange, are impersonal, and dangerous. They lack a sense of community which reduces access to impo social networks and causes families to live in isolation.

As cities expand, single-family homes are replaced with multiple-family developments, causing the population density to increase in order to accommodate an increasing population. According to the US Census Bureau (1995), African-American households in central cities were larger and were more likely to be crowded (more than one person per room) as compared with white households. This crowding brings with it poor living conditions, and a sense of being trapped in dirty and unacknowledged areas. People tend to live near their families, creating culturally homogeneous ghettos where there is a common language, religion, and set of culturally sanctioned norms. Isolation from, or rivalry against, surrounding neighborhoods or ethnic groups creates tension based on ignorance and fear, as well as segregation, which is common in many inner cities. Social segregation acts as a protective measure, but creates a debilitating lack of exposure and ignorance of other people. As disadvantaged neighborhoods spread, people from surrounding, more affluent communities begin to leave the city limits in what has been termed "white flight". In their search for safer schools and neighborhoods, they take with them a strong economic base.

Gale, Rothenberg-Pack and Potter (2002) describe the opposite phenomenon of gentrification, which is defined as being "the influx of upper-middle class or wealthy households into previously poor neighborhoods" (p.6). People wanting to live in culturally rich and economically thriving areas tend to move back into cities, causing rents and real-estate prices to sky-rocket. Landlords and real-estate developers capitalize on this influx, raise rents for existing tenants, and purchase old buildings to replace them with luxury condominiums. This causes many inner city residents to be driven from their homes, causing the disintegration of many inner city communities. As the demographics of inner cities change, more disadvantaged residents are forced to live in more isolated areas with fewer resources, and reduced economic opportunities. Transience becomes the norm, causing insecurity and a lack of strong community ties.

According to Koball and Douglas-Hall of the National Center for Children in Poverty (November 2003), children in low-income families are twice as likely to have moved within the space of a year as children in higher-income families. The reasons for moving are eviction, to find better housing, to buy a home, to find cheaper housing, or to find a better neighborhood.

As low-income families are forced to relocate, children are required to change schools. Jason et al. (2001) found that when high-risk children transfer to a new school during their elementary school years, they often fail at the tasks of gaining peer and teacher acceptance, learning school rules, and meeting academic standards. Major changes in peer group and neighborhood familiarity cause decreases in self-esteem, extracurricular involvement, and grade-point average. Moving is a stressor that may prevent at-risk children from focusing on the demands of a new setting. A sense of stability is a crucial element to normal child development and success.

b. Education

Home and school environments are the locations where children spend most of their time. Schools are often described as being microcosms of the larger society. Students will therefore receive their impressions of society from the lessons learned in these locations. How children are treated in schools will inform them as to how society views them. What teachers expect of them will inform them as to what they can achieve. Unfortunately, getting good teachers to work in inner city schools is difficult. Teachers in these schools are often under-qualified, have low expectations for their students, hold racial stereotypes, and are unable to manage behavioral and emotional issues that many students bring with them. Inner city children may enter school with sometimes debilitating conditions, owing to past experiences which affect the quality of their lives and their ability learn. Behavioral disturbances and academic deficits often result in at-risk children receiving a special education label.

As summarized by McLoyd (1998), academic achievement and cognitive functioning as determined by test scores, grade retention, failure, placement in special education, expulsion, graduation rates, and drop-out rates, are influenced by many factors that are directly related to living in poverty. Children living in poverty are more at risk of having unemployed or uneducated parents. These children receive less cognitive stimulation such as verbal interactions with parents and access to literacy materials. This prevents children from being academically ready to succeed in school.

As described by Druian and Butler (2001), at-risk children often attend schools or programs with few resources, low achievement expectations and inconsistent management procedures. Owing to a lack of oversight and resources, poor teaching conditions, and a lack of teacher training, these students are often taught by uninvolved and unaccountable teachers who do not engage their students in the learning process. There is often a high teacher turnover, and a lack of consistent and passionate leadership. Resources such as computers, arts classes, and extra-curricular activities – which positively engage children, keep them off the streets, improve their academic performance, and reduce the chance of early drop-out – are usually lacking in inner city schools. Parental involvement is low, as is administrative support for often overburdened teachers. Owing to the demographic layout of inner city communities, schools in these locations tend to be racially and socio-economically homogeneous. As described by Gale et al. (2002), an environment of predominantly low-income and less educated classmates can negatively affect student performance.

Of the roughly 16 per cent of all school-age children living in poverty, 24 per cent reside in central cities (US Department of Education 2003). These children typically reside in homes where access to literate adults, books and other literacy tools are lacking, and they generally demonstrate lower reading skills and knowledge when they enter kindergarten than children from homes where the literacy environment is richer. Not only is educational preparedness lacking for these children, but often they don't have access to an education that is as rich and motivating as do children who live in the suburbs.

Owing to lower property taxes in the inner city, and a less affluent tax base, per capita local expenditure for public school students in urban environments is much lower than in suburbs. As a result, schools in inner city neighborhoods are underfunded and understaffed. Qualified teachers have few incentives to work in inner city schools, thanks to a lack of resources and support, over-crowding, and the potential for danger. Teachers working in the inner city are often inexperienced, lack training and supervision, and are poorly paid.

Because life in the inner city can be tenuous, it is difficult for children to understand that completing their education is a way to plan for the future. The US Census Bureau (2002) reports that of those people 18 years and over living in central cities, 34 per cent of blacks, 27 per cent of whites, and 27 per cent of Hispanics had completed high school. Priorities in the inner city revolve around survival in the present without forethought for the future. Students in inner city schools are therefore more likely to skip school, get suspended, drop out, or get expelled. US Department of Education statistics from the year 2000 indicate that young adults living in families with incomes in the lowest 20 per cent were six times as likely to drop out of high school as their peers from families with incomes in the top 20 per cent. Reasons for dropping out include not understanding the work, not liking school, failing, not getting along with teachers and peers, having disciplinary problems such as suspension, not feeling safe, having to get a job to support a family, becoming a parent, or having a substance abuse problem.

Dropouts from high school are more likely to be unemployed or to earn less when they do become employed, and are more likely to receive public assistance. Potential dropouts can be identified early and have characteristics such as living in poverty, having low academic skills, poor school attendance, low parental academic achievement, being raised by a single parent, having a negative self-perception, and being enticed by alternatives such as employment or pregnancy (Druian and Butler 2001). Schools where a significant number of students don't graduate can be characterized as having low expectations, poor disciplinary and classroom management strategies, a lack of curricular focus, and very little technical and financial support (Druian and Butler 2001). This combination of poor schools and lack of parental and community support predisposes students to avoid schooling in favor of other, less desirable activities.

c. Healthcare

The physical health of residents in a given community depends not only on demographics and exposure to common risk factors such as violence and pollution, but also on insurance coverage, and availability of and access to healthcare services.

As we have seen, often families living in inner cities are headed by single females of minority background. Many lack substantial education, are unemployed, and live in poverty. Children living in these families have shown a high incidence of infant mortality, asthma, allergies, learning disabilities and missed days of school owing to illness or injury (US Department of Health and Human Services 2003). One reason for this may be a lack of consistent health insurance, which in the United States comes from consistent employment. According to Eberhardt et al. (2001), one-third of low-income residents in central cities are uninsured. Lack of health insurance prevents many inner city families from having a regular source of healthcare and receiving regular preventive treatment such as prenatal care, vaccinations, dental care, and mammography, all of which can reduce the risk of disease and mortality.

As summarized by McLoyd (1998), children living in poverty are often born prematurely or with physical complications owing to inadequate prenatal care, poor nutrition, and prenatal exposure to drugs. Perinatal complications often result and can create longer-term developmental problems, given that poor families have less access to social, education, and material resources to assist them.

Adding to the difficulty of receiving adequate healthcare is the fact that physicians and dentists are in lower supply in urban areas than in suburban areas (Eberhardt et al. 2001). Owing to a weak infrastructure and poor transportation networks in disadvantaged neighborhoods, hospital accessibility is often challenging for families who do not own vehicles.

Living in the inner city additionally exposes children to environmental hazards such as air pollution, hazardous waste sites, lead paint, and pesticides. Landrigan et al. (1999) describe the frequent necessity of using pesticides to combat insects and rodents in old and poorly maintained housing projects. Children living in such overcrowded homes or apartments are at risk of increased exposure to toxic products, which can cause neurological, endocrine, and other developmental disabilities.

d. Employment

Employment provides financial and emotional security for families. Being able to pay the bills allows for a sense of control and achievement, without which disintegration of the family can occur. As McLoyd (1998) states, "family income positively affects child outcomes not so much for what it can buy, but for what it represents" (p.193). Employed parents act as role models for their children, instilling values such as achievement and responsibility. This in turn influences child motivation and academic success.

Employment in the inner city is difficult to secure owing to a scarcity of jobs, and hard to maintain owing to the personal histories of job-seekers, a lack of return for low-paying jobs and the degree of hardship for the employee. Many blue-collar jobs are moving out of inner cities or overseas owing to labor and real-estate costs. This leaves more administrative jobs in inner cities that require higher educational attainment. New businesses are not tempted to set up in inner cities owing to lack of a financially secure customer base, lack of transportation, difficult access for suppliers, high cost of real-estate, and lack of basic security.

As stated by the US Census Bureau (May 2001), 16 per cent of inner city families are headed by a single female, and 10 per cent of these families have children under the age of 18. It is left to these single mothers to provide financial security for their families. Single mothers themselves often lack basic schooling and professional skills, which makes it difficult for them to search for and sustain reliable jobs. A lack of educational attainment limits opportunities for employment, thereby leaving single mothers with few options.

Another issue facing many single mothers is that of childcare. Mothers raising children on their own must secure safe and affordable childcare for young children while they are at work. It is often unrealistic for a mother to pay for suitable childcare, and so, unless family members are willing to contribute to this task, she has no option but to settle for inadequate childcare, or to stay home. This leaves her dependent on welfare and government agencies. Dependency on welfare is often passed on through the generations. Having parents on welfare teaches an attitude of passivity and takes away a sense of self-reliance and motivation for higher educational and economic attainment.

A study conducted by the US General Accounting Office (November 1998) on the prevalence of domestic violence found that 20 per cent of welfare recipients were victims of domestic violence in the 12 months prior to receiving welfare, and 65 per cent had been victims of domestic violence at some time in their lives. The study describes how the effects of domestic abuse can filter into a woman's ability to find employment and remain employed. Women who are victims of domestic violence are more likely to have been repeatedly unemployed and have a greater job turnover. The research indicates that often an abuser will prevent a woman from attending job interviews or job training for fear that financial independence from him will provide her with opportunities to leave the abusive relationship. Because of this threat, abusers will try to thwart employment attempts by refusing to take care of children, preventing the woman from buying the appropriate clothing, or inflicting visible signs of abuse such as bruises or cigarette burns so that the woman will be uncomfortable attending an interview. Some abusers will attempt to sabotage employment prospects of a woman who has a job by frequently calling the workplace, coming to the workplace unannounced, or attempting to disrupt the work day. This clearly jeopardizes her ability to retain her job. Being a victim of domestic violence often prevents a woman from performing adequately in the workplace, making it difficult for her to sustain her job and work towards promotion. She may show up late, or not at all, owing to physical illness or injury, emotional distress (depression, low self-esteem, post-traumatic stress disorder), or practical issues (lack of childcare or necessary material items). Domestic violence is one of the many obstacles that single mothers face in the inner city while trying to secure employment in order to raise their families.

Apart from obtaining illegal income from selling drugs or prostitution, often the only option for a single mother is to get a minimum-wage job in a service industry such as fast food or retail, which forces her to work many hours for little pay. Such jobs often require rote tasks that provide little intellectual challenge, or personal satisfaction. In her detailed study of the working poor in New York city, Newman (1999) describes how if you do secure a minimum-wage job, your salary will often not be enough to live on, given the high cost of living in cities. Because there are so many people looking for jobs in the inner city, employers can afford to keep wages low. This causes employees to take on extra shifts or to take on second jobs, thus decreasing their quality of life, and preventing them from spending time with their families.

As described by Kamerman *et al.* (2003), when mothers take on extra shifts at their workplace (often overnight), this takes them away from parenting time, which decreases supervision and the ability to assist with academic assignments. Kamerman *et al.* found that this causes academic problems in their children such as low cognitive scores, and increased suspensions from school. Furthermore, they describe how maternal employment can negatively affect adolescents. They report poor school performance, a high rate of grade repetition, and a high use of special education services for these children. The causes seem to be linked to the fact that mothers who work full-time leave their adolescent children largely unsupervised after school hours, and depend on them to take over family responsibilities such as caring for younger siblings.

Han, Waldfogel and Brooks-Gunn (2001) found that maternal employment in the first year of a child's life has more detrimental effects on children in low-income families than on children in financially secure households. They suggest that this may be owing to other circumstances in low-income families such as poor and inconsistent childcare, as well as strain and hardship on mothers.

Marital discord has also been linked to parents being overworked, which in turn can affect parenting style and the home atmosphere. Minimum-wage jobs offer little hope of promotion, and often take a physical and mental toll on employees. Employees who experience unpleasant job environments may return home to their families feeling tired or frustrated. This in turn may affect parenting behaviors, and may create an unfavorable home climate.

In some circumstances, maternal employment has been shown to have favorable outcomes for children. Moore and Driscoll (1997) studied families who moved from welfare dependency to employment and found that children whose mothers earned more than $5.00 per hour had better outcomes than children of mothers who earned the minimum wage. Specifically, they showed that behavioral problems in children decreased as maternal wages increased.

Unemployment is pervasive in inner city families. This is owing to dependence on welfare, lesser education, lack of labor market skills, and racism. McLoyd *et al.* (1994) examined the effects of maternal unemployment and work interruption on adolescent socio-emotional functioning. They found that maternal unemployment negatively affected children's functioning owing to the effect that unemployment had on parenting. Mothers who became unemployed were more at risk of developing depressive symptoms and cognitive distress, which negatively affected their parenting. These mothers became more punitive and less emotionally available. Their children in turn showed higher anxiety, more cognitive distress and lower self-esteem.

Employment ensures income and stability, which provide basic necessities and security to families. Unemployment and ensuing financial strain take away a sense of well-being, independence and responsibility from adults. Making a living in the inner city requires families to circumvent obstacles and to prioritize elements in their lives such as education versus employment or family versus work. These decisions are often detrimental to the quality of life of both adults and children.

3.3 Domestic stressors

a. Parenting

The effect of the family on outcomes for inner city children can go both ways. A positive family environment can act as a protective or moderating factor against the ills of living in the inner city. A negative family environment can exacerbate already existing conditions, creating negative outcomes for children. Parenting includes not only providing the basics such as supervision, food and clothing, but also helping children when they are in need, providing consistency and structure, listening to them, and engaging them in conversations. Whether or not effective parenting is occurring is determined by exposure to chronic stress, undesirable life events, socio-economic status, educational attainment of the parent, parents having had good role models themselves, age of the parents, parental mental health, parental employment, family support, and much more.

Families living in inner cities are faced with consistent stressors such as poverty and violence. Parents in these situations can themselves become emotionally distressed or impaired, which reduces their capacity for being supportive, expressive, and responsive parents. Poor parenting as manifested by emotional unavailability or instability, harsh disciplining, low supervision, lack of structured family life, and weak parent–child attachment has been shown to have devastating effects on child outcomes.

Gorman-Smith, Tolan, and Henry (2000), studied the effect of family functioning on patterns of delinquency in children. They found that, depending on neighborhood configurations, different parenting skills were necessary to prevent negative outcomes in children. Specifically they found that children living in stressful neighborhoods were most at risk of exhibiting patterns of delinquency in households where there were high levels of discipline, structure, and parental monitoring, but low levels of family cohesion, emotional closeness and dependability. Children who were the least at risk of exhibiting delinquent behavior were raised in families that emphasized emotional cohesion, had a strong family orientation, provided consistent parenting, and had clear organization of familial roles and responsibilities. These families were most frequently found in communities that had greater structural resources and social networks.

Gorman-Smith et al. (1996) studied the family histories of 362 male adolescents living in the inner city to determine whether domestic context had an effect on delinquent outcomes for children. They classified subjects according to their histories into non-offenders, non-violent offenders, and violent offenders. They found that those adolescents in the violent offender group had poorer discipline in the home, less family cohesion, and less parental involvement than the other two groups. This would suggest that a lack of consistent consequences for inappropriate behavior, instability in the home, and the lack of parental supervision can lead to negative outcomes for children.

Sagrestano et al. (2003) found that an increase in conflict in the home and a decrease in parental monitoring were associated with increases in child and adult depressive symptoms. It was hypothesized that owing to peer-like relationships between these adults and children, there was a lack of clear boundaries and role definitions. Children often took on parental roles, which could become burdensome and could lead to depressive symptoms. Many inner city families are headed by single females who have to work. Many work long hours or have several jobs. This leaves little if any time to monitor children, so that often older siblings are required to watch younger ones. This lack of parental supervision leaves children to fend for themselves. Lack of parental supervision was found to increase the likelihood of violent behavior in children by Singer et al. (1999). They describe how parental monitoring should include knowing where children are, knowing the peer group, setting expectations about completion of tasks and curfews, and following through with consequences, should rules be broken.

Tolan and McKernan-McKay (1996) identified family characteristics that have a negative impact on future outcomes for children. They have divided them into two categories: parental management skills such as lack of organization, lack of supervision, and harsh discipline practices, and family relationship patterns such as marital discord, poor communication patterns, negative affect, lack of affection, lack of compromising abilities, power struggles, and no differentiation between the role of parent and child. They found that all of these have resulted in antisocial behaviors such as aggression or isolation in children.

Parents often lack basic parenting skills owing to a lack of appropriate role models in their own lives, lack of education, and little sense of responsibility. The unstable nature of life in the inner city makes helping and protecting your own child a constant strain and an overwhelming undertaking. Living in the inner city can be exhausting for parents, leaving them with little physical or emotional energy to attend to their child's developmental needs.

b. Domestic conflict

Domestic conflict occurs most commonly as a result of physical or emotional assault of a father against a mother. Children who witness violence between adults in their own homes do so through sight, or by hearing a violent act. Children in these situations are either bystanders, or become involved in some way owing to their own desire to protect a parent, or by being used by one of the parents against the other (hostage situation, forcing the child to watch, using the child as a spy). No matter what the situation, children are often left in caretaking situations after a conflict by having to provide physical care or having to call for help.

As described by Edelson (1999), witnessing domestic conflict has far-reaching implications for children. He divides these outcomes into two categories: impairment of behavioral and emotional functioning such as aggression, antisocial behavior, withdrawal, anxiety and depression and impairment of cognitive functioning, and attitudes such as justification of their own use of violence. He further discusses long-term developmental problems for domestic violence witnesses, such as adult depression, low self-esteem, and adult criminality. Henning et al. (1996) studied the effects of witnessing domestic violence in a sample of adult women. Those women who had witnessed domestic violence during childhood were found to demonstrate higher levels of psychological distress and greater social maladjustment (less perceived social support, low attachment to others, and lack of social integration) than those who had not.

Deardorff, Gonzales, and Sandler (2003) found that family stress (such as single-parent homes and marital conflict) directly impacted on depressive symptoms in inner city adolescents. Such symptoms included anxiety, suicidal ideation, academic deficits, and substance abuse. It was suggested that because family stress is something that children cannot control, they develop a feeling of hopelessness regarding their ability to effect change or to impact on their futures. This hopeless outlook can lead to the development of depressive symptoms.

Family stress caused by interpersonal conflict was also found to increase the likelihood that male African-American adolescents would exhibit violent behavior, in a study conducted by Paschall and Hubbard (1998). They found that neighborhood poverty added to family stress and conflict, which in turn affected adolescent tendencies towards violence and having a negative self-worth.

Romero-Daza, Weeks, and Singer (2003) studied 35 impoverished women involved in street-level prostitution. Nearly all of the women had used drugs at some point in their lives. Fifty per cent of them describe how, as young girls, owing to lack of alternatives, they started using drugs to escape from violent home environments. In their homes, they were either victims of, or witnesses to, regular verbal or physical abuse. This demonstrates how the cycle of violence and poverty starts at a very early age, and how domestic factors can lead to severe consequences for children.

c. Parental mental health

Garbarino (2001) reports that when exposed to traumatic situations, children get cues on how to react from the adults around them. If the surrounding adults take charge and demonstrate a calm and positive reaction, children will retain a sense of relative safety. If, on the other hand, the adults begin to panic, they become emotionally unavailable to give their children what they need. It is important that adults provide messages of safety so that children feel a sense of protection and authority. Parents are not always able to provide this to their children as they are often traumatized themselves.

Parents living in neighborhoods with chronic violence describe a feeling of helplessness and frustration owing to their inability to protect their children effectively from negative influences such as gangs and violence. This leads some parents to becoming overly protective and authoritarian in their methods of disciplining, sometimes using physical punishment, preventing children from going outside or being extremely restrictive. On the other hand, some parents react by becoming depressed. Parents who are depressed are not psychologically available to their children. This prevents developmentally appropriate early attachment and can lead to instances of neglect and poor parenting. For children whose parents are not physically or psychologically available, their peer group becomes an alternative support system.

Maternal depression and anxiety have been seen to negatively affect outcomes for children, as depressed mothers are often not as affectionate, do not respond with appropriate affect, and are less sensitive to the needs of their children. A study conducted by the National Institute of Child Health and Human Development (1999) found that depressed mothers were the least sensitive when observed playing with their children. Children growing up with a depressed mother were found to be less cooperative, had more behavior problems, and scored lower on school tests. This would suggest that mothers who are responsive and provide a home environment that encourages pro-social behaviors such as helping and communication, enable their children to become more socially adjusted.

Parents who feel frustrated and stressed by having to care for their children are described as having a high level of parental aggravation. This can manifest as harsh disciplinary techniques, interpersonal conflict, and abandonment of responsibilities. As shown by McGroder (2000), children being raised by highly aggravated adults are more likely to have cognitive and socio-emotional difficulties. Furthermore, low-income children and children being raised by a single parent are more likely to have a highly aggravated parent.

Emotional distress in parents such as anxiety and depression as well as beliefs of parental ineffectiveness have been found to be increased under economic pressure, or during marital conflict (Elder *et al.* 1995). They found that White parents in their sample tended to live in communities with adequate social resources and a shared sense of vigilance amongst the neighbors. Parental distress was lower in these situations. African-American parents, on the other hand, tended to live in neighborhoods where social cohesion was low and poverty was high, causing high levels of parental distress. In unsafe neighborhoods, parents must be vigilant and proactive to ensure that their children are not exposed to negative influences. This unending task can become burdensome as parents struggle to provide safety.

d. Child abuse

Child abuse is an extreme form of poor parenting and can take the form of physical, sexual, emotional, or educational abuse. The outcomes for children are devastating and can cause far-reaching emotional, behavioral, and cognitive impairment. As summarized by McLoyd (1990), child abuse cases are found in disproportionately high numbers within disadvantaged families, especially when combined with other risk factors. Child abuse is often associated with frustration and depletion of emotional resources that result from financial and family stress. Negative life events such as job loss, moving, or death create stressful situations that parents often don't have the resources to cope with. Children often become the victims of parental anger, disillusionment, or marital discord.

Child abuse and neglect cases can vary in severity from cases of children not being adequately clothed, fed, or brought to school, to cases ending in severe injury or death. No matter what the circumstance, these situations are a result of parental desperation, the outcome being child victimization.

References
Anderson, R.N. and Smith, B.L. (2003) *Deaths: Leading Causes for 2001.* National Vital Statistics Reports, 52(9). Washington DC: US Department of Health and Human Services, Center for Disease Control and Prevention, National Center for Health Statistics.

Brooks-Gunn, G.J. and Duncan, G.J. (1997) 'The effects of poverty on children.' *The Future of Children, 7*, 2, 55–71.

Campbell, C. and Schwarz, D.F. (1996) 'Prevalence and impact of exposure to interpersonal violence among suburban and urban middle school students.' *Pediatrics, 98*, 3, 396–403.

Cooley-Quille, M., Boyd, R.C., Frantz, E., and Walsh, J. (2001) 'Emotional and behavioral impact of exposure to community violence in inner city adolescents.' *Journal of Clinical Child Psychology, 30*, 2, 199–207.

Deardorff, J., Gonzales, N.A., and Sandler, I.N. (2003) 'Control beliefs as a mediator of the relation between stress and depressive symptoms among inner city adolescents.' *Journal of Abnormal Child Psychology, 31*, 2, 205–217.

Druian, G. and Butler, A. (2001) *Effective Schooling Practices and At-risk Youth: What the Research Shows.* Northwest Regional Educational Laboratory, School Improvement Research Series. Accessed August 2004 at www.nwrel.org/scpd/sirs/1/topsyn1.html.

Duncan, G.J., Yeung, W.J., Brooks-Gunn, J., and Smith, J.R. (1998) 'How much does childhood poverty affect the life chances of children?' *American Sociological Review, 63*, 3, 406–423.

Eberhardt, M.S., Ingram, D.D., and Makuc, D.M. (2001) *Health United States 2001: Urban and Rural Health Chartbook.* Washington DC: US Department of Health and Human Services, Center for Disease Control and Prevention, National Center for Health Statistics.

Edelson, J.L. (1999) 'Children's witnessing of adult domestic violence.' *Journal of Interpersonal Violence 14*, 8, 839–870.

Elder, G.H., Eccles, J.S., Ardelt, M., and Lord, S. (1995) 'Inner-city parents under economic pressures: Perspectives on the strategies of parenting.' *Journal of Marriage and the Family 57*, 3, 771–785.

Farrell, A.D and Bruce, S.E. (1997) 'Impact of exposure to community violence on violent behavior and emotional distress among urban adolescents.' *Journal of Clinical Child Psychology, 26*, 2–14.

Fitzpatrick, K.M. and Boldizar, J.P. (1993) 'The prevalence and consequences of exposure to violence among American youth.' *Journal of the American Academy of Child and Adolescence Psychiatry 32*, 424–430.

Gale, W.G., Rothenberg-Pack, J., and Potter, S.R. (2002) *Problems and Prospects for Urban Areas.* Policy Brief, Conference Report #13. Washington, DC: The Brookings Institution.

Garbarino, J. (2001) 'An ecological perspective on the effects of violence on children.' *Journal of Community Psychology 29*, 3, 361–378.

Garbarino, J., Kostelny, K., and Dubrow, N. (1991) 'What children can tell us about living in danger.' *American Psychologist 46*, 376–383.

Garrett, P., Ng'andu, N., and Ferron J. (1994) 'Poverty experiences of young children and quality of their home environments.' *Child Development 65*, 331–345.

Gorman-Smith, D., Tolan, P.H., Zelli, A., and Heusmann, L.R. (1996) 'The relation of family functioning to violence among inner city minority youth.' *Journal of Family Psychology 10*, 2, 115–129.

Gorman-Smith, D., Tolan, P.H., and Henry, D.B. (2000) 'A developmental-ecological model of the relation of family functioning to patterns of delinquency.' *Journal of Quantitative Criminology 16*, 2, 169–198.

Guo, G. (1998) 'The timing of the influences of cumulative poverty on children's cognitive ability and achievement.' *Social Forces 77*, 1, 257–288.

Halpern, R. (1992) 'The role of after-school programs in the lives of inner city children: A study of the "Urban Youth Network".' *Child Welfare 71*, 3, 215–231.

Han, W., Waldfogel, J., and Brooks-Gunn, J. (2001) 'The effects of early maternal employment on later cognitive and behavioral outcomes.' *Journal of Marriage and Family 63*, 2, 336–354.

Henning, K., Leitenberg, H., Coffey, P,. Turner, T., and Bennett, R.T. (1996) 'Long-term psychological and social impact of witnessing physical conflict between parents.' *Journal of Interpersonal Violence 11*, 1, 35–51.

Jason, L.A., Filippelli, L., Danner, K., and Bennet, P. (2001) 'Identifying high risk children transferring into elementary schools.' *Education 113*, 2, 325–330.

Kamerman, S.B., Neuman, M., Waldfogel, J., and Brooks-Gunn, J. (2003) *Social Policies, Family Types and Child Outcomes in Selected OECD Countries.* Paris, France: Organisation for Economic Co-operation and Development.

Knitzer, J. (2000) *Promoting Resilience: Helping Young Children and Parents Affected by Substance Abuse, Domestic Violence, and Depression in the Context of Welfare Reform.* National Center for Children in Poverty, Child and Welfare Reform, Issue Brief 8. New York, NY: Columbia University School of Public Health.

Koball, H. and Douglas-Hall. (November 2003) *Where do Children in Low-income Families Live?* National Center for Children in Poverty. New York, NY: Columbia University School of Public Health.

Landrigan, P.J., Claudio, L., Markowitz, S.B., Berkowitz, G. S., Brenner, B.L., Romero, H., Wetmur, J.G., Matte, T.D., Gore, A.C., Godbold, J., and Wolff, M.S. (1999) 'Pesticides and inner city children: exposures, risks and prevention.' *Environmental Health Perspectives Supplements 107*, S3, 431–437.

McGroder, S.M. (2000) 'Parenting among low-income, African-American single mothers with preschool-age children: Patterns, predictors, and developmental correlates.' *Child Development 71*, 3, 752–771.

McLoyd, V.C. (1990) 'The impact of economic hardship on black families and children: Psychological distress, parenting, and socioemotional development.' *Child Development 61*, 311–346.

McLoyd, V.C. (1998) 'Socioeconomic disadvantage and child development.' *American Psychologist 53*, 2, 185–204.

McLoyd, V.C., Epstein Jayaratne, T., Ceballo, R., and Borquez, J. (1994) 'Unemployment and work interruption among African-American single mothers: Effects on parenting and adolescent socioemotional functioning.' *Child Development 65*, 562–589.

Moore, K.A. and Driscoll, A.K. (1997) 'Low-wage maternal employment and outcomes for children: A study.' *The Future of Children 7*, 1, 122–127.

National Center for Children in Poverty (1996) *One in Four: America's Youngest Poor.* New York, NY: Columbia University School of Public Health.

National Center for Children in Poverty (August 2003) *Low-income Children in the United States.* New York, NY: Columbia University School of Public Health.

National Institute of Child Health and Human Development (1999) 'Chronicity of maternal depressive symptoms, maternal sensitivity, and child functioning at 36 months.' *Developmental Psychology 35*, 5, 1297–1310.

Newman, K.S. (1999) *No Shame in My Game: The Working Poor in the Inner City.* New York: Vintage Books.

Osofsky, J.D., Wewers, S., Hann, D.M., and Fick, A.C. (1993) 'Chronic community violence: What is happening to our children?' *Psychiatry 56*, 36–45.

Paschall, M.J. and Hubbard, M.L. (1998) 'Effects of neighborhood and family stressors on African-American male adolescents' self-worth and propensity for violent behavior.' *Journal of Consulting and Clinical Psychology 66*, 5, 825–831.

Proctor, B.D. and Dalaker, J. (September 2003) *Poverty in the United States: 2002.* Current Population Reports: Consumer Income, P60-222. Washington, DC: US Census Bureau.

Romero-Daza, N., Weeks, M., and Singer, M. (2003) 'Nobody gives a damn if I live or die: Violence, drugs, and street-level prostitution in inner city Hartford, Connecticut.' *Medical Anthropology 22*, 233–259.

Sagrestano, L.M., Paikoff, R.L., Holmbeck, G.N., and Fendrich, M. (2003) 'A longitudinal examination of familial risk factors for depression, among inner city African-American adolescents.' *Journal of Family Psychology 17*, 1, 108–120.

Sheley, J.F., McGee, Z.T., and Wright, J.D (1992) 'Gun related violence in and around inner city schools.' *American Journal of Diseases of Children 146*, 877–882.

Simons, R.L., Murry, V., McLoyd, V., Lin, K., Cutrona, C., and Conger, R.D. (2002) 'Discrimination, crime, ethnic identity, and parenting as correlates of depressive symptoms among African-American children: A multilevel analysis.' *Development and Psychopathology 14*, 371–393.

Singer, M.I., Miller, D.B., Guo, S., Flannery, D.J., Frierson, T., and Slovak, K. (1999) 'Contributors to violent behavior among elementary and middle school children.' *Pediatrics 104*, 4, 878–884.

Tatum, B.D. (1997) *Why are all the Black Kids Sitting Together in the Cafeteria? And other Conversations about Race.* New York: Basic Books.

Tolan, P.H. and McKernan-McKay, M. (1996) 'Preventing serious antisocial behavior in inner city children: an empirically based family intervention program.' *Family Relations 45*, 148–155.

US Census Bureau (1995) *Housing in Metropolitan Areas–Black Households. Statistical Brief, SB/95-5. Washington, DC: US Department of Commerce, Economics and Statistics Administration.*

US Census Bureau (May 2001) *Profiles of General Demographic Characteristics: 2000 Census of Population and Housing.* Washington DC.

US Census Bureau. (March 2002) *Educational Attainment of People 18 Years and Over.* Washington, DC.

US Department of Education, National Center for Education Statistics (2000) *Dropout Rates in the United States: 2000.* Washington, DC.

US Department of Education, National Center for Education Statistics (2003) *The Condition of Education 2003.* NCES 2003-067/68. Washington DC.

US Department of Health and Human Services (November 2003) *Summary Health Statistics for US Children: National Health Interview Survey, 2001. Vital Health Stat 10(216).* Washington, DC: National Center for Health Statistics.

US Department of Justice (2002a) *Victim Characteristics.* Office of Justice Programs. Washington, DC: Bureau of Justice Statistics. Accessed August 2004 at www.ojp.usdoj.gov/bjs.

US Department of Justice (2002b) *Crime Characteristics.* Office of Justice Programs. Washington, DC: Bureau of Justice Statistics.. Accessed August 2004 at www.ojp.usdoj.gov/bjs.

US Department of the Treasury and US Department of Justice (June 1999) *Gun Crime in the Age Group 18–20.* Washington, DC.

US General Accounting Office (November 1998) *Domestic Violence: Prevalence and Implications for Employment Among Welfare Recipients.* Report to Congressional Committees, GAO/HEHS-99-12. Washington, DC: Health, Education and Human Services Division.

Weist, M.D., Acosta, O.M., and Youngstrom, E.A. (2001) 'Predictors of violence exposure among inner city youth.' *Journal of Clinical and Child Psychology 30*, 1, 187–198.

Wellman, D. (1977) *Portraits of White Racism.* Cambridge: Cambridge University Press.

Zinsmeister, K. (June 1990) 'Growing up scared.' *The Atlantic Monthly 265*, 6, 49–66.

CHAPTER 4

Outcomes for At-risk Children in the Inner City

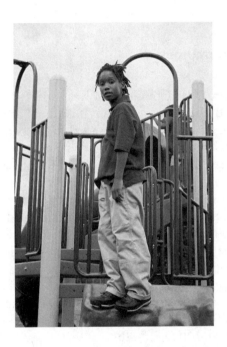

Living in the inner city creates many opportunities for exposure to often traumatic events at home, in school, or in the neighborhood. Witnessing or being a victim of violent crime, abuse, eviction, or illegal substance use can leave permanent scars on the impressionable mind of a child. The circumstances described in the preceding chapter can accumulate in a child's life to create serious and debilitating physical, emotional, behavioral, social, and academic outcomes such as anxiety, learning difficulties, and poor social skills. These outcomes have been described as "externalizing consequences" such as inappropriate aggressive behaviors and drug use, or "internalizing" ones such as depression and post-traumatic stress disorder. Externalizing symptoms are typically more disruptive and visible, whereas internalizing symptoms in the absence of disruptive behaviors are often more difficult to detect. The range and degree to which a child develops one or a combination of these outcomes depends on the interaction between stressors and moderating factors present in the child's life.

School is the location where maladaptive outcomes are usually observed, academic failure and discipline problems being the primary red flags. If properly diagnosed, necessary academic and mental health interventions can be implemented. Often, however, low academic achievement is assumed to be caused by a learning disability. Many inner city children receive a special education label that affords them academic and counseling support, but often fails to address more pervasive problems affecting psychological and family functioning.

4.1 Behavioral outcomes

a. Delinquency

Delinquency in its broadest definition involves antisocial behavior such as acts of defiance, destructiveness, or aggression (Buka and Earls 1993). Depending on the breadth and consistency of these exhibited behaviors, children can develop conduct disorders which manifest as physical aggression, property damage, deceitfulness, theft, or serious violations of the rules (American Psychiatric Association 1995). Taken to the extreme, delinquency may require law enforcement intervention, and subsequent court action.

The profile of a child under the age of 18 incarcerated for a violent offense in the United States is that of an African-American or Hispanic male living in poverty. The profile of an incarcerated adult is typically that of a male of minority background, who has not completed his education, is unemployed, has a history of physical or sexual abuse, or has been treated for a mental or physical disability. Exposure to negative circumstances and antisocial peers and adults during childhood are a common indicator of adult criminality (US Department of Justice, 2002a, 2002b).

When exploring the backgrounds of juvenile delinquents many stressors were found to be similar to those faced by inner city children. They include poor health and neurological functioning (prenatal complications, head injuries), poor early academic skills and success (low IQ, learning disability), and dysfunction in the family and parenting style (lack of supervision, abuse). No single factor causes delinquency in a child, however exposure to multifactor pathways leads to optimal circumstances for delinquent behavior (Buka and Earls 1993).

In attempting to understand the reason for high levels of delinquent behavior exhibited in inner city children, Guerra et al. (1995) studied the effects of economic disadvantage, stressful events, and individual beliefs on aggressive behavior. They found that children living in poverty were more likely to be exposed to stressful home and neighborhood situations which instill a culture of violence, and a necessity to respond with violence in order to stay alive. In addition, children living in poverty adopted beliefs that were accepting of aggressive behavior, owing to the normalized and sometimes idealized view of aggression in urban communities. Success through other channels wasn't visible in these communities, making violence the most immediate means of obtaining respect and material rewards.

Early aggressive behavior in urban boys is highly predictive of later delinquent behavior and other antisocial behavior such as substance abuse and smoking. In researching the consequences of exposure to stressful life events on urban elementary school children, Attar, Guerra and Tolan (1994) found that life stressors such as exposure to violence, moving to a new home, a death in the family, or violent crime victimization increased peer-reported aggressive behavior, and this behavior increased during the following year. This is further supported by Jones and Forehand (2003), who suggest that past behavior is the best predictor of future behavior, especially when multiple samples of behavior are examined.

b. Psychosocial adjustment

Between the ages of six and twelve, children develop or fail to develop basic academic and social skills necessary to survive and succeed in their environments. Psychosocial adjustment relates to a child's ability to develop appropriate social skills such as relationship formation, communication skills, and self-esteem. Psychosocial adjustment is affected by surrounding elements such as family, community, and school. Many at-risk children develop inappropriate social responses such as aggression or withdrawal, as a result of poor role-modeling, poor parenting, or traumatization. When adults are unable or unavailable to provide support in dealing with stressors, children must rely on their own resources, which are often maladaptive.

As described by Osofsky et al. (1993), children who have been exposed to violence demonstrate a variety of socially inappropriate behaviors. Some children become aggressive in their play patterns with peers as an attempt to imitate behaviors they have witnessed, or simply because they view such activities as 'normal'. Some children 'act tough' or uncaring in order to protect themselves from fear, anxiety, or grief. Such posturing serves as a way to distance themselves from difficult emotions and 'untrustworthy' people. In an attempt to avoid negative feelings or stimuli associated with a negative event, children shut down their emotional reactions and demonstrate consistently flat affect. Inappropriate emotional responses prevent children from fully understanding and communicating about events in their lives. When children aren't able to express themselves appropriately, often their needs go unmet.

Bolger *et al.* (1995) found that children, especially boys growing up in families experiencing persistent family economic hardship were more likely to exhibit difficulties with peer relations, show inappropriate behaviors at school, and report low self-esteem, than children in financially secure families. In addition, when the study began, the children living in poverty were academically behind their peers, and did not catch up during the years of the study.

c. Teenage pregnancy

According to Sawhill (2001), despite the fact that teenage pregnancies have declined sharply since the 1990s, motherhood at a young age continues to cause costly and debilitating circumstances for families and children. The causes of teenage pregnancy are complex and include a combination of domestic deterioration, lack of education, lack of access to healthcare and birth control, lack of future orientation, a need to be loved, and a breakdown in social responsibility.

Most single mothers face major challenges in raising their children alone, and being a teen mother brings additional obstacles. Teen mothers typically drop out of school and are unemployed. Going on welfare is often the only way to support themselves. Very few teen mothers marry or receive financial support from the child's father, and most remain on welfare and live in poverty for extended periods of time.

An, Haveman and Wolfe (1993) studied the role of childhood events and economic circumstances on teenage pregnancies and welfare receipt. They describe a number of possible pathways leading to teenage pregnancy. The first is living in a welfare-dependent family where the primary caregiver is a single mother on welfare. Aspects of a welfare family include lack of a male presence, dependence on government support, patterns of unemployment and an environment where out-of-wedlock childbearing is acceptable. The second is living in an isolated community lacking information and connections. The third is family socio-economic status, which is related to levels of maternal education and maternal employment. The fourth is the experience of stressful events during childhood such as changes in family structure or moving, which can create feelings of insecurity and lack of control. Having a child is seen as a way to assuage those feelings and replace them with ones of being needed and loved. The final pathway leading to teenage pregnancy is the consideration of financial benefits of having a child. Teenage mothers often lack labor market skills and opportunities and see childbearing as a way to gain economic independence. Giving birth brings access to welfare benefits, social services, health insurance, job training and education. It also offers independence from parental control and reduced pressure to attend school. An, Haveman and Wolfe's study shows that daughters who have experienced stressful events, live in welfare-dependent families, and have mothers with low educational attainment are most at risk of becoming teenage mothers.

d. Academic failure

Schools in inner city neighborhoods are often lacking in resources and qualified teachers. However, this is only partly why many children in inner cities
experience academic failure. Growing up in homes with few books and illiter-
ate adults provides an academically poor learning environment. Chaotic homes
often prevent children from reading, studying, or completing their homework,
and adults are often unavailable or unable to assist. In addition, children living
with stressors such as violence and poverty often demonstrate low academic
performance, owing to psychological conditions that impair their ability to
succeed academically.

As summarized by Warner and Weist (1996), children who are exposed to
violence often demonstrate cognitive deficits such as memory loss or poor
concentration, which hinder the learning process. These may occur owing to
sleep disturbances (nightmares), fatigue, anxiety, intrusive thoughts and
traumatizing memories (flashbacks).

Perez and Widom (1994) studied the long-term academic and intellectual
effects of childhood abuse or neglect. They found that children who had been
abused or neglected often faced substantial emotional and environmental
disruptions during their development. These affected their academic performance and readiness to learn. This study showed that children who were
abused or neglected had a lower IQ and a lower reading ability than the control
group, and that these deficits persisted into adulthood. Academic failure as
manifested by failure to complete or attend school has far-reaching implications for future success. Lack of education can cause humiliating adult
outcomes such as illiteracy and unemployment, which in turn have devastating
effects on self-worth and achievement.

4.2 Emotional outcomes

a. Depression

Depression is a broad term used to describe a vast number of differentiated disorders. Length of symptoms and functional impairment caused by symptoms
determines the severity of the disorder. As described by the DSM-IV (American
Psychiatric Association 1995), typical symptoms include decreased interest in
activities, flat affect, inability to sleep or concentrate, anxiety and depressed
mood. More severe outcomes such as conduct disorder, delinquency, low
academic achievement, early pregnancy, substance abuse, eating disorders, and
suicidal ideation have been linked to depression.

There is an unusually high incidence of depression in inner city children.
Living in poverty predisposes children to develop depressive symptoms, owing
to constant exposure to uncontrollable stressful conditions such as domestic
conflict and violence. Deardorff, Gonzales and Sandler (2003) demonstrated
that economic, family, and peer stress reduce the sense of control that children

need in order to feel safe. A belief in there being an external locus of control over life events and the accompanying feeling of incompetence can lead to children feeling hopeless. These feelings are high predictors of depression in children and can impact on the way they behave and view the future.

As summarized by Bolland (2003), hopelessness is an abundance of negative expectations concerning the self and the future. The belief is that desirable outcomes will not occur and that negative outcomes will occur, and that this state of affairs cannot be modified. Owing to an expectation of failure or even death at an early age, at-risk children see little point in being careful or law-abiding. Because their negative fate is inevitable in their eyes, they often engage in hazardous activities, putting themselves in danger and making their outlook self-fulfilling. Bolland reported a high prevalence of hopelessness in a high poverty, inner city adolescent population. He further demonstrated that feelings of hopelessness were associated with increased levels of violence, drug use, promiscuity, and accidental injury, especially in males.

The effect of family risk factors such as domestic conflict and parenting style was examined by Sagrestano et al. (2003). They found that high domestic conflict and low parental monitoring were associated with high levels of depressive symptoms in children. Exposure to conflict in the home not only generated stress from living in a hostile family environment, but reduced access to protective factors that positive parenting may present. Lack of parental monitoring often occurred owing to a blurring of roles between parents and children. Children were often required to take on parental duties such as childcare and housework, creating a heavy burden to carry.

The effect of exposure to violence on depressive symptoms was studied by Fitzpatrick (1993). He found that victimization increased the likelihood that young children, especially females, would develop depressive symptoms. He also found that witnessing violence had no significant effect on depression. He accounted for this unusual finding by theorizing that young children chronically exposed to violence become desensitized to daily stressors. They have developed highly sophisticated coping mechanisms in order survive their daily ordeals. Emotional numbing or disassociation result, which themselves have mental health implications.

b. Anxiety

Often found in conjunction with depression in inner city children are various forms of anxiety. Osofsky et al. (1993) describe children exposed to violence demonstrating separation anxiety and fear of being without their mothers at all times, including while sleeping. Hurt et al. (2001) discussed how exposure to violence caused school-age children to develop depression and anxiety, which manifested as extreme worrying that they might get shot or die, fear of going outside, and wishing they were dead. In addition these children demonstrated low self-esteem, poor academic performance, and high levels of absence from school.

Living in inner cities can be stressful owing to the unpredictable nature of often chaotic neighborhoods. Schwab-Stone *et al.* (1995) studied a large sample of children in an urban public school system and found that 74 per cent of these children felt unsafe in one or more contexts such as home or school. They describe how constant imminent danger causes a state of chronic threat, which requires children to adjust their personal behaviors and outlook in order to cope. Often these adjustments come in the form of a greater willingness to use physical aggression, diminished perception of risk, lowered personal expectations for the future, antisocial behavior, and diminished academic achievement. These often self-injurious behaviors prevent healthy development and the realization of individual potential.

Kliewer *et al.* (1998) found that levels of anxiety and depression were mediated by levels of maternal and social support. Specifically they found that witnessing (hearing about or seeing) violence was related to high levels of internalizing symptoms such as intrusive thoughts, especially in children with inadequate social or maternal support. Having a reliable adult to confide in decreased the likelihood that the child would develop depression or anxiety.

c. Post-traumatic stress disorder (PTSD)

Post-traumatic stress disorder is defined by the DSM-IV (American Psychiatric Association 1995) as the development of characteristic symptoms (intense fear, helplessness, disorganized or agitated behavior) following personal exposure to or witnessing of an extreme traumatic stressor such as sexual or physical assault, death in the family, or a serious accident. Results of PTSD include persistent re-experiencing of the traumatic event, persistent avoidance of stimuli associated with the trauma, and numbing of general responsiveness. These persist over time and cause clinically significant distress or impairment in social or occupational functioning. Some outcomes of PTSD in children include difficulty in concentrating, conduct disorders, dissociation, reliving the event, loss of acquired developmental skills such as bowel and bladder control or motility, sense of doom for the future, personality changes, separation anxiety, and higher risk of adult psychiatric disorders. Children often lose interest in previously enjoyed activities, avoid talking about their emotions, and are unable to feel close to people.

Parson (1994) describes trauma as a violent intrusion into the self which destabilizes our sense or organization and integrity, and disrupts our functioning. A sense of powerlessness and insecurity can cause children to withdraw into isolation, or compensate for their vulnerability by becoming aggressive. A belief that nothing matters causes traumatized children to engage in dangerous and often impulsive behavior as a way of transforming their damaged self-esteem. Parson goes on to describe how many traumatized inner city children feel internally fragmented. Dissociative reactions act as defense mechanisms to protect against dangerous and frightening conditions, and can lead to a breakdown of internal systems, thus impairing sensory, perceptual, affective and conceptual functioning. This can interfere with academic functioning as well as the normal development of peer and parental relationships.

As described by Garbarino (2001), experiencing a threatening event requires children to reframe their view of the world. To make sense of traumatic events, children need to adjust their already existing responses and develop alternative cognitive frameworks in order to cope.

A common predictor of PTSD in children is exposure to violence. Children in the inner city are at constant risk of being a victim of, or a witness to, violent events, with consequent high rates of PTSD in inner cities. Schools with high rates of murder, assault, or robbery, have a high incident of PTSD amongst the student body, especially in girls (Berton and Stabb 1996). Whether or not PTSD symptoms develop depends on a number of factors such as gender, familial support, and coping mechanisms.

Foster, Kuperminc and Price (2004) examined gender differences in development of PTSD and related symptoms such as anxiety, depression, anger, and dissociation. They found a higher incidence of depression and anxiety symptoms in girls than in boys. They also found that girls showed the same incidence of symptoms, as either a witness or a victim of violence. Boys, on the other hand, showed more distress when they were victimized than as bystanders.

References

American Psychiatric Association (1994) *Diagnostic and Statistical Manual of Mental Disorders, Fourth Edition.* Washington, DC: American Psychiatric Association.

An, C., Haveman, R., and Wolfe, B. (1993) 'Teen out-of-wedlock births and welfare receipt: The role of childhood events and economic circumstances.' *The Review of Economics and Statistics 75*, 2, 195–208.

Attar, B.K., Guerra, N.G., and Tolan, P.H. (1994) 'Neighborhood disadvantage, stressful life events, and adjustment in urban elementary school children.' *Journal of Clinical Child Psychiatry 23*, 391–400.

Berton, M.W. and Stabb, S.D. (1996) 'Exposure to violence and post-traumatic stress disorder in urban adolescents.' *Adolescence 31*, 122, 489–499.

Bolland, J.M. (2003) 'Hopelessness and risk behavior among adolescents living in high-poverty inner city neighborhoods.' *Journal of Adolescence 26*, 145–158.

Bolger, K.E., Patterson, C.J, Thompson, W.W., and Kupersmidt, J.B . (1995) 'Psychosocial adjustment among children experiencing persistent and intermittent family economic hardship.' *Child Development 66*, 4, 1107–1129.

Buka, S. and Earls, F. (1993) 'Early determinants of delinquency and violence.' *Health Affairs,* Winter 1993.

Deardorff, J., Gonzales, N.A., and Sandler, I.N. (2003) 'Control beliefs as a mediator of the relation between stress and depressive symptoms among inner city adolescents.' *Journal of Abnormal Child Psychology 31*, 2, 205–217.

Fitzpatrick, K.M. (1993) 'Brief report: Exposure to violence and presence of depression among low-income African-American Youth.' *Journal of Consulting and Clinical Psychology 61*, 3, 528–531.

Foster, J.D., Kuperminc, G.P., and Price, A.W. (2004) 'Gender differences in posttraumatic stress and related symptoms among inner city minority youth exposed to community violence.' *Journal of Youth and Adolescence 33*, 1, 59–69.

Garbarino, J. (2001) 'An ecological perspective on the effects of violence on children.' *Journal of Community Psychology 29*, 3, 361–378.

Guerra, N.G., Heusmann, L.R., Tolan, P.H., Van Acker, R., and Eron, L.D. (1995) 'Stressful events and individual beliefs as correlates of economic disadvantage and aggression among urban children.' *Journal of Consulting and Clinical Psychology 63*, 4, 518–528.

Hurt, H., Malmud, E., Brodsky, N.L., and Giannetta, J. (2001) 'Exposure to violence: Psychological and academic correlates in child witnesses.' *Archives of Pediatric Adolescent Medicine 155*, 1351–1356.

Jones, D.J. and Forehand, G. (2003) 'The stability of child problem behaviors: A longitudinal analysis of inner city African-American children.' *Journal of Child and Family Studies 12*, 2, 215–227.

Kliewer, W., Lepore, S.J., Oskin, D., and Johnson, P.D. (1998) 'The role of social and cognitive processes in children's adjustment to community violence.' *Journal of Consulting and Clinical Psychology 66*, 1, 199–209.

Osofsky, J.D., Wewers, S., Hann, D.M., and Fick, A.C. (1993) 'Chronic community violence: What is happening to our children?' *Psychiatry 56*, 36–45.

Parson, E.R. (1994) 'Inner-city children of trauma: Urban violence traumatic stress response syndrome.' In Wilson, J.P. and Lindy, J.D. (eds) *Countertransference in the Treatment of PTSD*, 157–178. New York: Guildford Publications, Inc.

Perez, C.M. and Widom, C.S. (1994) 'Childhood victimization and long-term intellectual and academic outcomes.' *Child Abuse and Neglect 18*, 8, 617–633.

Sagrestano, L.M., Paikoff, R.L., Holmbeck, G.N., and Fendrich, M. (2003) 'A longitudinal examination of familial risk factors for depression, among inner city African-American adolescents.' *Journal of Family Psychology 17*, 1, 108–120.

Sawhill, I. (2001) What can be Done to Reduce Teen Pregnancy and Out-of-wedlock Births? Welfare Reform & Beyond Brief #8. Washington DC: The Brookings Institution, Center on Urban & Metropolitan Policy.

Schwab-Stone, M.E., Ayers, T.S., Kasprow,W., Voyce, C., Barone, C., Shriver, T., and Weissberg, R.P. (1995) 'No safe haven: A study of violence exposure in an urban community.' *Journal of the American Academy of Child and Adolescent Psychiatry 34*, 10, 1343–1352.

US Department of Justice (2002a) *Victim Characteristics*. Office of Justice Programs. Washington DC: Bureau of Justice Statistics. Accessed August 2004 at www.ojp.usdoj.gov/bjs.

US Department of Justice (2002b) *Crime Characteristics*. Office of Justice Programs. Washington DC: Bureau of Justice Statistics. Accessed August 2004 at www.ojp.usdoj.gov/bjs.

Warner, B.S. and Weist, M.D. (1996) 'Urban youth as witnesses to violence: Beginning assessment and treatment efforts.' *Journal of Youth and Adolescence 25*, 3, 361–377.

CHAPTER 5

Moderating Factors

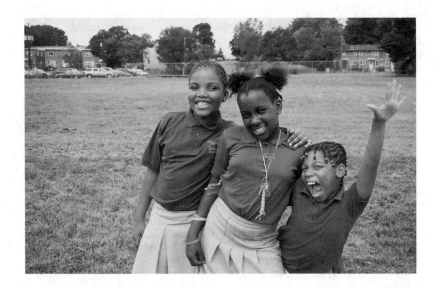

Moderating, or protective, factors are elements that protect children from the possibly debilitating stressors that they face. When these factors are present, children will avoid developing negative outcomes despite exposure to stressors. When these factors are absent, negative consequences can be expected especially when coupled with living in the inner city. Moderating factors have a strong influence over child outcomes and are instrumental in determining whether a child will thrive or decline in the inner city.

Living in the inner city does not necessarily lead to negative outcomes. Children who successfully thrive in potentially harmful environments are said to be resilient (Luthar, Cicchetti, and Becker 2000). These children have managed to adapt to potentially debilitating circumstances with little or no impact on their development or functioning. Many resilient children benefit from some or all of the moderating factors below.

As summarized by Bogenschneider, Small, and Riley (1994), most risk factors can be countered with associated moderating factors. Therefore, by studying risks, we inevitably discover avenues of entry for prevention. By encouraging the development of moderating factors, we counteract risks and address possibly devastating outcomes for children.

5.1 Social support

Many studies have shown the importance of social support as a mediator between stressful inner city circumstances and child outcomes (Dubow, Edwards, and Ippolito 1997; Perkins-Quamma and Greenberg 1994; Youngstrom, Weist, and Albus 2003). High levels of social support have been shown to be indicative of more positive outcomes for children. The more a child feels loved, cared for, valued, and accepted by those around her, the better she will feel about herself and the more effective her coping mechanisms will be. The more social support available in inner city communities through agencies, religious organizations, community centers, or schools, the more resources will be accessible to inner city families to help in the development of their children.

Yoshikawa (1994) showed that social support for parents had a strong protective element against delinquency and antisocial behavior in their children. Services such as parenting classes, provision of pre- and post-natal care, and educational and vocational training positively affected parenting quality and therefore child outcomes.

Dubow and Ullman (1989) describe three measures of social support: peer, family, and teacher. Peer support involves whether a child is made fun of or left out; family support includes whether a child feels valued as an important family member, close family relationships, positive discipline strategies, and extended family support; teacher support includes whether a child feels close to his teachers and acknowledged by them. Each of these influences how a child will feel about himself and therefore how he reacts to his circumstances.

5.2 Parenting

Homes that are organized and predictable, with clearly outlined rules and responsibilities, will act as strong moderators against the often chaotic surrounding neighborhoods. Positive, caring, and stable parental presence provides a degree of protection from stressors in the inner city. Having a strong relationship with an adult who is supportive, engaging and attentive to child responses and ideas allows a child to grow and learn in a positive and nurturing environment. Overstreet et al. (1999) found that the presence of a mother in the home decreased the development of internalizing symptoms in children. They also found that the larger the family, the less at risk the children were of becoming depressed, owing to the important protective nature of having a large family support network.

Parental involvement such as supervision, monitoring peer groups and school performance, increases the likelihood that an at-risk child will succeed in the inner city (Bolger *et al.* 1995). Jarrett (1995) describes five family characteristics that will ensure positive child outcomes as determined by social mobility. She lists having a supportive adult network structure, restricted family–community relations, stringent parental monitoring strategies, strategic alliances with mobility-enhancing institutions and organizations, and adult-sponsored development. Such families engage in activities and relationships that will develop access to positive mainstream opportunities for their children and limit inappropriate influences from the neighborhood or family. They have set and clearly communicated high academic and behavioral expectations and created avenues for achievement.

An important determinant of outcome for children who have been emotionally or physically traumatized is the degree of emotional support from parents, as manifested by parental reaction and stability. Irwin (1996) described how, when parents of sexually abused children were consistently supportive, caring and emotionally available after a traumatic event, the risk of the child developing a dissociative disorder decreased.

5.3 Education

Schools that provide stable, safe and intellectually stimulating environments encourage attendance and engage students in learning. Schools with a positive climate and high social and academic expectations develop a sense of purpose and belonging in students and make their learning meaningful. In addition, clearly defined structures and policies allow children to feel secure. By providing children with diverse opportunities for involvement through academics, the arts, or sports, schools are in a unique position to capture a child's attention and focus him or her away from potentially dangerous activities. When children feel that they have responsibilities and commitments, and that the adults around them have an authentic interest in them and high expectations for their success, they will often respond by rising to the occasion. Children in these types of school are shown to demonstrate higher academic achievement. In addition these schools report less aggression and substance abuse, thanks to strong anti-substance abuse norms and information, structured discipline policies, and opportunities for positive social involvement (O'Donnell, Hawkins, and Abbott 1995).

Children who are encouraged and challenged in the educational setting will develop motivation and curiosity, which will propel them to high levels of academic achievement. Academic self-esteem increases chances of high-school completion and post-secondary education. In addition, access to positive adult role models provides inner city children with a view of what is possible and an avenue to get there.

Yoshikawa (1994) showed that enrollment in high-quality educational infant day-care or preschools had positive outcomes for children. Child-centered programs that focused on the promotion of social, emotional, intellectual and physical development made children ready for school and likely to succeed.

5.4 Ethnic identity

Living in a neighborhood where racial identification and pride are strong, provides a sense of community and shared values, which give children a feeling of meaning and belonging (Simons *et al.* 2002). When minority children are provided with a positive view of their reference-group, their self-concept becomes more positive, influencing their view of who they are and what they can achieve. For African-American children, it was found that the internalization of Afrocentric values was positively associated with self-esteem and psychosocial adjustment (Thomas, Townsend, and Belgrave 2003). Ethnic identification allows for positive self-identification, counters fear and demoralization, and is an important coping mechanism for minority children.

5.5 Child characteristics

Factors such as gender and age mediate outcomes for at-risk children, depending on the circumstances. In general, girls tend to develop internalizing outcomes and boys tend to develop externalizing ones. Younger children are more at risk of developing more debilitating long-term consequences than older children. Intrinsic moderating skills that children develop or are born with will either support or prevent success in the inner city and will determine how children react to stressors.

a. Social skills

How he or she interacts with peers and adults will influence success for an inner city child. When a child is responsive, compassionate, and has good communication skills she will be more apt to develop positive and sustaining relationships. These become her support network that she can rely on in times of need.

b. Conflict resolution

A child's ability to resolve conflict using positive strategies such as apologizing, compromising, or seeking help, rather than negative ones such as threatening, fighting, or yelling, goes a long way to protecting a child from negative outcomes.

c. Problem-solving

Appropriate social problem-solving skills such as the ability to plan, to think abstractly, to reflect, to be flexible, and to attempt alternative solutions, have been shown to decrease behavior problems and increase academic success (Dubow and Tisak, 1989; Perkins-Quamma and Greenberg 1994). These skills help children to negotiate the complex demands of their environment and prepare them to react and effect change in difficult situations.

d. Emotional management

How children manage difficult and often intense emotions such as anger and grief will influence how they deal with stressors. An ability to communicate their needs effectively and to seek out help from trustworthy adults will help them to get any counseling or support that they need.

e. Self-concept

How a child views herself and the events in her life impacts on how she will react to stressful situations. If a child has a sense of power and independence, she will feel that she has some control over her actions and choices. This self-confidence gives her a sense of responsibility and helps her to believe in herself and her abilities. Self-concept is influenced by self-esteem, external reflections of self, and treatment by others. Kliewer and Sandler (1992) theorize that children with high self-esteem view stressors in a more positive light, which influences their choice of coping strategies. For example, a child with low self-esteem may view a failing grade as a reflection of her inability to succeed and may give up studying, whereas a child with high self-esteem may decide to study harder and try to improve her grade.

f. Future expectations

Having positive expectations for the future includes an expectation of attaining certain goals such as achieving in school, getting a job, and having positive relationships with family and peers. This outlook is influenced by parenting, educational expectations, and access to positive role models. Children with a sense that these goals are achievable were found to be less likely to develop problem behaviors and are less influenced by negative peer influences (Dubow et al. 2001). These children tend to show higher levels of school involvement, have more family and social support, and more positive internal resources such as problem-solving skills and high self-esteem. These children can be described as having a sense of purpose that gives them something to live and work for.

DuRant et al. (1994) found that urban children of employed parents of a higher socio-economic status, and who attended religious services regularly, had a higher sense of purpose and fewer feelings of hopelessness. These children were less likely to develop depressive symptoms and use violence, and had a higher belief that they would be alive at age 25 than children living in more disadvantaged situations.

5.6 Access to mental health professionals

Whether a child and his family have access to mental health professionals in the school or community will influence how he deals with stressors and copes with outcomes. As described in Chapter Six, therapeutic interventions with an inner city, at-risk child population go a long way towards preventing negative outcomes and healing existing ones.

References

Bogenschneider, K., Small, S., and Riley, D. (1994) *An Ecological, Risk-focused Approach for Addressing Youth-at-risk Issues.* University of Wisconsin-Madison/Cooperative Extension, Wisconsin Youth Futures, Technical Report #1. Accessed August 2004 at www.cyfernet.org/research/youthfut1

Bolger, K.E., Patterson, C.J, Thompson, W.W., and Kupersmidt, J.B. (1995) 'Psychosocial adjustment among children experiencing persistent and intermittent family economic hardship.' *Child Development 66,* 4, 1107–1129.

Dubow, E.F. and Tisak, J. (1989) 'The relation between stressful life events and adjustment in elementary school children: The role of social support and social problem-solving skills.' *Child Development 60,* 1412–1423.

Dubow, E.F. and Ullman, D.G. (1989) 'Assessing social support in elementary school children: The survey of children's social support.' *Journal of Clinical Child Psychology 18,* 52–64.

Dubow, E.F., Edwards, S., and Ippolito, M.F. (1997) 'Life stressors, neighborhood disadvantage, and resources: A focus on inner city children's adjustment.' *Journal of Clinical Child Psychology 26,* 2, 130–144.

Dubow, E.F., Arnett, M., Smith, K., and Ippolito, M.F. (2001) 'Predictors of future expectations of inner city children: A 9-month prospective study.' *Journal of Early Adolescence 21,* 1, 5–28.

DuRant, R.H., Cadenhead, C., Pendergrast, R.A., Slavens, G., and Linder, C.W. (1994) 'Factors associated with the use of violence among urban Black adolescents.' *American Journal of Public Health 84,* 4, 612–617.

Irwin, H.J. (1996) 'Traumatic childhood events, perceived availability of emotional support, and the development of dissociative tendencies.' *Child Abuse and Neglect 20,* 8, 701–707.

Jarrett, R.L. (1995) 'Growing up poor: The family experiences of socially mobile youth in low-income African-American neighborhoods.' *Journal of Adolescent Research 10,* 1, 111–135.

Kleiwer, W. and Sandler, I.H. (1992) 'Locus of control and self-esteem as moderators of stressor-symptom relations in children and adolescents.' *Journal of Abnormal Child Psychology 20,* 393–411.

Luthar, S.S., Cicchetti, D., and Becker, B. (2000) 'The construct of resilience: A critical evaluation and guidelines for future work.' *Child Development 71,* 3, 543–562.

O'Donnell, J., Hawkins, J.D., and Abbott, R.D. (1995) 'Predicting serious delinquency and substance use among aggressive boys.' *Journal of Consulting and Clinical Psychology 63,* 4, 529–537.

Overstreet, S., Dempsey, M., Graham, D., and Moely, B. (1999) 'Availability of family support as a moderator of exposure to community violence.' *Journal of Clinical Child Psychology 28,* 2, 151–159.

Perkins-Quamma, J. and Greenberg, M.T. (1994) 'Children's experience of life stress: The role of family social support and social problem-solving skills as protective factors.' *Journal of Clinical Child Psychology 23,* 3, 295–305.

Simons, R.L., Murry, V., McLoyd, V., Lin, K., Cutrona, C., and Conger, R.D. (2002) 'Discrimination, crime, ethnic identity, and parenting as correlates of depressive symptoms among African-American children: A multilevel analysis.' *Development and Psychopathology 14,* 371–393.

Thomas, D.E., Townsend, T.G., and Belgrave, F.Z. (2003) 'The influence of cultural and racial identification on the psychosocial adjustment of inner city African-American Children in school.' *American Journal of Community Psychology 32*, 3/4, 217–228.

Yoshikawa, H. (1994) 'Prevention as cumulative protection: Effects of early family support and education on chronic delinquency and its risks.' *Psychological Bulletin 115*, 1, 28–54.

Youngstrom, E., Weist, M.D., and Albus, K.E. (2003) 'Exploring violence exposure, stress, protective factors and behavioral problems among inner city youth.' *American Journal of Community Psychology 32*, 1/2, 115–129.

CHAPTER 6

Therapy with Inner City, At-risk Children

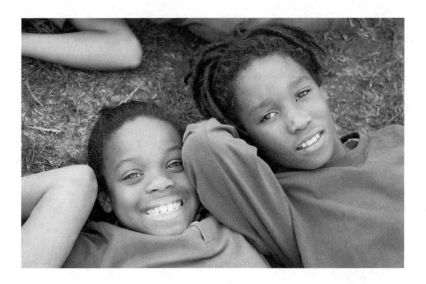

Inner city, at-risk children and their families often manifest an array of needs that require multi-faceted and simultaneous mental health interventions to restore a sense of organization and cohesion (Erwin 1994). The goal of therapy in this context is to assist a child to integrate her experiences and to effectively cope with subsequent ones. Coordination of services between a variety of mental health professionals and social services agencies is often the most direct and effective way of encouraging healing and improved functioning. Owing to the individual nature of circumstances and reactions, mental health professionals need to approach therapy with this population with an open mind and an ability to adapt. There is no prescribed method of treatment, but rather an array of possible interventions that professionals can adopt to suit the situation at hand.

Therapy with this population can take the form of prevention, support, or in-depth psychotherapy to address a presenting need. As described by Buka and Earls (1993), mental health interventions that work with this population occur early in life, are comprehensive, are flexible, involve parents and children, and are continuous rather than discrete. Owing to the vast range of issues faced by this population, interventions need to occur at the physical, social, emotional and cognitive levels.

The Metropolitan Area Child Study Research Group (2002) further agreed that comprehensive intervention is necessary for at-risk children. They emphasize the importance of initiating interventions in the classroom (through social-cognitive curricula delivery, effective classroom management, and encouragement of prosocial behavior), in small groups (for targeted high-risk children to develop social skills, to minimize negative peer reinforcement, and to change cognitive and behavioral norms), and with the family (through parenting classes that develop communication and provide a support network). They also note that the earlier the intervention, the more positive the outcomes will be. Interventions have a cumulative effect, with children receiving more interventions showing the most positive outcomes. The authors emphasize that these interventions are the most effective when the settings have ample resources and support.

The topics addressed in this chapter are designed to further describe mental health treatment with inner city, at-risk children. Specific interventions, therapist qualities, and relevant therapeutic issues for this population are discussed. In addition the creative arts therapies are introduced, with an emphasis on common goals and processes.

6.1 Interventions

a. Individual therapy

Mental health interventions for at-risk children are aimed at managing emotional reactions, improving behavioral functioning, and encouraging developmentally appropriate interactions. Pynoos and Nader (1988) describe treatment goals for working with children who have been exposed to chronic violence. Because these children often demonstrate a variety of outcomes such as PTSD and grief, the therapist must be flexible and capable of addressing them simultaneously. The authors discuss the encouragement of emotional expression, normalizing of emotional reactions, decreasing cognitive distortions, facilitating the use of social support systems, and providing a supportive atmosphere in which emotions can be expressed. The interventions described here aim to bring a sense of normalcy to the life of a child, while at the same time providing support and encouragement.

Therapists often take on different roles depending on the circumstances faced by the child (Garbarino 2001). Garbarino describes how, when a child has been a victim of a violent crime that violates normal reality, she will need help in regaining a sense of normalcy and integrating the traumatic event into her understanding of reality. Through reassurance and support from loving adults in her surroundings, assimilation of the traumatic event and regaining a sense of security will slowly occur. If, on the other hand, a child is exposed to chronic violence, she may manifest severe outcomes such as PTSD and alterations in personality and behavior. In these situations she will need help redefining her understanding of a dangerous world and her reactions to it, through the strengthening of primary relationships which can counteract feelings of insecurity, distrust, and self-worth.

b. Group therapy

Group therapy by its very nature provides a sense of belonging that inner city children often do not experience in their families and seek out in gangs. Participation in group therapy can fill this need to be identified as part of a group in order to develop a sense of identity. As group norms develop, clear messages about values and expectations are instilled. As routines and rules emerge, alternative behavioral expectations develop, which will hopefully generalize to other contexts (Halpern 1992). Depending on how groupings are determined, group members often share similar experiences (abuse) or obstacles (depression or anger management). This gives the groups a focus, allows for feelings of understanding and helps children to feel that they are not alone. By creating opportunities for acceptance, group therapy often helps children to develop confidence and mastery over the difficult situation.

Therapeutic groups go through stages of development (Yalom 1995) which provide indicators as to what possible client reactions will be and what therapeutic interventions may succeed. Moving from an orientation stage, during which structure and goals are established with much focus on the therapist, to a conflict stage, where interpersonal dynamics and issues of leadership are addressed, to group cohesiveness, where group members commit to the personal and group process, therapeutic groups provide a unique microcosm of group situations that children will experience in other contexts.

Bilides (1992) describes group-work with inner city adolescents which revolved around four different types of groups: support, theme, education, and responsibility. Each had a clearly defined purpose and method. All required structure, limit setting, support, and containment of difficult emotions on the part of the therapist, through techniques such as restating, giving instructions, refocusing, making parallels, modeling, and emphasizing strengths. As group members shared problems, they were often called upon to role-play, brainstorm, and provide constructive criticism in order to develop a network of mutual help and group cohesion. By giving voice to individuals within the group setting, the children developed a sense of importance and confidence. Bilides (1992) developed a series of guiding principles that emerged from his work and were shown to be effective with this population. He describes how groups should be long-term, well defined, structured, provide clear limits, strive towards developing normalcy, and respect all contributions as long as they are within the established group norms.

Some organizations are able to target groups of children who would be considered at risk for particular behaviors, and to provide interventions geared to addressing specific issues. Eargle, Guerra and Tolan (1994) describe a small group intervention that aimed to prevent aggression in urban boys through changes in cognitions, social skills, and behavior. In their approach, constructive anger outlets and non-aggressive methods of coping with violence were addressed through structured skill development. Techniques such as "stop and think" were learned through role-play, script and action plan development, and conversations about consequences. The advantage of group-work in this context was that group members were asked by the therapists to monitor one another's behavior as a method of positive reinforcement.

Stein *et al.* (2003) developed a school-based intervention program for reducing children's symptoms of PTSD and depression that were the result of chronic exposure to violence. Their approach involved cognitive and behavioral interventions which were delivered by clinicians over the course of ten sessions. Through education, relaxation, emotion management (combating negative thoughts), creative expression (drawing and writing), and social problem-solving they found a decrease in PTSD and depression symptoms. Success in this case can be mainly attributed to the intense collaboration between teachers and clinicians. Frequent consultations ensured the sharing of information and the addressing of student needs.

c. Family Therapy

Families in inner cities often demonstrate dysfunctional patterns arising out of chaotic environmental and domestic situations, which require intervention at the family level. In addition, traumatic events occurring to an individual affect the entire family. Family therapy treats the family system as a whole, rather than treating a specific person, and is often required in addition to individual therapy. Attention is paid to family patterns of interaction and individual roles within the family unit. Family therapy attempts to identify and modify maladaptive family dynamics and relationships, with the aim of improving overall and individual functioning (Goldenberg and Goldenberg 1995).

In addition to specific family therapy interventions, parents often require their own guidance in the form of individual therapy or group counseling. Because adults are often suffering from their own issues, many inner city parents are uninvolved and unengaged in the process of therapy for themselves or their children. Families are often required to care for children who have been traumatized. While dealing with their own emotions and reactions to a situation, adults often need guidance as to how to best support the child. Through support groups or parenting classes, parents can receive information about how to manage their own reactions, what to expect from their children, and how best to support recovery.

d. School counseling

Many schools implement specific preventive curricula that aim to provide children with targeted information and skills. These are typically delivered to entire classrooms as part of the school curriculum. Topics such as violence prevention, bullying, sex education, and conflict management are addressed, to provide children with concrete experience of ways to cope. While increasing awareness and knowledge about these topics, such programs help children and teachers to identify risk factors in children and avenues for seeking help.

Atkins *et al.* (1998) describe how schools often serve as the most consistent institutions available to inner city families. They therefore provide a unique opportunity for access and mental health delivery. They discuss the importance of integrating mental health goals in ongoing school routines and school culture. By developing vocabulary and activities around topics such as respect, discipline, communication, and responsibility, children will develop these notions by living them. This moral development will counteract negative temptations and will instill in children coping mechanisms and the confidence necessary to make positive choices. It is important to involve all adults such as administrators, teachers, and parents, as well as students, in the promotion of prosocial behaviors. This will ensure that consistent messages are being communicated that will become integral to school and personal functioning.

The growing field of social and emotional learning (SEL) is fast coming to the forefront of innovative educational practices (Cohen 2001). The comprehensive infusion of social and emotional competencies in schools develops socially and academically successful individuals. Ideally, SEL is infused into all aspects of a school, from school culture to delivery of instruction, to behavioral expectations. It is becoming clear that when the social and emotional needs of children are addressed, learning capabilities are enhanced (Zins *et al.* 2004).

6.2 Therapist qualities

Therapists take on many roles when working with inner city children. They often act as parents, teachers, and therapists, providing not only therapy, but basic needs such as food and clothing as well. It is important to maintain clear boundaries with this population and to provide positive experiences of appropriate child–adult relationships, as well as appropriate separation. A therapist must be available to develop a strong therapeutic relationship with a child, as this will allow the child to be heard and supported and to experience a corrective emotional experience. This in itself promotes healing and works to correct an injured sense of trust (Crenshaw *et al.*1986). The more a therapist gets to know the child, the better she will be able to determine and address the child's needs. The therapist is responsible for defining the scope of this relationship and sticking to it.

Many of these children present overwhelming histories, which can become burdensome to a therapist. Establishing a purpose and goals will help a therapist to more effectively manage the therapeutic process and will combat feelings of ineffectiveness. Retaining a focused and present demeanor will improve the quality of service and will help the therapist see progress, no matter how minute.

Working with inner city children requires daily contact with traumatized children and families and associated cognitive, emotional and physical damage. Maintaining an unconditional stance of support and containment, sustaining empathic responses, and establishing meaning and purpose, enables children to trust the therapist, allowing healing to occur. By correcting cognitive distortions and normalizing emotional reactions, the therapeutic process enables children to integrate their experiences into the course of their development. At the same time, the role of a therapist is not to teach values but to "facilitate the normal process of moral differentiation" (Aigen 1991, p.123).

Eargle, Guerra and Tolan (1994) discuss the importance of a therapist knowing her population and the specific circumstances under which her clients live. This will allow interventions to be realistic and suited to the particular reality of the client. If interventions are not relevant or suitable for a particular situation, the value of the intervention will be discounted and the child's needs will not be met.

Bilides (1992) states that therapists act by default as role models. Children watch a therapist and learn not only from what they hear, but from what they see. It is important that a therapist be authentic and stable in her interactions. Children can sense when a therapist is emotionally unavailable or misguided by preconceptions. To aid in this process, it is essential that therapists have a clear sense of their own identities and beliefs. By being self-aware a therapist is able to be authentic, available, empathic, and connected (Camilleri 2001). This is often accomplished through professional supervision and knowing where to get support when in need.

Being aware of cultural differences and needs is an important competence for a therapist to develop. Working in inner cities requires in-depth knowledge of different cultural norms of interaction, communication, gender identity, and authority. A therapist who is aware of these will be adept at identifying moments of racial conflict or assumption that occur within the therapeutic process (Bilides 1992). Celebrating cultural differences rather than maintaining a "color-blind" approach creates avenues for connecting and forming relationships. A "color-blind" approach can overlook valuable information and aspects of the self, and in so doing may prevent therapeutic work from being accomplished.

As described by Batmanghelidjh (1999) it is essential that a therapist be a consistent and stable presence in the lives of these children. To counteract previous experiences of adult unreliability, it is essential to maintain a predictable therapeutic pattern of attendance and structure. Likewise, structure within sessions will go a long way towards gaining the trust of inner city children and providing a safe and supportive atmosphere. Reliable session structure will send a clear message to a child that therapy is very different from the often chaotic "real world".

Access to mental health professionals is often challenging and delivery of services is often prevented owing to a lack of insurance. Persistent out-reach is often required to get children the services that they need. McKernan-McKay *et al.* (1998) found that a high degree of out-reach on the part of therapists and agencies was necessary to get families to attend intake appointments and to continue services on an on-going basis. They found that a telephone call and an initial interview showed significant increases in on-going attendance and use of services. When therapists reach out to families by being sensitive to scheduling, transportation and informational needs, the children will get the services they need. A suspicious and uniformed parent is often the most difficult barrier to overcome for a child to receive therapy.

In order for a therapist to maintain the characteristics mentioned above, it is essential that he or she be committed to continued learning and personal care. Not only is it important to have received necessary training, but on-going professional supervision, individual therapy, and an ability to take care of personal needs will allow a therapist to work with patients in an authentic and informed manner.

6.3 Therapeutic issues

a. Cultural differences

Very often mental health professionals are from a different cultural background than their clients. A therapist must be aware of her own assumptions and stereotypes if a trusting relationship is to develop. Negative stereotypes going in both directions can affect the quality of the therapy and can act as a roadblock to growth. A therapist should enable her client to understand and deal with the outside world, while maintaining a realistic and empathic view of her client's reality (Bilides 1992).

b. Transference

Transference is the tendency of a client to project onto a therapist feelings that have nothing to do with that person. Yalom (1995) describes this as being "a specific form of interpersonal perceptual distortion" (p.44). For example, feelings about people from a child's past can emerge and influence how that child interacts with a therapist. When identified as transference by a sensitive therapist, it can be used as an important therapeutic tool.

c. Countertransference

Countertransference, defined as a therapist's unusually intense emotional reaction to a client, can manifest in a variety of ways. When the therapist's personal motivation or past experiences influence his or her decisions, then he or she is often working in a way that is self-protective and counterproductive for the client. Examples described by Erwin (1994), such as avoidance of a therapeutic issue, racial stereotyping, pitying, or "passionate parenting", are clear indications of countertransference that may be detrimental to the therapeutic process. Erwin goes on to say that a therapist who is self-aware in her reactions will monitor them and use them in such a way that they inform, rather than distort, her therapeutic decisions.

d. Diagnosis

Many at-risk children have unmet mental health needs. Owing to a lack of trained professionals and attentive parents, many mental health problems go undiagnosed, especially if a child has an internalizing symptom such as depression or anxiety, which is not immediately evident (Bickham *et al.* 1998). Misdiagnosis is another concern. For example, when children exhibit academic deficiencies they often receive a special education label, rather than recognition and investigation of potential mental health needs that may be hindering learning.

e. Access

Availability of mental health services is often lacking in inner city neighborhoods because of lack of funding and infrastructures. Available services may be inaccessible, due to a lack of transportation or a lack of insurance coverage. In addition, some parents are only available in the evenings or on weekends and require childcare in order to bring one of their children to an appointment.

f. Attendance

Children who need mental health interventions often don't have the resources to know what they need, and rely on adults to provide for them. Many adults don't have the education or the resources to inquire about services, or are unable to take their children to consistently attend.

g. Normalization

Children who are exposed to chronic violence and other stressors demonstrate behaviors and emotional reactions that become normal and expected. Among people who are experiencing the same emotions, these become part of life and are not viewed as needing treatment (Warner and Weist 1996).

h. Stigmatization

Some individuals discourage expression of emotions because it is viewed as unnecessary and weak. Some people believe that depending on someone else to talk to and to seek help from demonstrates vulnerability and is humiliating, as it is assumed that individuals in such cases cannot take care of themselves. Mental health intervention is stigmatizing in some communities. Batmanghelidjh (1999) describes how some members of the African-American community view White mental health professionals as ruining or spoiling their children by catering to them through mental health interventions for problems that should be dealt with independently.

i. Fear of blame

Some parents fear that if their child receives a mental health intervention, the problem will be acknowledged publicly. Parents sometimes fear that they will be criticized for being ineffective parents and blamed for child outcomes (Bickham *et al.* 1998). Many adults are suspicious of the mental health system and fear that their children will be "taken away" from them.

j. Defensiveness

Many inner city children are resistant to or leery of treatment. Because they lack stable and reliable adults in their lives, it often takes a long time for children to trust and open up to a therapist. They have had to adopt a defensive attitude to protect themselves from their environments, and this stance is often so ingrained that it becomes a therapeutic issue or barrier to progress. Crenshaw *et al.* (1986) describe how in work with abused children, breaking the silence requires attention to therapeutic timing, preparation, empathy, and supportive responding. Resistance to disclosure is a means of protection and often manifests as denial or magical thinking.

k. Fear of intimacy

Inner city children have often lacked affectionate and loving relationships with adults. Because of past disappointments these children have difficulty opening up to a therapist and trusting them for fear of abandonment. Experiencing affection is often a new thing for these children, who often confuse love with receiving material items from (for example) absent fathers.

6.4 Creative arts therapies

As stated by the National Coalition of Creative Arts Therapists (2004) creative arts therapies such as music, dance, art, drama, poetry, and psychodrama

> use arts modalities and creative processes during intentional interventions in therapeutic, rehabilitative, community, or educational settings to foster health, com-

munication, and expression; promote the integration of physical, emotional, cognitive, and social functioning; enhance self-awareness; and facilitate change.

Creative arts therapies interventions are grounded in specific psychological theories (behaviorist, cognitive, humanistic, developmental, psychoanalytic) which inform methods and goals. They can be provided in a variety of contexts and formats to meet the needs of diverse populations.

In describing music therapy from a humanistic perspective, Boxill (1985) explains how music is used as a therapeutic tool to restore, maintain, and improve psychological, mental, social, and physical health within the context of a client–therapist relationship. Although every creative arts therapies field is unique in materials and methods, they all employ similar processes to attain goals that ensure client well-being.

The creative arts therapies provide unique avenues for working with children. Expression through the arts is socially acceptable and, when used in mental health interventions, makes therapy less stigmatizing for children (Wengrower 2001). Presenting children with familiar and culturally relevant media makes them less reluctant to engage in therapeutic interactions. More important, participation in the arts is fun, playful, and intrinsically gratifying – which increases motivation, investment, and participation in therapy. The arts provide an "aesthetic context" (Aigen 1991, p.113) in which to support, connect, and heal.

Using examples from each creative arts therapies field, shared goals and processes in terms of their advantages for use with inner city, at-risk children are described below.

a. Processes

(I) PARALLEL PROCESSES

What sets the creative arts therapies apart from more conventional methods of psychotherapy is the use of artistic and therapeutic processes simultaneously. This twofold approach broadens opportunities for connection between therapist and client and enhances the therapeutic experience. When processes occur simultaneously within the therapeutic relationship, healing can occur on multiple levels.

Art-making and Words

Use of the arts in therapy allows therapists to engage clients in purposeful creative experiences that promote growth through the process of art-making, as well as through the artistic product that is created. Engagement in creative expression employs emotional, cognitive and physical functions, allowing for a multidimensional experience and creating many opportunities for growth and connection with the therapist. Arts experiences connect the therapist to the client by acting as "fields for interaction" (Aigen 1991, p.125).

In some cases meaning is derived through the hands-on creative experience alone, and in other cases through the addition of a cognitive experience. Depending on the child, a verbal element may elucidate important feelings that arise during therapy. Creative arts therapies interventions may jumpstart verbalizations by triggering memories or dislodging feelings (Camilleri 2002). By creating an emotional reaction, creative arts therapies experiences have the capacity to circumvent defenses and access the unconscious realm. In her description of poetry therapy to address issues of racism, Stepakoff (1997) describes how poetry therapy not only recovers buried memories, but enables recognition, naming, and reintegration of previously submerged aspects of the self.

In some cases verbalization within the creative arts therapies realm adds a dimension to the therapeutic process. As described by Frisch (1990) in her discussion of the music therapy process, "words can increase the music's effectiveness when they are used in a way that structures, that directs or highlights the musical activities of the session" (p.20). Camilleri (2005) describes her use of verbal questioning within the music therapy context as an integral part of her social skills development approach. Discussions following music therapy experiences guide children towards finding meaning and making connections. Children are encouraged to identify skills that they used during the music-making and to share examples of times in their lives when these skills are necessary. Words in this context act as a bridge between the music therapy session and the children's lives outside the session. The point at which students can make the connection between "musical production and internal process" (Frisch 1990, p.20) is the point at which therapeutic growth takes place. Kruczek and Zagelbaum (2004) discuss how the success of their psycho-educational drama interventions with at-risk youth was amplified through subsequent discussions which allowed for both affective and cognitive engagement.

Child and Therapist

The creative arts therapies enable the child and therapist to engage in a simultaneous process that allows for flexible, ever-changing and in-the-moment responses. Engaging in an artistic activity with a child engages processes similar to those in interactions between a child and a caregiver (Bannister 2003). This familiar mode of interaction makes the process of therapy less daunting if it can be assumed that the child has experienced positive relationships with adults in the past. If not, the therapeutic interaction can repair negative relationships from the past.

Process and Product

Creative arts therapies offer benefit not only from therapeutic and artistic processes, but from the artistic products that are created. Therapeutic growth in areas such as relationship formation and communication occurs in the process of creation with peers or the therapist. At the same time, individual therapeutic growth occurs in the revelation and integration of the content that is expressed through the creative product.

(II) SYMBOLIC REPRESENTATION

Creative arts therapists working within a psychoanalytic frame of reference encourage the use of "transitional objects" (Winnicott 1971), items that a child becomes attached to that represent something or someone from their lives. Whether using stories, instruments, paint, scarves, space, or puppets, the materials act as a container for the child to use symbolically. Creating emotional distance by projecting stories and feelings onto an outside medium is often the only way a child can manage and share devastating emotions. There is safety in the distance, which will pave the way for integration of negative emotions and experiences as therapy progresses. Transitional objects act as the point of connection between the child and the therapist, through which repressed feelings can be evoked, content can be disclosed, and a therapeutic relationship can emerge.

Through symbolic representation and use of different media, children can re-experience or recreate events in their lives in ways that may be more manageable. In this way, the creative arts therapies allow children to experience a "corrective emotional experience" (Friedlander 1994, p.97). Haen and Brannon (2002) describe how, in drama therapy, outcomes and reactions can be modified through "corrective enactment" (p.37). These reparative experiences emerge based on changes initiated by the child or the therapist.

(III) FLEXIBILITY AND STRUCTURE

While being flexible and encouraging creative play, the creative arts therapies use structured and predictable arts processes that develop a sense of safety. Whether creating a mural or a play, there are specific artistic steps to be taken which the therapist can use to organize and channel the often chaotic energy that a child presents (Camilleri 2000). The combination of freedom and structure provided in creative arts therapies has been explored by Moreno (1985), who describes how the structured and unstructured qualities of musical instruments provide a dual potential for therapeutic intervention.

(IV) USE OF THE BODY

Some at-risk children have been physically violated, suffering not only psychological damage, but physical damage as well. These children are often unable to describe their feelings, which tend to manifest as bodily reactions such as tension or weight fluctuations. As noted by Farr (1997), affect is often disclosed through movement. To address physical traumas, therapies that utilize the body to address its reactions are best suited. Bannister (2003) suggests that children who have been physically abused retain their traumatizing memories in a sensory way. These impairments can therefore only be accessed in a sensory modality.

Use of the body enables children to avoid "intellectualization" and allows for a connection between mind and body to occur. Through hands-on activities and action a child can work through negative life events and develop physical techniques to cope with negative situations. Stress management techniques such as relaxation and breath control can be taught to help a child deal with scary and anxiety-provoking situations.

b. Goals

(I) SELF-EXPRESSION

Creative arts therapies provide appropriate verbal and nonverbal means of self-expression as alternatives to maladaptive ones. In their description of an arts-based violence-prevention program, Long and Soble (1999) describe how the children "created vivid imagery and powerful enactments as a way of expressing and sublimating…feelings and thoughts arising from this sharing" (p.344). Through art and drama exercises the children developed concrete problem-solving methods, appropriate communication skills, and action plans to be used when dealing with difficult situations.

Children often lack the vocabulary to converse freely, have lost the capacity to speak, or avoid speaking in order to protect themselves from re-experiencing negative emotions (Batmanghelidjh 1999). Creative arts therapies provide alternative opportunities for expression and communication through symbolic representation in art, music, role-playing, or movement. Hands-on therapeutic arts experiences have often been described as providing opportunities for catharsis, as difficult emotions or relationships are made evident in the experience and reintegrated in more manageable forms.

(II) EMOTIONAL GROWTH

Over time, creative arts therapies experiences guide children towards health. Emotions or behaviors can be identified, expressed and worked through with the aim of gaining mastery over them, modifying them, and ultimately integrating them into the self as a whole. The creative arts therapies provide developmentally appropriate interventions that help children to connect with their true emotions, as well as to people around them, in nurturing and healing relationships.

(III) SOCIAL SKILLS DEVELOPMENT

Creative arts therapies provide hands-on experiences that enable children to develop important social skills such as team-work, sharing, communication, and self-discipline, which work to improve academic performance and reduce instances of violence (Camilleri and Jackson 2005). These opportunities allow children to work towards mastery of skills by repeatedly using them appropriately in a structured environment and by engaging in healing and reparative experiences. The hope is that with guidance, children will generalize what they have learned to other aspects of their lives.

(IV) PLAY

Some inner city children have lost their capacity to be playful and to experience joy (Bannister 2003) because traumatic experiences have shut them down or circumstances have forced them to rapidly "grow up". Creative arts therapies have the capacity to encourage children to play and to use their creative imaginations, often aiding a child to regress to a more appropriate developmental age. Bannister (2003) describes how many traumatized children are unable to discuss their issues but enjoy reading or making up stories that consciously or unconsciously relate to their trauma. She discusses how these children use the "play space, area of illusion, or space between" (p.20) to work through their situations metaphorically.

Axline (1947) described play therapy as a comprehensive method of treatment for children. She describes the importance of introducing play when children are unable to overcome obstacles or to express themselves with words alone. Her formulation of play therapy is based on self-directed play interactions with a therapist in order to reach self-actualization and self-realization.

(V) ROLE-DEFINITION: ART IMITATING LIFE

As in most therapy situations, the creative arts therapy context often mirrors home or classroom situations in that children fall into similar roles and exhibit similar behaviors. How children manipulate materials and interact with group members and the therapist gives important information about their functioning outside of sessions. The session acts as a context within which to address roles and modify behaviors for the purpose of improving interactions outside of a session.

As described by Yalom (1998), feelings elicited from an immediate therapeutic experience are often similar to those experienced in life. By addressing them in the safe context of a therapy session, children are enabled to better cope with them should they occur again. As Camilleri (2006) states, "As they control the music, they are in essence controlling themselves and their impulses. The music therapy context becomes a template for their lives, and learning that occurs through the music will over time translate into changes occurring in their behaviors" (p.210).

As roles become clearer, children slowly build up a sense of themselves as essential participants in a larger picture. They refine their interactions and reactions which contribute to early identity formation.

(VI) CREATIVITY

Creative arts therapies allow children to tap into their creative imaginations and use this resource for connection, growth, and healing. Both therapist and child meet in the creative process where one seeks repair and the other offers guidance. Through intimate artistic sharing the child is welcomed as a sum of many parts which need to be integrated into a whole. Because creativity lies within each of us, all children have the capacity to self-heal when supported by the safety of the therapeutic process.

References

Aigen, K. (1991) 'Creative fantasy, music and lyric improvisation with a gifted acting-out boy.' In K.E. Bruscia (ed.) *Case Studies in Music Therapy*. Gilsum: Barcelona Publishers.

Atkins, M.S, McKernan-McKay, M., Arvanitis, P., London, L., Madison, S., Costigan, C., Haney, P., Zevenbergen, A., Hess, L., Bennett, D., and Webster, D. (1998) 'An ecological model for school-based mental health services for urban low-income aggressive children.' *Journal of Behavioral Health Services and Research 25*, 1, 1094–3412.

Axline, V.M. (1947) *Play Therapy*. Boston, MA: Houghton Mifflin.

Bannister, A. (2003) *Creative Therapies with Traumatized Children*. London: Jessica Kingsley Publishers.

Batmanghelidjh, C. (1999) 'Whose political correction? The challenge of therapeutic work with inner city children experiencing deprivation.' *Psychodynamic Counseling 5*, 2, 231–244.

Bickham, N.L., Pizarro, L.J., Warner, B.S., Rosenthal, B., and Weist, M.D. (1998) 'Family involvement in expanded school mental health.' *Journal of School Health 68*, 10, 425–428.

Bilides, D.B. (1992) 'Reaching inner city children: A group work program model for a public middle school.' In *Group Work Reaching Out: People, Places and Power*. The Haworth Press, Inc.

Boxill, E. (1985) *Music Therapy for the Developmentally Disabled*. Rockville, MD: Aspen Publications.

Buka, S. and Earls, F. (1993). 'Early determinants of delinquency and violence.' *Health Affairs*, Winter 1993.

Camilleri, V.A. (2000) 'Music therapy groups: A path to social-emotional growth and academic success.' *Educational Horizons*, Summer, 184–189.

Camilleri, V.A. (2001) 'Therapist self-awareness: An essential tool in music therapy.' *The Arts in Psychotherapy 28*, 79–85.

Camilleri, V.A. (2002) 'Community building through drumming'. *The Arts in Psychotherapy 29*, 261–264.

Camilleri, V.A. (2006) 'Music therapy with inner city, at-risk children: From the literal to the symbolic'. In S.L. Brooke (ed.) *Creative Therapies Manual: A Guide to the History, Theoretical Approaches, Assessment, and Work with Special Populations of Art, Play, Dance, Music, Drama, and Poetry Therapies*. Springfield, IL: C.C. Thomas.

Camilleri, V.A. and Jackson, A.D. (2005) 'Nurturing excellence through the arts: A charter school focused on arts and technology helps urban students' talents bloom.' *Educational Leadership*, March 2005, 60–64.

Cohen, J. (2001) *Caring Classrooms / Intelligent Schools: The Social-Emotional Education of Young Children*. New York: Teachers College Press.

Crenshaw, D.A., Rudy, D., Triemer, D., and Zingaro, J. (1986) 'Psychotherapy with abused children: Breaking the silent bond.' *Residential Group Care and Treatment 3*, 4, 25–38.

Eargle, A.E., Guerra, N.G., and Tolan, P.H. (1994) 'Preventing aggression in inner city children: Small group training to change cognitions, social skills, and behavior.' *Journal of Child and Adolescent Group Therapy 4*, 4, 229–242.

Erwin, P.A. (1994) 'Inner-city children of trauma: Urban violence traumatic stress response syndrome (U-VTS) and therapists' responses.' In J.P. Wilson and J.D. Lindy (eds) *Countertransference in the Treatment of PTDS.* New York: Guilford Publications, Inc.

Farr, M. (1997) 'The role of dance/movement therapy in treating at-risk African-American adolescents.' *The Arts in Psychotherapy 24*, 2, 183–191.

Friedlander, L.H. (1994) 'Group music psychotherapy in an inpatient psychiatric setting for children: A developmental approach.' *Music Therapy Perspectives 12*, 92–97.

Frisch, A. (1990) 'Symbol and structure: Music therapy for the adolescent psychiatric inpatient.' *Music Therapy 9*, 1, 16–34.

Garbarino, J. (2001) 'An ecological perspective on the effects of violence on children.' *Journal of Community Psychology 29*, 3, 361–378.

Goldenberg, I. and Goldenberg, H. (1995) 'Family therapy.' In R.J Corsini and D. Wedding (eds) *Current Psychotherapies.* Itasca, IL: F.E. Peacock publishers, Inc.

Haen, C., and Brannon, K.H. (2002) 'Superheroes, monsters, and babies: Roles of strength, destruction and vulnerability for emotionally disturbed boys.' *The Arts in Psychotherapy 29*, 31–40.

Halpern, R. (1992) 'The role of after-school programs in the lives of inner city children: A study of the "Urban Youth Network".' *Child Welfare 71*, 3, 215–231.

Kruczek, T., and Zagelbaum, A. (2004) 'Increasing adolescent awareness of at risk behaviors via psychoeducational drama.' *The Arts in Psychotherapy 31*, 1–10.

Long, J.K., and Soble, L. (1999) 'Report: An arts-based violence prevention project for sixth grade students.' *The Arts in Psychotherapy 26*, 5, 329–344.

McKernan-McKay, M., Stoewe, J., McCadam, K., and Gonzales, J. (1998) 'Increasing access to child mental health services for urban children and their caregivers.' *Health & Social Work 23*, 1, 9–15.

Metropolitan Area Child Study Research Group. (2002) 'A cognitive-ecological approach to preventing aggression in urban settings: Initial outcomes for high-risk children.' *Journal of Consulting and Clinical Psychology 70*, 1, 179–194.

Moreno, J. (1985) 'Music play therapy: An integrated approach.' *The Arts in Psychotherapy 12*, 17–23.

National Coalition of Creative Arts Therapies Associations. 'Factsheet on the creative arts therapies.' Accessed August 2004 at www.nccata.org.

Pynoos, R.S. and Nader, K. (1988) 'Psychological first aid and treatment approach to children exposed to community violence: Research implications.' *Journal of Traumatic Stress 1*, 445–473.

Stein, B.D., Jaycox, L.H., Kataoka, S.H., Wong, M., Tu, W., Elliott, M.N., and Fink, A. (2003) 'A mental health intervention for schoolchildren exposed to violence: A randomized controlled trial.' *Journal of the American Medical Association 290*, 5, 603–611.

Stepakoff, S. (1997) 'Poetry therapy principles and practices for raising awareness of racism.' *The Arts in Psychotherapy 24*, 3, 261–274.

Warner, B.S. and Weist, M.D. (1996) 'Urban youth as witnesses to violence: Beginning assement and treatment efforts.' *Journal of Youth and Adolescence 25*, 3, 361–377.

Wengrower, H. (2001) 'Arts therapies in educational settings: An intercultural encounter.' *The Arts in Psychotherapy 28*, 109–115.

Winnicott, D.W. (1971) *Playing and Reality.* London: Tavistock Publications Ltd.

Yalom, I.D. (1995) *The Theory and Practice of Group Psychotherapy.* New York: Basic Books.

Yalom, I.D. (1998) *The Yalom Reader.* New York: Basic Books.

Zins, J.E., Weissberg, R.P., Wang, M.C., and Walberg, H.J. (2004) *Building Academic Success on Social and Emotional Learning.* New York: Teachers College Press.

Part II

Healing the Inner City Child

CHAPTER 7

"Hear Me Sing"

Structured Group Songwriting with Inner City, At-risk Children

Vanessa A. Camilleri, MA, MT-BC

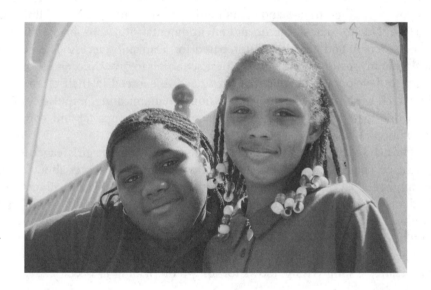

A structured group songwriting experience for at-risk children in school settings in New York City and Washington DC is described. It emphasizes the importance of the process and the benefits of the song product. The music therapy group process often mirrors dynamics that children experience in their lives, while song topics can reflect very real hopes, dreams, or fears. This provides two levels for therapeutic intervention: the interpersonal songwriting process, and the personal expression contained in the song product. Structured group songwriting allows children to express themselves, develop a sense of pride and ownership, and contribute to a collaborative effort that culminates in a celebrated accomplishment.

Prelude

From the chaos of a typical day in an inner city elementary school emerge five pre-teenage girls, laughing, shoving, bursting with energy and craving attention. They tumble into the music therapy room, dump their belongings on the floor, and fall heavily onto chairs and beanbags. Slowly they settle, shedding their toughness, leaving their edge at the door, shrinking slowly into their real selves. Suddenly they are less bold, and more vulnerable, more authentic in their presence as ten- and eleven-year-olds. As they listen to the opening chime, some close their eyes, trusting the ritual that begins their weekly music therapy session. Their task is to listen to the sound and raise their hand when the sound disappears. This moment of transition allows them to leave the rest of the day behind and to focus for an instant on themselves.

The children described here are regular education children who attend two charter schools in New York City and Washington DC. Both are located in inner city neighborhoods with few resources, deteriorating buildings, and struggling families. The children face daily interactions with violence, drugs, and poverty in their homes and communities, often coming to school unfed or un-clean. Due to toxic domestic and environmental situations, many children are not socially and emotionally prepared for academic success. The goal of music therapy sessions conducted at these schools is to give children the opportunity to develop social skills that they need to succeed in their classrooms. Skills such as sharing, listening, expression, communicating, impulse control, and working together are targeted through in-depth musical and cognitive exploration.

The need to be heard and acknowledged is evident in the girls' eagerness to share their chaotic stories and confused emotions. As one shares about losing her mother, a succession of stories about relatives lost to murder, illness, and accidents ensues, with incidental mention of shootings, theft, and illegal activity. The normalcy of these conversations reflects the prevalence of their content. Songwriting has emerged as a natural avenue for jump-starting the therapeutic process in this context. By encapsulating the essence of endless conversations, songwriting allows for long-term healing to occur.

Songs

Popular, client-composed, or improvised songs have been used by music therapists working with a variety of populations such as abused adolescents (Lindberg 1995), bereaved adolescents (Dalton and Krout 2005), emotionally impaired adolescents (Edgerton 1990), reading and language impaired children (Gfeller 1987), special education students (Nordoff and Robbins 1995), spinal-cord injured patients (Amir 1990), traumatic brain-injured patients (Baker, Kennely and Tamplin 2005; Robb 1996), schizophrenics (Silverman 2003), cancer patients (Magill-Bailey 1984; Logis and Turry 1999), borderline personality disorder patients (Dvorkin 1991) chemically dependent adults (Freed 1987; Jones 2005), psychiatric adults (Ficken 1 and HIV patients (Cordobes 1997).

Songs have been described by music therapists as a means to contain often difficult and terrifying emotions. As described by Dvorkin (1991), songs can be used as transitional objects by absorbing and communicating dangerous feelings. Acting as a bridge between patients and their issues, a healthy distance is created through which patients can gain perspective and insight. The structure of a song can capture the essence of a conversation, bring order to an often chaotic mixture of experiences, and help to organize confusing and overwhelming information.

In a detailed account of her singing journey through music therapy, a cancer patient and her music therapist describe how songs helped her to express, identify, and contain feelings that threatened her emotional stability. The songs gave her something to hold on to and to control in a life where her physical condition was beyond her control (Logis and Turry 1999). Songs literally give voice to expressions of pain or joy, and give those involved a sense of being heard and validated. As described by Amir (1990), songs can "serve as a vehicle for...thoughts, feelings, and sensations and their integration" (p.70). They are transportable pieces of poetry that children in music therapy sessions can own, bring with them when they leave, and use to their benefit when in need.

Songs provide a mode of communication and create opportunities to use the human instrument, the voice. As Magill-Bailey (1984) states, the voice "is an instrument through which we express feelings and thoughts and extend important parts of ourselves" (p.7). Singing is an intimate mode of self-expression which can improve mood (Kenny and Faunce 2004) and encourage human contact and relationship formation. As Austin describes,

> When we sing, we are intimately connected to our breath, our bodies, and our emotional lives... When we sing, we can give voice to and find relief from intense pain, fear, and anger. When we sing, we can celebrate and express joy... We can connect with each other and we can build and strengthen community. (Austin 1998, p.316).

Songwriting

While allowing for exploration of important content material, songwriting can address a variety of additional needs (Robb 1996). It allows participants to self-disclose, express themselves, verbalize, master emotions, create alternative realities, seek productive solutions, gain insight, see multiple perspectives, bring feelings to the surface, and recover repressed material (Cordobes 1997; Ficken 1976; Freed 1987; Robb 1996). Because songs can be written down or recorded, they are a source of immediate feedback for clients (Ficken 1976). Songs can be kept at a distance from a child, making their content more palatable and easier to handle. The structured nature of a song condenses often confusing emotions into simple and more manageable statements. The song validates and honors a child's self-expression in a form that can be shared and transported. As Robb (1996) states "The song-writing process is one that harnesses the creative abilities of individuals and empowers them to express their experiences and emotions in a way that many have never before experienced" (p.14).

At the same time, the process of group songwriting is an excellent way to develop self-esteem and social skills such as group cohesiveness, social interaction, communication, problem-solving, listening, and respect. Songwriting is an active process that requires a responsive and energetic interplay between the people engaged in the process. It is a flexible experience that can be adapted to a wide range of ability and interest levels.

The songwriting process

The songwriting process described here outlines the essential steps necessary to create a song for the purpose of self-expression and social interaction. The songs described here are developed over time through a structured process rather than being improvised in the moment. Depending on the needs of the group, the order of steps may change. Both process and product remain essential elements of this therapeutic work.

The process of songwriting with children opens up opportunities to work on skills such as listening, team-work, risk-taking, and respect. The tasks that the children are required to fulfill in order to create a song help them to understand the value of working together towards a final accomplishment. Edgerton (1990) describes a similar group songwriting process and outlines the learning that occurs during each step. As shown in the case studies below, the final products are often expressions of hurt, growth, or hope which have been consolidated into structured compositions that give meaning to difficult experiences and a glimmer of possible alternatives.

Opening

The songwriting project can be introduced by having children share recordings of their favorite songs and identifying the singer or group, the genre, what the song is about, and what the message of the song is. A reminder is given about appropriate language for school. Most children know what is appropriate and what is not; however, they are encouraged to check in with the therapist if they are unsure. Many times children will sing along to popular songs as they are presented. As song themes are identified it becomes clear that the songs are about very familiar topics such as relationships, feelings, family, and friends. As the children recognize these similarities, it becomes clear that they too have material to write about.

Themes

Very often conversations at the beginning of a session revolve around a particular theme. Whether the theme is anger about teachers, sadness about a relative who has passed away, or fear about being jumped, such themes often thread themselves into conversations from week to week. A skilled therapist will pick up on these recurring themes and use them to establish a purpose for the songwriting project.

A theme that is self-developed and relevant to the children in the group will ensure buy-in, stimulate creativity, promote high interest, and will have direct value for the children involved. As Nordoff and Robbins (1995) state, "the children must be able to believe in each song they sing and identify not only with its content, but with the words that are used to express it" (p.24). Themes build group cohesion as the children see that they share common concerns. Once a group theme or themes are identified, children either vote on one if there are several, or agree to the one that stands out. This in itself can take much negotiating and is a good way to develop problem-solving skills and prepare the children for what is to come.

Once a topic is selected, a brainstorm is conducted on that theme. Typically the topic is written in the center of a large piece of paper and the children contribute words, sentences, or thoughts associated with the topic. They are surprised when the therapist writes down all suggestions, including words such as 'sex' or 'guns'. Every idea that is expressed is written down within the parameters of setting rules. If the word used is considered inappropriate for school, the group comes up with another way of communicating that idea. This method of free association gives the children a chance to explore and express real feelings and thoughts in a safe and structured environment. Writing down their words honors their contributions.

The chorus

Moving forward, the theme or "hook" for the song is clarified. The children must identify what they want the song to be about. In thinking about popular songs, often children will remember the chorus rather than the lyrics in the verses. The group is asked to identify songs that they all know, and to sing the chorus as a group. This demonstrates that the chorus should contain the "take away message" of the song. Children circle items on their brainstorm that are of particular importance to them, and from these the theme of their song emerges.

Verses

The content of individual verses is broken down so that each verse contains a specific message. Verses build upon the central theme and work towards the culminating message, often working through difficult situations towards a more positive message at the end. Songwriting gives children a sense of control as they can re-experience events through lyric-writing or manipulate them to create different outcomes in a socially acceptable manner. Working either in pairs or alone, each verse is developed based on more brainstorming. Children are required to listen to each other, share ideas, and ultimately compromise with their peers. After each brainstorming session the children are encouraged to take a risk and to share their often personal lyrics with the group. Constructive feedback and suggestions are given after the therapist has modeled the format. Lyrics are typed up for the following week. The children enjoy this aspect of the process, as the typed-up sheet gives their words importance. The therapist and children work to shape the verses so that the words make rhythmic sense without changing any content.

The final verse is developed as a group as a way to summarize the main idea of the song and to end on a positive note. Many times this last verse turns into a celebration of what the children want in life. Working on the last verse as a group helps to develop group cohesion and pride. Children are encouraged to cooperate, and to act in a way that is for the good of the group. If the need of the group is to remain in a more negative state, lyrics do not necessarily have to lead towards a positive outcome. However, it is important to realize that the children will remember these songs and take them with them no matter where they go. The hope is that the songs will help them to overcome difficult situations in the future.

The music

When working on the music for songs the therapist can give suggestions to choose from. The group considers the instruments, the tempo, the style, and how it should be performed. Children are encouraged to negotiate and compromise through this process. Many rehearsals help to iron out the details of the work in progress. The process is recorded from week to week so the children can listen back and provide suggestions for improvement. As the song takes on form and structure, group members encourage and support each other as they experiment with singing and playing the instruments. A title for the song and a name for the group are determined by discussing different suggestions.

The performance

The songwriting process can take many weeks and the children gain a sense of pride and protectiveness over their accomplishment. A performance can be arranged and children can invite guests to attend. With the audience assembled, lyrics are distributed, the songwriting process is described, the group members are introduced, and the song is performed. This culminating activity is a joyous event that children and teachers alike will always remember. In a life full of disappointment and failure, writing and performing a song has been shown to bring a sense of accomplishment and pride to children who often have nothing to be proud of. Their success is made even more vital as it is witnessed by adults and peers.

Case examples
1. "Teachers and kids": Songwriting as an expression of hurt

A group of six Fifth-grade girls consistently came to music therapy sessions angry. Some of them sat turned away from the group and some of them actively engaged in the opening rap, banging almost violently on the drum. The girls rarely discussed their feelings, but enjoyed putting their names on post-it notes and sticking them on colorful feeling faces displayed on the wall. Typically the girls were angry, annoyed, or frustrated. One week the girls were picked up early from their class by the therapist and a disturbing interaction with their female teacher was witnessed. There was clearly a power struggle going on between the girls and their teacher. The teacher seemed to speak at their level, using 'street gestures' and mannerisms to intimidate the girls. Instead of being a calming influence, the teacher engaged the girls in yelling matches that escalated into inappropriate behavior on the part of the girls.

Without mentioning the teacher directly, the therapist reflected how it must be difficult to be around adults who are constantly putting children down and yelling. Obviously surprised that talking about adults was acceptable, one of the girls said, "She talks like us." This opened up a long conversation in which the girls described how their teacher spoke to them in a "mean" way and never listened to what they had to say. Some compared her to siblings whom they constantly fought with. They described hating being in her classroom and being scared to ask questions because she would yell at them. As the conversation continued, the girls clearly stated that teachers should be people who respect you and whom you can trust. The underlying message was that the girls needed love and someone to look up to. Their classroom teacher embodied all adults in their lives who had disrespected and disappointed them. In this case it was important to allow the girls to "vent" so that they could then focus on the task at hand. The girls owned up to being disrespectful to their teacher, but, true to the message that these children have grown up with in their neighborhoods, "What she does to me, I will do back to her." We took this ingrained message and incorporated it into the chorus of a song:

Chorus

How I treat you
You should treat me
Working together
Is the way to be.

As the songwriting process developed there were occasions when the girls criticized each others' contributions and made fun of ideas. Putting each other down was a way to gain respect from peers. This culture of negativity showed toughness and seemed to be a way for the girls to survive in school and in their neighborhoods. They were taught how to hide their feelings, and to "act tough". Any sign of weakness made them a target for violence or teasing. The girls were reminded that this song about respect between children and teachers should be applied to any situation, including the task at hand of writing the song as a group. As time went on and the girls became more committed to the process, the group members began to remind each other of the song theme.

Many initial ideas involved the things that teachers had done to them. These were honored in two verses, which could have become four verses, had the therapist not shifted the focus to writing about their roles in these interactions. Reluctantly the girls composed a verse about how children should interact with teachers and how both parties were responsible for classroom interactions. The last verse was a summary of what the girls hoped for in a relationship with teachers, which represented how they wanted to be treated in general.

The girls had few positive adult role models in their lives. They were searching for an adult who would be different from others in their lives. The girls invited their teacher to hear the song. She initially refused. However, instead she invited the girls to perform the song in front of their entire class. Not only did this allow the girls to gain positive reactions from their peers, but the teacher was able to see what they were capable of, rather than assuming that they were "bad kids".

Teachers and Kids

Verse 1

Some teachers think they can always be mean
Some teachers move their heads and scream
Some teachers yell at us all day long
Some teachers grab and you know that's wrong.

Chorus

How I treat you
You should treat me
Working together
Is the way to be.
How I treat you
You should treat me
Working together
Is the way to be.

Verse 2

Teachers should not disrespect us kids
Teachers should never roll their eyes at kids
Teachers should not talk back to kids
Teachers should not argue with us kids.

Chorus

Verse 3

Kids should give respect to teachers
Just like they should give to us
Kids really should be kind to teachers
'Cause a little bit of love is never enough.

Chorus

Verse 4

Kids and teachers should just get along
Working together really makes us strong
Respect and learning we should share
The truth is that we really care.

Chorus

2. *"Let's Get Along": songwriting as an expression of growth*

Five notorious boys had been attending music therapy sessions for four months. During that time each of them had lost their recess, had parents called, had meetings with the principal and the dean of students, and had been suspended repeatedly for fighting and insubordination. Clearly the discipline system in the school was not working for them. Consequences had no impact on their behavior and many adults were at a loss as to how to reach them.

Music therapy sessions were often chaotic as the boys struggled to express themselves and competed for attention. There was very little listening, sharing, or respect. To address this, sessions had to become extremely structured with clear rules about whose turn it was. A routine was established that began with a pre-composed opening rap, followed by a group improvisation, and ending with turn-taking on the microphone to "freestyle". The freestyle rapping turns were extremely popular and gave the children an opportunity to express themselves, share lyrics, and get positive attention. Soon the boys wanted to skip the improvisation and wanted to freestyle during the entire session. Owing to the use of inappropriate language as well as negative comments about loved ones,

"Rules for rapping" were developed by the children – and adhered to, once they were typed up and hung on the wall:

1. No cussing.

2. No bad words.

3. Don't talk about people in the room.

4. Don't talk about relatives or friends.

5. Don't mention names.

6. Don't say inappropriate things like "I'm gonna shoot you".

Raps were recorded, and listening back to the previous week became part of the session routine.

Over time, themes in the freestyling emerged. The boys created unlimited lyrics about violence and fighting. Some used similar lyrics from week to week. Lyrics were typed up to facilitate this process and this organically developed into a songwriting project. At first all lyrics were typed up in one long list. The boys then divided the lyrics up into three sections which became the three verses for their song: witnessing a fight, being threatened, and making the decision not to fight. The boys worked in dyads to develop each of the three verses. Their task was to organize the lyrics into a coherent message. Ideas were shared and recorded.

The first few weeks were focused on verse development and discussion about fights they had witnessed or been involved in. It was difficult to determine which stories were accurate and which were embellished. During this time a few of the boys missed sessions because they were suspended for fighting. This became problematic because often decisions were made about their lyrics without them being present. Attending music therapy sessions quickly became an excellent motivator to stay in school.

The group began to make the connection between the song and their actions. Conversations began to revolve around alternatives to fighting and reasons not to fight. From these conversations the boys determined that they wanted to call their song "Let's Get Along". The chorus emerged swiftly as the song content became clear:

Chorus

I know we must not fight
We must get along
But we always get along
When we hear this song
So it's alright, OK
Sing it every day
We can get along
Even today.

Because they all wanted to rap, the lyrics were divided up and the therapist provided the beat on a drum. This also avoided conflict over who would play the drum and kept the boys focused on their song. All the boys knew the entire rap and initially wanted to rap the whole thing together. They were encouraged to each rap a few lines to give them a chance to take a risk and to give them a sense of ownership and responsibility. At first the boys were intolerant when a peer "messed up", which resulted in altercations. With guidance and a reminder about the song, the boys came to be more tolerant of mistakes. Every time the rap was rehearsed the boys got extremely excited. They would use much expression while they rapped and usually danced and jumped as they sang, especially during the chorus, which they all sang together.

A performance was arranged which included selected teachers and the dean of students. The boys were nervous but focused. After a fantastic performance and a conversation about the songwriting process and the song content, the music teacher invited the boys to record their rap on the school CD. Going to the recording studio, seeing their names on the CD jacket, and making their song available to peers, families, and teachers was an added bonus to this highly rewarding songwriting project.

Let's get along

Verse 1

I saw two people fighting
There's fighting every night
I said "Oh no don't fight tonight"
I was mad, sad, feeling really bad
What is it like to just feel glad?
Don't you want to live to see another day?
Do you want to go to jail,
And have to write mail?
Dear mom, I'm gonna be OK
And maybe if I'm lucky I'll be home some day.

Chorus

I know we must not fight
We must get alone.
But we always get along
When we hear this song
So it's alright, OK
Sing it every day
We can get along
Even today.

Verse 2

I was walking to the store
With my brother and my friend
They were waiting in the alley
Will this be the end?
They picked on my sister and talked about my mother
They tried to fight me and my little baby brother
They hit me in the head
Making sure I was dead
And tried to take my bread
And this is what I said
"Let's get along and help me with this song."

Chorus

Verse 3

I ain't gonna be the one who busts your lip
I'm gonna be on the mic make·it hip
I'm gonna be the one who's right I'm so tight
If I like school I'm not gonna fight
Better do the right thing
All day long
Stay out of trouble
STAY STRONG!

Chorus

3. "Making Your Way in the Ghetto": songwriting as an expression of hope

A co-ed group of fifth-graders set up the drums and cymbals at the beginning of each music therapy session. Their musical improvisations were energetic, loud, and often chaotic. This is how they related to each other. There was very little connection at first, but as the weeks progressed, patterns emerged and they began requesting of each other to "do the beat you did last week". The group began to organize itself musically, but when it came to conversations and discussion of the music, all positive patterns of interaction broke down. They put each other down, made negative comments, and made fun of each other. Despite their improved musical process they had a hard time speaking to each other respectfully. It seemed that when the music stopped, their guards went up immediately.

Songwriting emerged as way to use the music to involve the children in a positive form of communication. Beginning the process by having them talk to the therapist directly, rather than to each other, the children brainstormed about possible song topics. They began by saying things like "friends", "parties", and "love". More topics emerged such as "guns", "violence", and "gangs". The more bold the topics, the more "props" or compliments they received from their peers. Topics became more risky such as "sex" and "molestation". It became a competition as to who could come up with the most shocking idea. Every idea was written down, much to their disbelief.

As the project continued it was clear that their ideas were specific to where they lived and what they had witnessed in their lives. They soon realized that not all children live with violence and drugs in their neighborhoods. They agreed that what they were describing was life in the ghetto.

As they gathered lyric ideas, conversations deteriorated quickly into teasing and negativity. Any idea that was suggested was criticized. The process was getting nowhere because it was too public. The children continued to posture for each other and to "act cool". They were each given a piece of paper to write down their ideas privately. The only rule for the project was written on a poster: "NO PUT-DOWNS". Appropriate feedback was modeled and children commented on each others' work.

One child disregarded the procedure completely. Harry was the largest, loudest, and most talented person in the group. He intimidated his peers, and they often looked to him for approval. Every time someone shared lyrics, his response was negative and rude. As sharing progressed, however, it was clear that Harry was impressed with some of their ideas. As his peers cheered each other on, he saw how other children were receiving positive attention for their efforts. Harry did not share his lyrics, for a few weeks. When he finally did, he asked someone else to read them.

Harry's verse

Walking down the street

Guys pulling out their heat

When I'm outside, all I see is violence

When I go to sleep, all I want is silence

Instead all I hear is bang, bang

An old lady getting mugged by a young gang.

He was not satisfied with the way his lyrics were presented so he ended up rapping them himself. The group cheered as they had done for others. From this day on Harry was a focused and active participant in the songwriting process. He asked to come to the music therapy room during recess to work on his verse, and was integral in developing the music for the song.

Song lyrics seemed to fall into two categories. Some described the horrors of the ghetto such as muggings and drugs. Other lyrics included messages about getting your education in order to get out of the ghetto and succeed in life. It was important to include these two sides of their reality in their song.

The children could not agree on who would sing what, so it was decided that each person would sing their own verse and that the entire group would sing the chorus. In this case the chorus was developed after the verses. It was clear that the children wanted to believe that despite the circumstances of their neighborhoods, their future was still in their hands. They had received positive messages about completing their education from teachers at the school, and they used this in the song as a way to combat the ills of the ghetto. They seemed to want to reinforce this in their song, and created the following chorus:

Chorus

Dream high
You're gonna reach the sky
Your dreams can be real
You know the deal.

As the song took shape, so did the music. The boys in the group were uncomfortable singing, so they decided that they would rap the verses individually and sing the chorus as a group. This created a dichotomy between the harshness in the verses and a more peaceful sound for the chorus. The song was rehearsed and revised from week to week based on recordings of their work.

The children decided to perform their song. They made invitations and invited their favorite teachers. On the day of the performance four out of five of the group members were absent. The performance was cancelled. This was discussed during the next session. Some said that they were sick and others said they were scared. The children were encouraged to realize how hard they had worked and how important it would be to share this process with their teachers. The performance was rescheduled. On that occasion only two children showed up. They performed as well as they could and were applauded by the audience. They were commended for being brave enough to perform. It was clear that despite great gains through the songwriting process, these children remained extremely fragile. Despite a tough exterior, they were vulnerable and struggled with having the confidence to do something new and positive. They each received a copy of their song lyrics to take with them over the summer.

Making your way in the ghetto

Verse 1
It's so hard seeing murders and pain
People playing the wrong game

Selling drugs in a gang, using slang
Can't you feel the pain?
You should be ashamed.

Chorus

Dream high
You're gonna reach the sky
Your dreams can be real
You know the deal.

Verse 2

Walking down the street
Guys pulling out their heat
When I'm outside, all I see is violence
When I go to sleep, all I want is silence
Instead all I hear is bang, bang
An old lady getting mugged by a young gang.

Chorus

Verse 3

Doctors, lawyers, policemen
They grew up in the ghetto
They found a way to go
They made it by being real
By making the most of their deal.

Chorus

Verse 4

If you wanna pass in life
You got to get an education
Stop faking
And all that hating
That's if you wanna make it to your graduation.

Chorus

Verse 5

I thank God for paving the way
'Cause he made me what I am today

A talented youth
With dreams and the truth
Just believe and you can be one too.

Chorus

Conclusions

These examples illustrate the parallel process that occurs during the songwriting process. Not only are children learning important social skills (team-work, sharing, listening, respect) through the hands-on process, but they are at the same time working through important content material using original song lyrics. In this case the process and the product are essential therapeutic elements for growth.

The songwriting process constantly encourages children to listen to each other and respect each others' contributions. Since many children have lacked appropriate examples of positive social interactions, the therapist acts as a role model to guide the children through negotiations for sharing time and space. Countless opportunities are provided to practice collaboration and to correct inappropriate interactions.

The exploration of personal issues through composing songs allows children to express and give voice to concerns and hopes. By creating original lyrics, they are able to control and manipulate their experiences, often gaining mastery over difficult emotions and circumstances. As they internalize new approaches, behaviors and reactions can be modified, making improved outcomes possible for the future. Through this process, they are heard, and validated.

References

Amir, D. (1990) 'A song is born: Discovering meaning in improvised songs through a phenomenological analysis of two music therapy sessions with a traumatic spinal-cord injured young adult.' *Music Therapy 9*, 1, 62–81.

Austin, D. (1998) 'When the psyche sings: Transference and countertransference in improvised singing with individual adults.' In K.E. Bruscia (ed.) *The Dynamics of Music Psychotherapy.* Gilsum: Barcelona Publishers.

Baker, F., Kennely, J., and Tamplin, J. (2005) 'Themes within songs written by people with traumatic brain injury: Gender differences.' *Journal of Music Therapy 42*, 2, 111–122.

Cordobes, T.K. (1997) 'Group songwriting as a method for developing group cohesion for HIV-seropositive adult patients with depression.' *Journal of Music Therapy 34*, 1, 46–67.

Dalton, T.A. and Krout, R.E. (2005) 'Development of the grief process scale through music therapy songwriting with bereaved adolescents.' *The Arts in Psychotherapy 32*, 131–143.

Dvorkin, J.M. (1991) 'Individual music therapy for an adolescent with borderline personality disorder: An object relations approach.' In K.E. Bruscia (ed.) *Case Studies in Music Therapy.* Gilsum: Barcelona Publishers.

Edgerton, C.D. (1990) 'Creative group songwriting.' *Music Therapy Perspectives 8*, 15–19.

Ficken, T. (1976) 'The use of songwriting in a psychiatric setting.' *Journal of Music Therapy 13*, 4, 163–172.

Freed, B.S. (1987) 'Songwriting with the chemically dependent.' *Music Therapy Perspectives 4*, 13–18.

Gfeller, K. (1987) 'Songwriting as a tool for reading and language remediation.' *Music Therapy 6*, 2, 28–38.

Jones, J.D. (2005) 'A comparison of songwriting and lyric analysis techniques to evoke emotional change in a single session with people who are chemically dependent.' *Journal of Music Therapy 42*, 2, 94–110.

Kenny, D.T. and Faunce, G. (2004) 'The impact of group singing on mood, coping, and perceived pain in chronic pain patients attending a multidisciplinary pain clinic.' *The Arts in Psychotherapy 41*, 3, 241–258.

Lindberg, K.A. (1995) 'Songs of healing: Songwriting with an abused adolescent.' *Music Therapy 13*, 1, 93–108.

Logis, M., and Turry, A. (1999) 'Singing my way through it: facing the cancer, the darkness, and the fear.' In J. Hibben (ed.) *Inside Music Therapy: Client Experiences*. Gilsum: Barcelona Publishers.

Magill-Bailey, L. (1984) 'The use of songs in music therapy with cancer patients and their families.' *Music Therapy 4*, 1, 5–17.

Nordoff, P. and Robbins, C. (1995) *Music Therapy in Special Education*. Saint Louis: MMB Music Inc.

Robb, S.L. (1996) 'Techniques in song writing: Restoring emotional and physical well-being in adolescents who have been traumatically injured.' *Music Therapy Perspectives 14*, 30–37.

Silverman, M.J. (2003) 'Contingency songwriting to reduce combativeness and non-cooperation in a client with schizophrenia: a case study.' *The Arts in Psychotherapy 30*, 25–33.

CHAPTER 8

Lifesongs

Music Therapy with Adolescents in Foster Care

Diane Austin

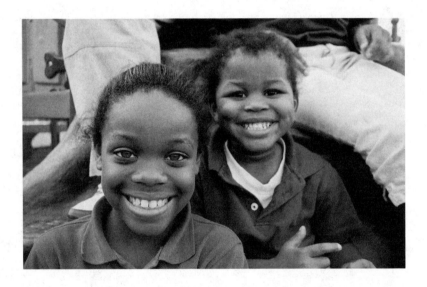

This chapter describes a music therapy program for adolescents in foster care that was started in 1991 at Turtle Bay Music School in New York City. Initially, a grant provided weekly music therapy services for a maximum of sixteen girls. Over time the program's success brought in additional funding, which allowed for the inclusion of boys. The adolescents in the program came from group homes in the area. When the group homes were shut down because of budget cuts, the foster care agency began referring teens from individual foster homes. Music listening, singing, songwriting and playing improvised music proved effective in facilitating self-expression and non-violent communication, and in creating a safe and playful environment in which relationships could grow and community could flourish.

Introduction

Darryl's rap

Tried to stay alive
At the age of five
For a young black boy
That's no surprise.

Took us from our mother
Cause she was doing drugs
We all felt worse
Than we ever was.

Sent us to a stranger
For a long time
She had her own kids
Paid us no mind.

Sent us back to our mother
Time for round two
It was the same old story
So what else is new?

Days go by
At the new foster home
Surrounded by people
Yet I'm still all alone.

Adolescence is a time of transition. One's identity is vulnerable and in flux. The many biological, psychological, social, and cognitive changes that are occurring are confusing and challenging. This is a time of great emotional lability, a time of testing boundaries and limits, and a time of rebellion and ambivalence. "All or nothing" thinking defends against a sense of identity confusion (Blos 1962; Erikson 1968; Novello 1979).

These problems are exacerbated for adolescents in foster care because they reach this stage of identity formation and increased independence without having successfully completed earlier stages of development. They consequently lack the necessary tools to face the increased responsibilities and expectations of their environments. Because of neglect or inadequate parenting, basic physical, emotional and psychological needs have not been met, leaving these children with limited social, emotional and financial support. They have great difficulty tolerating feelings and their underdeveloped egos can get overwhelmed by sexual and aggressive energy. Lacking the ego strength to contain or express their emotions, they can end up acting them out in self-destructive ways (Berkovitz 1995).

Many adolescents in foster care have suffered early childhood losses such as the death or incarceration of a parent. Childhood trauma such as physical, sexual or emotional abuse is common, and sadly this abuse is sometimes repeated in foster homes. As a result, these adolescents have great difficulty trusting others and forming attachments. They often suffer from intense feelings of anxiety, rage and depression. Unconsciously they may blame themselves for the situation they are in. Many of these teens are moved from one foster home to another, which only intensifies their feelings of abandonment and adds to their feelings of hopelessness (Berkovitz 1995; Herman 1992).

Music therapy is a logical form of treatment for these clients. Music plays a central role in the lives of adolescents. It can provide them with a form of object constancy (Hartmann 1952), in that their music and favorite singers are always available to them in ways that their parents and foster parents are not. With the flip of a switch they can be enveloped in sounds that are familiar and reliable, sounds that can energize and comfort, and rhythms, melodies, and harmonies that can create a cocoon of safety which allows them to block out the harsh realities of their lives.

Adolescents identify strongly with their musical choices and their favorite singers often become role models. These identifications can bolster a compromised sense of self and play a part in building peer relationships. The songs they gravitate towards are most revealing in the ways in which they mirror, reflect and validate the inner and outer worlds of the adolescent.

Adolescents are generally very resistant to verbal psychotherapy (Berkovitz 1995; Frisch 1990). Listening to music, singing, rapping, songwriting and improvising music as part of a group or in an individual music therapy session provides adolescents with a safe and creative outlet for their feelings. The nonverbal and symbolic aspect of music makes it an indirect and therefore non-threatening way to communicate.

The structure inherent in music can offer stability to adolescents who have an unstable psychic structure, and can provide them with a strong, resilient container for intense affects. Music therapy can help adolescents increase self-awareness, build self-esteem, strengthen their identities and solidify their connections to others (Clendenon-Wallen 1991; Frisch 1990; Haines 1989; Henderson 1983; Lindberg 1995).

Beginning

On a rainy Saturday afternoon in October 1991, I sat waiting for my first group of girls to arrive. I was very anxious. I had never worked with adolescents before. As an analytically oriented music therapist in private practice, my clients were all self-referred adults. This was the work I had been doing for ten years, that I was trained for and that I was comfortable with. Although I had been preparing for this day by reading and receiving supervision, I realized, as I rearranged the instruments for the fifth time, that I did not feel as confident as I would have liked.

I thought about the girls who were being bussed into New York City from two group homes in Brooklyn. This would be a new experience for them as well. I was told that they hated therapy and were only coming because they liked music. It was strongly suggested that I should avoid any reference to therapy.

This day was also a first for Turtle Bay Music School. The school, located on New York City's East side, was one of the oldest community music schools in the United States and had never run a music therapy program before. I wondered what the impact of teens from the inner city would be on the Turtle Bay music teachers, their students and the staff.

I don't remember much about that first day, but when it was over, I sat exhausted at my desk, making notes and trying to process what had happened. Images flashed through my mind of angry African-American and Latino girls. Many had been told that they had to attend this program, and they were not happy about it. Some seemed interested but did not want to appear "uncool" in front of their peers. My initial assessment was that some of these girls would benefit from music therapy, but that others were not appropriate for a group setting. I also realized that they would need a lot of structure and that I had taken this job with unrealistic expectations. My fantasy had been that we would create songs and poems about their lives that would culminate in a musical drama. The reality was, I couldn't even get them to sit together in a circle.

First month

I had a new plan. After talking to my supervisor I decided to cut the group time to 45 minutes. An hour was too long. After meeting with the Turtle Bay staff, I was able to secure additional funds to hire three second-year master's music therapy students to teach piano, voice and guitar. The school had an excellent drum teacher who liked working with adolescents and was available on Saturdays.

I would continue to run two music therapy groups, one for girls 11 to 13 years old, and one for girls 14 to 18. Each group would consist of six to eight members. My primary goal was to establish group cohesion. This would allow them to work on creative self-expression, non-violent communication and issues surrounding identity and self-esteem. These children were not used to doing things collaboratively and cooperatively. They were more comfortable fighting or insulting each other or myself, because that behavior was familiar.

Every client would also have an individual, half-hour therapeutic music lesson during which they could learn to sing, learn an instrument of their choice, or use the time for private music therapy sessions. The private session would provide extra support and individual attention as well as the opportunity to develop musical skills. The hope was that self-esteem and confidence would build so that playing music in groups would not be as threatening.

Adolescents are very sensitive to the values and judgments of their peers. This often manifests as resistance to singing, playing music, or engaging in meaningful dialogue within a music therapy group. Being in a group brings up family dynamics, and for children in foster care even sitting in a circle can be too intimate and therefore threatening.

Resistance is a natural part of the therapeutic process and relates to all the defenses evoked by clients to protect themselves from exposure and change. Resistance may take the form of non-participation, and attitudes, verbalizations, or actions that prevent connection, self-awareness and insight. Adolescents often fear judgment and rejection from peers if they express themselves authentically in music and words. They may also defend themselves against an adult authority system that they have learned to distrust. Sharing music with peers and group leaders is an intimate experience and therefore one they may want to avoid (Austin and Dvorkin 1993; Milman and Goldman 1987).

Crisis

By the end of the first month I felt like quitting. It was difficult to keep a consistent group of girls from week to week and I never knew if someone had dropped out, was sick, or had run away. Different caseworkers brought the girls each week and most of them were not acquainted with every girl's history and current status.

One week, very tall twins appeared in my group. Within minutes they were banging on the drums, smashing the cymbals, and screaming. I tried to get them back to their seats. When that failed I tried to take the drumsticks away from them, and at some point I lost it and screamed, "Shut up, shut up!" I was horrified by my behavior. I had never yelled at a client before.

I had heard that adolescents could induce rage in even the most seasoned therapist. It was true. In my first group I had managed to control my anger, despite being told I couldn't play the piano, had bony feet, and that my voice "sucked". By the second group, I was exhausted and I left the school in tears.

On Monday I arranged for a meeting with the director of Turtle Bay and the clinical coordinator and staff in charge of Graham-Windham group homes. The clinical coordinator and I wondered how the referrals were being made. I had naturally assumed that after our planning meetings in September, a referral system was put into place. I was wrong. I realized that I had to be in closer contact with the agency. A weekly phone meeting was arranged with the senior social worker, who would act as the liaison between Graham-Windham and Turtle Bay. The caseworkers would make referrals and the social workers would follow up on their suggestions. As a further incentive to maintain consistent attendance, each week when they left Turtle Bay the caseworkers would take

the girls out to dinner and a movie. We hoped that Saturday would bec
day for self-expression, learning, play and community building. The results ot
the meeting were positive and I left feeling encouraged. The twins and several
other participants were deemed inappropriate for the program.

Moving forward

By the fourth month I had a fairly consistent group of 14 girls attending the
program. The combination of group music therapy and individual lessons was
proving to be effective. Most of the girls looked forward to their individual
sessions and tolerated the group. In their private sessions they had the undiv-
ided attention of the therapist and felt freer to explore music and to discuss
personal problems, safe from the competition and judgment so prevalent in
group. Different aspects of their personalities often emerged when they were
away from their peers.

For example, Shanise only wanted to hear rap music in group. It matched
her tough persona. In her individual sessions, however, she began to improvise
on the piano. Her improvisations were described as consonant and melodic.
One week, her music therapist brought in some different kinds of songs for
Shanise to listen to. Shanise chose to learn a song by a contemporary "New
Age" singer. She learned to play the left hand and the right hand separately and
eventually played the parts together. She said that she liked the way the chords
sounded as they were spread out across the piano's keyboard. Shanise was very
proud of her accomplishment and eventually agreed to allow me to come to her
lesson to listen to her play the new song.

The music conveyed a tender and soft side of Shanise that she had never let
me see before. Her willingness to let me hear this music indicated her increasing trust in me. My acceptance and approval of this part of her personality
seemed to help her accept it. Shanise still appeared withdrawn in group, but she
began to engage in small ways, such as turning the pages of the sheet music
while the group sang. Gradually she became more tolerant of other members'
music and more engaged during group activities. By her second year in the
program, Shanise functioned as more of an ally than an adversary during group
music therapy sessions. She told the group that she still loved rap but was
learning some classical music and enjoyed it. Looked at symbolically, just as
Shanise had learned to play "the two parts together" and to enjoy two different
kinds of music, she was beginning to weave together two parts of herself into a
more integrated personality.

Clinical interventions

During that first year, I became even more aware of the need for consistency
and structure with this population. I did not want to be a cop but sometimes felt

like one, as I struggled to establish and maintain rules and guidelines to make the group a safe place for everyone.

I realized that we might avoid an unnecessary power struggle if each group made their own rules. It was interesting to observe the final results. Their rules were stricter than mine would have been and included things I might not have thought of, such as "no spitting", "no cursing", and "no dissing each other". I attributed this to the primitive, harsh super-ego that is often part of the make-up of the abused or neglected child (Blos 1962).

In the beginning, music improvisation usually led to chaos so I opted for more structured musical experiences. For example, each person would have an opportunity to begin a rhythm and the rest of the group would follow. These teens were poor listeners because they were rarely listened to themselves. This exercise was useful in improving their ability to listen to themselves and each other, but they soon tired of it.

The girls enjoyed conducting the group, which gave them a way to work through their resistance to the music and to eliminate their tendency to rebel against me as an authority figure. The conductor would decide who would play what instrument and when they would play. She would also determine the tempo and dynamics of the improvisation. The girls allowed their peers to control the music, when they would have given me a hard time. Working with changes in tempo and dynamics as well as starting and stopping the music was helpful for improving impulse control as well as empowering the girls.

People with histories of trauma feel disempowered because they have been in situations when neither resistance nor escape is possible. Traumatic events overwhelm the psyche and the victim is rendered helpless and terrified (Herman 1992). Interventions that give clients choices and a healthy sense of being in control are therefore therapeutic in that they provide opportunities for clients to assert themselves, recover a sense of power and autonomy, and become active participants in creating their own safe environment.

One week I asked the girls to bring in a favorite song on tape or CD. I told them that their song would be played if they wanted to participate and asked each of them to think of something that they liked about each song. If it was not the kind of music that they liked, they were asked to think about what that person might like about it and to say something positive without "dissing" it. Respect for each other's music was something we had talked about often.

I was proud of both groups. There was some teasing but ultimately they were each able to find something positive to say about every song. This was important because the girls strongly identified with their songs and their songs represented aspects of their personalities. The songs were also useful as projective devices. An example is when Karaar said, "I think T'challa likes this song because it's a slow jam and she seems like a shy person who could be romantic when she's with her man." The girls seemed to enjoy getting feedback about their songs, and indirectly about themselves. I hoped that this experience enabled the girls to take a small step toward being able to empathize with each other and gradually feel less threatened by people's differences.

During the last few months of that first year, the younger girls began singing together around the piano while I played. Their inspiration came from a large bag of sheet music of songs by their favorite artists. The older girls tended to sing only when the group was small. There were a few very strong singers in their group, and this may have intimidated the others.

Throughout the year I often found myself sitting on the floor and listening to CDs with my groups and my individual clients. During those moments I remember questioning if what I was doing was music therapy. It wasn't what I learned in school and wasn't the way I usually practiced, but something positive was happening. The girls were opening up to me and each other. They slowly began talking about difficult issues, like what it was like being in foster care.

I had one rule about CDs. "You can play anything as long as you're willing to talk about it." Of course, in the beginning, some of the girls tried to shock me by bringing in songs that were sexually explicit, and sometimes they succeeded. When we talked about the songs, however, some important discussions emerged. One discussion we had during the second year of the program was about their first sexual experiences. The conversation led to the discovery that every girl except one had been sexually abused. I suggested we write a group poem with each girl contributing one or two lines as a way to express and contain some of the feelings they were experiencing. This creative effort helped to break through the feelings of isolation and distrust so prevalent in this population.

Sometimes they brought in violent songs. Since they were listening to them, I believed it was better if they listened to them with me so that we could talk about the feelings that the songs evoked. I learned that Karaar's father was in jail for killing her brother, that Tania and her sisters had been brutally beaten by their mother, and that all of these girls had a legacy of pain and anger that made life incredibly difficult for them.

By the end of the first year the girls realized that they were getting more than music lessons. Shanequa confronted me, "This isn't music lessons, this is therapy!" I agreed with her and said that they should have been told the truth. Therapy was the topic of discussion in both groups. I explained music therapy to them and the concept that therapy is not just for "crazy people". We talked about what they had learned and experienced in the program. Several of the girls said they would be returning next year.

Major changes

Everyone involved felt that the first year had been a success. Turtle Bay had applied for several grants and we learned that there would be additional funds for the upcoming year. Both the Turtle Bay and Graham-Windham staff wanted to include boys in the program. Two mores music therapists would co-lead the boys' groups and I would continue to lead the girls' groups. The other music therapists would work exclusively with individuals, but we would all have private clients.

In March 1996, owing to budget cuts, Graham-Windham closed its group homes and relocated the residents, many of whom were participants in our music therapy program, to individual foster homes. Although many had to travel an hour or more on their own to get to Turtle Bay, 15 of our original 24 adolescents were motivated enough to continue coming to the music therapy program. Many of these teens had been with us for three or four years. Some of them eventually returned to their families or went on to independent living. Some went on to trade school and a few went to college. Some fell through cracks in the system.

In October 1996 the music therapy program would begin with an entirely new group of adolescents. The majority of these new participants would come from therapeutic foster homes that were limited to taking in only one or two adolescents who needed extra supervision owing to psychiatric diagnoses, were on medication or were required to attend psychotherapy sessions.

Starting the year with all new participants was daunting. Except for the first year, we had always had five or six teens who had been in the program for two or more years. These teens often became our allies or role models and helped to integrate new children into the program. They would usually speak at orientation and describe the program in language that newcomers could relate to. Now it was all up to us.

The director of Turtle Bay and I decided to hold an open house to introduce potential participants and new Graham-Windham staff to the music therapy program and the Turtle Bay Music School. Following the open house, my staff and I attended our first overnight retreat with adolescents who were interested in attending Turtle Bay. We spent two days with the group, talking, playing games and getting to know each other. We also ran music therapy groups and had individual sessions. It was helpful to get these teens away from the city and all that they associated with urban life. They were less resistant and defensive in this peaceful environment, and the amount of time available allowed us more opportunities to get acquainted with each other.

The program got off to a good start. As the year progressed, we all felt that there was a qualitative difference in the music therapy sessions. Resistance was still present, but not to the degree it had been in the past. Many of the adolescents from therapeutic foster care seemed more comfortable expressing their feelings musically and/or verbally and were more appreciative of what our program had to offer them. I attributed this difference to several factors. The majority of these teens had a better quality of life than the adolescents from group homes did. The group homes provided beds for many foster children but were understaffed and lacked adequate supervision. According to our clients,

the group homes and the neighborhoods they lived in felt unsafe. The therapeutic foster homes only took in several adolescents, providing these teens with
more privacy, in a more disciplined and less chaotic environment. Many of the
children were also required to attend psychotherapy and/or were taking medication that enabled them to function more effectively in the world.

By December, the boys' groups were improvising musically and the older
boys were beginning to talk about issues they were struggling with. The
younger girls' group was singing and occasionally playing music and the older
girls were talking about issues that emerged from the songs they brought into
the group. Things were going smoothly – until February, when we received
complaints from neighbors and Turtle Bay staff about "kids hanging out in
front of the school and throwing things." Apparently a delivery boy had nearly
been hit with a soda can.

An administrative meeting was held with the staff from Turtle Bay,
Graham-Windham and the music therapy program. One of the biggest
problems was that the program took place on the second and third floors and
the waiting room was on the first floor, where there was little to do while
waiting for the sessions to begin. The other problem was the lack of adequate
supervision in the waiting room.

After a creative brainstorming session some positive changes were implemented into the program. A new waiting room was created on the second floor,
where the groups and many of the private lessons took place. The room was
equipped with a CD player, a piano, games, and snacks, and was supervised by
two Graham-Windham counselors. This change centralized the music therapy
program and added a new dimension to it. We now had a community room
where we could gather informally before, in-between, and after music therapy
sessions. Over time, this room became the place where we ate, played, and celebrated birthdays and holidays together. This shared space increased the
amount of social and musical interaction between the girls and the boys, the
teens and the staff, and strengthened our sense of community. Our program
now utilized a three-tiered approach to music therapy: individual therapeutic
music lessons, group music therapy and community music therapy.

Rituals played an important role in creating community. Besides celebrating birthdays and holidays, we held graduation ceremonies, a tradition that
began with the programs' inception. Each year, participants received certifi-
cates stating the number of years they had completed. An outing to a play and
restaurant or an activity like bowling became part of the graduation celebration
as well.

In 1997, a new tradition began. One of the boys initiated a discussion in
his music therapy group about having a concert at the end of the year so that
everyone could share his/her music with the whole program. Almost everyone
wanted to be involved and wanted to invite parents, foster parents, teachers,
social workers and friends.

The concerts were held in the Turtle Bay theatre and were a huge success. The children sang or played in groups or alone and some performed original songs or poems. Maria didn't want to perform but was excited when she was asked to be the announcer for each act. Everyone seemed to revel in the attention and the positive reactions they received. Several teens who didn't want to perform initially, changed their minds when they heard the applause and felt the excitement in the theatre. The staff helped them to quickly pull something together, so that ultimately everyone was involved and felt a tremendous sense of achievement from being a part of this successful group effort.

Conclusions

In order to work effectively with adolescents, therapists need to be grounded in their bodies. They need to be conscious of and comfortable with their own sexual and aggressive energy. Clinical work with adolescents requires a high degree of self-awareness and self-observation because adolescents are able to "push buttons" in areas where a therapist is most vulnerable, either as a parent of a teenager or as a result of unresolved issues from one's own adolescence. Some of the most common forms of countertransference that emerge with adolescents are:

1.   the authoritarian need to dominate

2.   the wish for gratification by being the beloved, good parent

3.   the need to identify with the adolescents and win acceptance by becoming one of the gang

4.   induced rage or projective identification, in which the client splits off parts of the self – intense emotions like hate and rage and transference reactions – and projects them onto the therapist. The therapist identifies with the projected aspects and may unwittingly act out the feelings with the client (Berkovitz 1995; Davies and Frawley 1994).

It is also important to be aware of transference/countertransference reactions that stem from racial differences. I learned that until we discussed the "elephant in the room" (the fact that our staff was primarily White and the teenagers were African-American or Latino), we could not create trust or a cohesive group.

When the program started I was very empathic, but had difficulty being firm and using my aggression to enforce rules and boundaries. I learned by using the music. Before the children arrived my staff and I would often drum, sing and play music together. We all felt more present and embodied afterwards. Sometimes the staff would play together at the end of a difficult night to let off steam.

The way I work today as a music psychotherapist has been influenced by the years I spent working with the adolescents at Turtle Bay. Adolescents need the presence of the therapist's authentic self to reflect, interpret, model and educate in ways that are direct, active and involved. They need therapists who express their feelings appropriately but honestly. Adolescents know "phony" and they won't trust it.

During my third year at Turtle Bay, Shanequa confronted me. She said, "Tell me the truth. When you first met me, would you have left me alone in here with your pocketbook?" I was caught off guard and didn't know how to respond. I decided to tell the truth, "No." She answered, "You see, you are prejudiced!" and then added, laughing, "You're right, I wouldn't have either!"

The Turtle Bay Music Therapy Program ended in 2004 owing to massive cuts in government funding. Shanequa and her brother were in the audience for our final show. Their younger sister was performing that night. Over the years we had worked with several members of her family. They, like so many others, had come to think of our program as an antidote to the parents, foster parents and social workers who were there one day and gone the next. We were a community of caring people that would always be there for them. We and they had every reason to believe in the positive impact of the program.

References

Austin, D. and Dvorkin J.M. (1993) 'Resistance in individual music therapy.' *The Arts in Psychotherapy 20*, 423–429.

Berkovitz, I.H. (1995) *Adolescents Grow in Groups: Experiences in Adolescent Group Psychotherapy.* London: Jason Aronson Inc.

Blos, P. (1962) *On Adolescence: A Psychoanalytic Interpretation.* New York: The Free Press.

Clendenon-Wallen, J. (1991) 'The use of music therapy to influence the self-confidence of adolescents who are sexually abused.' *Music Therapy Perspectives 9*, 73–81.

Davies, J.M. and Frawley, M.G. (1994) *Treating the Adult Survivor of Childhood Sexual Abuse: A Psychoanalytic Perspective.* New York: Basic Books.

Erikson, E. (1968) *Identity, Youth and Crisis.* New York: W.W. Norton and Company, Inc.

Frisch, A. (1990) 'Symbol and structure: Music therapy for the adolescent psychiatric inpatient.' *Music Therapy 9*,1, 16–34.

Haines, J.H. (1989) 'The effects of music therapy on the self-esteem of emotionally disturbed adolescents.' *Music Therapy 8*, 1, 78–91.

Hartmann, H. (1952) 'The mutual influences in the development of ego and id.' In *Essays on Ego Psychology.* New York: International University Press.

Henderson, S. (1983) 'Effect of a music therapy program upon awareness of mood in music, group cohesion and self-esteem among hospitalized adolescent patients.' *Journal of Music Therapy 20*,1, 14–20.

Herman, J.L. (1992) *Trauma and Recovery.* New York: Basic Books.

Lindberg, K.A. (1995) 'Songs of healing: Songwriting with an abused adolescent.' *Music Therapy 13*, 1, 93–98.

Milman, D. and Goldman, G. (1987) *Techniques of Working with Resistance.* Northvale, New Jersey: Jason Aronson.

Novello, R.N. (1979) *The Short Course in Adolescent Psychiatry.* New York: Brunner/Mazel Publishers.

CHAPTER 9

"Can You Play With Me?"

Dealing With Trauma, Grief and Loss through Analytical Music Therapy and Play Therapy

Juliane Kowski

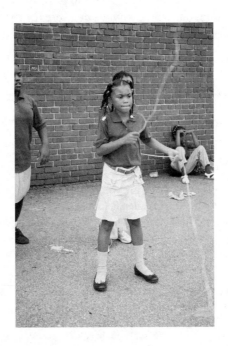

This chapter describes the case of a four-year-old boy who suffers from separation anxiety and adjustment difficulties owing to the loss of a loved one. He exhibits violent and disruptive behavior in his classroom and has difficulty during transitions and when separating from his parents. Analytical Music Therapy (AMT) and psychodynamic play therapy (PT) were used as treatment methods to meet his developmental needs. Half-hour sessions were held twice weekly during a period of five months at the Warren Street Center for Families and Children, a preschool facility sponsored by the Lutheran Medical Center in Brooklyn, New York. AMT and PT methods are described and issues of resistance, transference, and countertransference are explored.

The setting

Warren Street Center is a daycare facility that provides care for 120 chil
from low-income families. It is an ACD (Agency for Child Development)-funded
childcare center, with a preschool and an afterschool program. Children aged
three to five attend three groups a day and afterschool enrichment activities are
offered for school-age children.

A music therapy support program was established to offer individual and
group sessions. The main issues addressed were trauma, grief and loss but additional factors such as divorce, domestic violence, substance abuse, economic
instability, neglect, abandonment, inconsistent relationships and poor
parenting skills were also frequently explored. Children were referred to music
therapy by teachers and/or parents to address behavioral issues. The music
therapist also worked in classrooms and conducted drum circles to support the
therapeutic work undertaken during music therapy sessions.

Weekly case conference meetings were held by the team, which included a
social service coordinator, teachers, educational directors, the music therapist
and a clinical supervisor. Treatment goals, progress on cases, tools for use in the
classroom and current candidates for referral were discussed.

Theoretical framework and techniques

This chapter will demonstrate how combining AMT and PT techniques creates
new treatment opportunities for young children who suffer from trauma, grief
and loss. The cornerstone of this approach is based on the AMT work of Marie
Priestley and Benedikte Scheiby.

Children's feelings are often inaccessible at the verbal level. Music often
provides a more suitable vehicle for expression as it involves a form of playing.
Healing can occur within the "playing" with guidance from the therapist, who
is able to analyze the symbolic content of play. AMT with children can be
defined as the analytically informed, symbolically inspired use of improvised
music and songs, pre-composed songs, musical stories and musical accompaniment to explore the child's inner life (Priestley 1994).

Play has been used as a form of therapy since early psychoanalytical techniques were developed and is a universal tool that is used to facilitate communication, to build relationships and to advance health and growth (Winnicott
1971). Psychodynamic PT concentrates on introducing or reawakening the
child's ability to engage in self-healing play. Behavioral techniques are used to
explore the internal world of a child through analysis of environmental and
developmental factors and of defenses that the child has created. The therapy
seeks to establish an equilibrium of the id, ego and superego.

AMT and PT are well suited to being used together. Both depend on the
analysis of resistance, transference and countertransference. Emphasis is on
interpretation of the child's play and musicmaking to gain insight into inner
conflicts and traumas. Children use play and music symbolically as manifes-

tations of internal concerns. They can tolerate the expression of powerful feelings and experiences through these mediums in a safe way. The goal is for the child to process the traumatic event and to give it appropriate and realistic meaning so that it can be stored as a tolerable memory.

Children's ability to express feelings is limited by their undeveloped verbal skills and immature processing of fantasy and reality. The therapist analyzes needs, and uses this understanding to help the child overcome problems, thus shaping the movement of therapy. The goal is to improve the child's ability to control his or her environment. The therapist must remain playful while employing various techniques that encourage the child to be curious, spontaneous and willing to explore. The therapy is designed to use play and music to lead the child to acquiring coping skills and inner peace.

Traumatized children often replay an event or scene over and over again. Such play can be devoid of enjoyment or freedom of expression. Adding sound and music to this type of play helps children to master the frightening feelings caused by their traumatic experience. When the child is fixated on repetitive play or when their musical play seems stuck, the therapist must intervene in order to prevent the child from becoming re-traumatized.

Release is a crucial aspect of engaging in play and making music. In the reenactment of a traumatic event, the child is able to release pain and tension. Within the therapeutic environment the child is in control. By moving out of the role of the victim the child can become the one who is empowered. The therapist's role is to witness the play and, at times, to add verbal or musical effects to the child's scenario.

The combination of music and play builds a bond between the child and the therapist. This connection adds a unique dimension to the child's experience of human relationships. It permits closeness and a sense of deep satisfaction from creating music, as well as from the familiarity of playing with toys. Instruments can become transitional objects. They can serve as characters or toys with which children create stories.

Analytical music therapy techniques
Priestley (1994) developed the following groups of techniques to probe consciousness, access the unconscious and strengthen the ego.

CONSCIOUSNESS-PROBING TECHNIQUES
- **Holding**: the therapist acts as a container for all of the child's musical and sound expression.
- **Splitting**: the child is encouraged to role-play conflicts and projections musically in order to explore feelings that have been lost or become unconscious.

- **Investigation of emotional investment**: emotions are explored musically when words are counterproductive or seem illogical.

EGO-STRENGTHENING TECHNIQUES

- **Reality rehearsal**: the child practices changes and responses that have been learned or realized in therapy, which may be used to overcome problems that the child may encounter in the future.

- **Affirmations**: life, joy, and peace are celebrated.

- **Sub-verbal communication**: improvised music is created without the imposition of a title or a direction.

- **Patterns of significance**: Music improvisations create opportunities to discover feelings about a significant life event such as birth or death.

Play therapy techniques

Psychodynamic play therapy uses the concepts of resistance, externalization, transference and countertransference (Cangelosi 2004). Within this frame-work, a therapeutic alliance is established and maintained, child/parent relationships are explored, developmental deficits and needs are addressed, and internal conflicts are dealt with. These issues can be relieved by bringing them to the conscious level, increasing ego-resources, improving coping skills, and decreasing symptoms. A variety of play therapy techniques, as developed by Kaduson and Schaefer (1997, 2001, 2004), are described:

- **Use of metaphors and symbols**: Children often use metaphors and symbols to express their worries. The therapist decides whether to stay within the metaphor and use it to address underlying issues, or to make a direct connection to his or her understanding of reality.

- **Color your feelings**: The child identifies a variety of feelings and chooses colors to match them. The child then colors the location of the feelings on a drawing of an outlined body and talks about their origins.

- **Throw splat eggs**: The child and therapist take turns throwing fake, sticky eggs at a surface. Each time an egg is thrown, a like or dislike is identified. This physical release often allows the child to share information that otherwise might not be revealed.

- **Monster**: When children feel anxious, they often choose the symbol of a monster in their play. The monster can be fought, overcome and defeated in therapy sessions, thus developing courage and resourcefulness to help with mastering internal fears.

- **Pretend or role-play**: Children are encouraged to use role-playing to act out traumatic events in a safe way. Things happen to an imagined third person and the child is often able to develop a rescue intervention.

- **Broadcast news**: The child and therapist pretend to be delivering a news broadcast to imaginary children who call in and ask questions that the child, as the expert in the field, will answer. The therapist plays the role of a child caller and can raise issues that the child finds difficult to verbalize. The child may discover resources and problem-solving skills independently.

- **Blowing bubbles**: The child and therapist blow bubbles of different sizes, learning how to inhale and exhale deeply. This playful technique teaches breath and body control that can be used when feeling anxious, overwhelmed or angry.

- **Dollhouse play, handpuppet play, pretend play and use of playdough**: These create a playground in which the child has the opportunity to free-associate and share his or her world safely. The therapist can observe, challenge, or decide to intervene. In order to discover underlying issues, the therapist incorporates meaningful symbolic content into the child's choice of play. The therapist must maintain a balance between helping the child to express issues symbolically, without breaking down defensive barriers prematurely.

Cry for help – A case history

When I first met Bill (not his real name), a four-year-old African-American boy, he was very angry and was kicking, screaming, and spitting. His facial expression resembled that of a lost, hurt animal. I held him in a tight embrace and sat down in the hall outside his classroom. I felt somewhat frightened by this violent outburst from such a small child. Words didn't reach him, so I began to sing a lullaby. Eventually he calmed.

Before beginning my sessions with Bill, I met with his parents. Both were unemployed; however, the mother soon began working. His father was the primary care-giver. The mother seemed to be emotionally disengaged and was somewhat confrontational, while the father was less defensive and very concerned. It was immediately evident that the parents were unable to set limits for Bill. They did not understand the severity of their son's problems and were in denial.

Bill's babysitter, a woman who had taken care of Bill full-time for the first three years of his life, had died suddenly, six months before Bill was referred to music therapy. The parents had underestimated the long-lasting impact of this loss and had not observed any changes in his behavior until they were contacted by his school because of his unruly behavior.

Two much older siblings (his mother's children by a former partner), were members of the household. Bill was the "baby" of the house and was reported to get away with bad behavior. From the description of his home life, I concluded that Bill received little limit-setting, and that his parents were in need of help with parenting skills.

Some months after the babysitter died, Bill had changed classrooms and had been placed with older children. This involved meeting new peers as well as adjusting to a new teacher. All these factors had apparently triggered his aggressive behavior. He refused to follow directions, wasn't getting along with his peers, and used his body to resolve conflicts. He expressed anger, and acted unpredictably and violently. His teachers were unable to cope with his outbursts. On two occasions he had to be restrained. Bill asked for his dad repeatedly and behaved anxiously when he was dropped off in the mornings and during transitions. Bill was obviously crying out for help.

Based on my assessments, made through musical interactions and play, I concluded that Bill was primarily suffering from the loss of his babysitter, whose death had not been acknowledged or processed. In addition, his difficulty with transitions at school and anxiety about his mother's upcoming absence because of her new job triggered acting-out behaviors that indicated high separation anxiety and fear that his parents might disappear, as his babysitter had done. The following goals were established for Bill:

1. to increase feeling identification

2. to increase impulse control and anger control

3. to decrease anxiety

4. to identify feelings regarding the death of his babysitter

5. to develop coping skills

6. to increase frustration tolerance

7. to develop positive social skills

8. to increase his ability to accept limits.

Warming up

SESSION 1

Bill came into the room eager to explore and challenge limits. His verbal skills were good for his age and he was able to express himself clearly. Anticipating transition difficulties, I introduced an egg timer. Bill set the timer for 30 minutes and learned that when it would ring, it would be time to sing good-bye. I established some ground rules in order to keep Bill, the toys and the instruments safe. In this phase of treatment I encouraged him to share his feelings and to express himself with sounds and musical instruments.

SESSION 3

Bill arrived in a seemingly angry state. During the hello song he beat the xylophone so strongly that the bars went flying off, making it difficult to contain his musical expression. The volume was so high that I felt he wanted to tune me out. He moved to the piano and played clusters, at times forming repetitive, ongoing triplets. He then eased into a march-like rhythm:

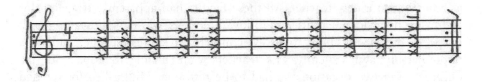

I played the guitar, first mirroring and containing his chaos, then slowly following his rhythm with F major and C minor chords. He sang loudly:

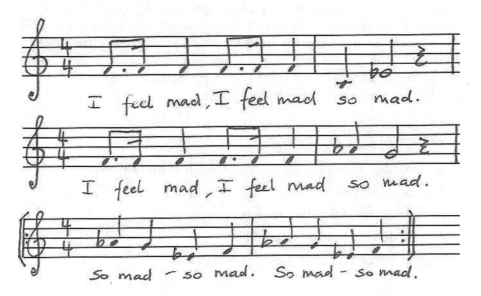

I mirrored his singing to make sure that he heard himself. Using an improvised song, I started to ask him why he felt so angry. He answered that his teacher would not let him see his dad. I assured him that his dad was going to come and pick him up at three o'clock. He pointed to the drum set and I asked him what he wanted me to play, making sure that he felt that he was in control. He chose a big drum for me to play, as if he wanted to make sure that I would be able to hold him musically. He began to play a strong quarter-note rhythm, which I followed. He chanted "Ms O makes me so mad" repeatedly. I repeated the same phrase and then added, "Because I can't see my dad. I miss my dad." I repeated these phrases. His drumming slowed and quieted down. Deep sadness emanated from his small body. I saw tears welling up in his eyes. I chanted "I feel sad, I miss my dad" repeatedly, holding him in his sadness. He stopped and pointed to one of the feeling chart pictures on the wall. He chose "lonely" and said, "That is me." I was amazed by his ability to make the connection between missing his father and feeling lonely.

Using the AMT techniques of *holding* and *investigation of emotional investment*, I tried to explore why he felt angry and attempted to connect with him through his sadness. I used my own countertransference and connected with my own lonely inner child. I still miss my father, having lost him twice through divorce and early death.

Bill picked up the rain stick, thunder tube and a stick. He wanted to play being in a thunderstorm, which was clearly an unconsciously used metaphor for the tumultuous and confusing feelings that he was experiencing. I supported him without making interpretations or clarifications.

Bill then switched to *pretend play* and took out a few rubber dinosaurs. He played hide-and-seek with them and developed a story in which one of them fell over the xylophone and got hurt. Bill became the doctor and treated the dinosaur, offering comforting words. Within this role-play he talked about his fear of doctors. I listened, validated his fear and asked if he had ever had a bad time at the doctor's office. He told me about the time his brother was hit by a car and was driven away in an ambulance. Bill's parents had not revealed these facts to me. Bill played out themes related to this accident over and over again, trying to master his feelings of fear. When he played the role of the doctor he was in control and practiced nurturing behavior, attempting to process, heal and recover from this trauma.

At the end of the session Bill became anxious about leaving. I took out the bubbles and showed him how to make a huge bubble with a deep breath. We practiced blowing a few times. When he felt happy about his ability to blow bubbles, I showed him how to inhale deeply and to exhale. Playing my guitar, I accompanied his deep breathing with this song:

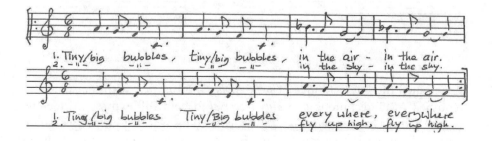

He left the room visibly less anxious.

During the session I switched back and forth between techniques derived from AMT and PT. They complemented each other and served the same objectives. The thunderstorm and dinosaur play allowed for the use of metaphor. In the thunderstorm play I allowed the metaphor to stand as it was, while in the dinosaur play I made a direct connection with Bill's life, referring to his brother's injury. At the conclusion of this session I used *blowing bubbles*, which taught Bill to use breathing in a playful way to lower his anxiety, and *affirmation,* which celebrated life and fun with the song.

Working through
SESSION 11

Bill started to play with the dollhouse. He told me that there was a dad and a boy. The dad climbed up on the roof, performing dangerous stunts but not quite falling off. I accompanied the scene on the guitar, rumbling and sliding between F and F# chords to match the danger of the situation. I asked Bill how the boy felt. He smiled and said that the boy followed his dad. I offered instruments to Bill because I felt that he was avoiding my question. I trusted that sound would connect Bill to his feelings. He shook the thunder tube wildly and then he walked over to the cymbal and hit it violently. I asked him to describe the sounds that he had made. "Scaaarrry," he said. He continued to make "scary" noises. I supported him by making scratching sounds on a drum.

It is very important for children to be heard and seen, for their feelings to be validated and for the therapist to stay with them in those scary places as long as is necessary. I asked Bill whether we could sing something to the imaginary dad. He started singing:

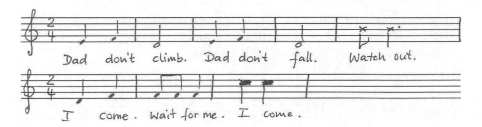

I combined the PT technique of *pretend play* and *role-play* with the somewhat modified AMT technique of *reality rehearsal* to help Bill express his feelings verbally. In the improvised song, Bill articulated his fear that his dad would get hurt and his wish to protect him. By creating and singing this song he rehearsed a possible talk with his dad.

SESSION 18

Bill told me that he was "mad at the class because everyone was mad at him." I used Bill's statement as an entry to work on feeling identification. We looked at a book of emotional expressions and started with the most basic feelings. We talked about when he felt happy, sad, angry or scared. I suggested that he find matching colors for the feelings and fill in an outlined body to illustrate where in his body he felt the feelings. He colored the entire body red for anger. Then he chose blue for sad, which he colored on the feet and hands. Bill identified happiness as orange, which he used on the face and chest, and green for feeling scared, which he scribbled all over the drawing. I suggested that we try to find matching instruments for each feeling. Bill ran over to the big gong, yelling "mad" and started beating it forcefully. I grabbed a stick and banged the cymbal, encouraging Bill to demonstrate the feeling with facial expressions. I experienced the sound that he made on the gong as pure bodily release, feeling that no words could better express the intensity of the emotion.

Bill chose the rain stick to represent feeling sad. I accompanied him on the guitar, playing D and G minor chords. I asked him what made him feel sad. He responded, "I don't know." I sensed his resistance and kept on playing (using the AMT technique of *holding*). He began to rock his body and slowly his resistance diminished. He suddenly stopped and said that his grandma (his babysitter) had died. I kept playing quietly and said that maybe his grandma dying made him feel sad. He nodded. Then he asked if we could sing for her. Bill chanted lines that invited answers, so I decided to respond for grandma:

Bill: Grandma, are you in heaven?	*Therapist:* Yes, I am.
Bill: Grandma, I miss you.	*Therapist:* I miss you too.
Bill: Grandma, I love you.	*Therapist:* I love you too.
Bill: Grandma, what do you do?	*Therapist:* I watch you.
Bill: But can you come visit?	*Therapist:* I can only come in your dreams.

Bill expressed deep sadness but also indicated that he had hope. He continued to ask questions about her death. Bill inspired my answers with facts that he had revealed in earlier sessions.

In the first part of the session, the PT technique *color your feelings* was used to address Bill's loss of his babysitter. I consider the subsequent musical interaction as an adaptation of the AMT *splitting* technique. We were both involved in role-playing, and Bill had the chance to explore his inner feelings and conflicts regarding the death of his babysitter.

SESSION 23

I showed Bill the splat eggs and invited him to throw them one at a time against the door, while saying something that he liked. I gave him an example: "I like spaghetti." He said, "I like ice cream." We took turns. He enjoyed this tremendously. He seemed to experience release while smashing the sticky eggs. Then I said, "I hate when someone lies to me." Bill told me about his own dislikes, which gave me information about events and relationships in his family.

Later in the session Bill said, "I hate monsters." He then picked up the thunder tube and started making loud noises. I encouraged him to play the monster with sound. He selected the washboard for me to play and I joined him in playing "monsters". Our music sounded ferocious and frightening. I wondered how long Bill could sustain this intensity of sound and I felt somewhat overwhelmed. It was imperative that I stay with him to enable him to communicate what he needed to express. Bill snatched a couple of sticks and started beating on the edges of drums, chairs, shelves and windowsills. Carefully, despite my concern that he might lose momentum, I introduced more rhythm. Slowly he joined me and we moved together in a steady beat. Suddenly he yelled, "We got you, monster. We caught you! We are going to put you away!" We repeated these phrases, shouting and marching around the room. His face reflected great pride.

The PT technique of *throwing splat eggs* gave Bill the opportunity to explore his fears, which we continued to work with through musical improvisation. Because monsters were a significant and reoccurring theme in Bill's therapy, I used and adapted the AMT technique of *pattern of significance* to address this issue. In the *dollhouse play*, monsters attacked "a mother". Bill played the role of the monster, using the thunder tube to scare the other handpuppets. The monster fought with the big dinosaur handpuppet and lost. Bill had created a book about monsters in which he drew images of the imaginary creatures. This gave him the courage to tie them up and "put them in jail." Bill worked hard to master his feelings of fear throughout this process. Monsters may be interpreted as symbols representing all the negative factors in a child's life. They also might stand for the overwhelming feelings of loss, anger and anxiety.

SESSION 27

Bill came into the room, seemingly upset. I asked him what had happened. He shook his head and moved close to the piano. He started playing clusters, while I answered on the guitar with sliding barre chords. His playing became very loud, chaotic and wild. Trying to contain him, I followed his expression, using the *holding* technique. Bill started to use his arms and elbows on the keyboard, looking at me to check whether this was allowed. He continued banging on the keyboard while I alternated between banging on the body of the guitar and playing sliding barre chords. His outpouring of anger made me decide not to use words, and instead, I made growling and howling sounds and encouraged

Bill to do the same. After some time he joined me and the playing reached a climax when Bill seemed to reach his physical limits. He ended the music and caught his breath. I felt exhausted, physically and emotionally, pausing to absorb what had just happened. Bill named the music "I Want my Dad". I was overcome by how much this music expressed not only anger, but anxiety, helplessness and despair.

I decided to incorporate these emotional issues into play by asking Bill if he wanted to play the *broadcast news* game. He seemed excited and took the telephones from the shelf. As we had played this game before, he knew that he would be the specialist who answers questions posed by imaginary child callers. I asked what a child can do when he or she feels anxious about separating from someone or losing parents or a family member. Bill described coping skills and he readily shared them with the "other" children.

In this case, the AMT technique of *subverbal communication* combined with the PT technique of *broadcast news* provided an opportunity for Bill to verbalize his feelings and coping mechanisms.

Termination

SESSION 33

Bill marched straight to the drums. He started beating the drum and developed a slow, steady rhythm. He shouted loudly that he was a butterfly. He picked up the butterfly handpuppet while I continued playing the rhythm that he had established. He turned the butterfly inside-out and it became a caterpillar that began to eat leaves and crawl around the room. Bill sang about how happy the caterpillar was to find all the leaves. I picked up the rhythm of his movements and reflected them on the drum. Bill decided that the caterpillar was full and that it had to go to sleep. He put the handpuppet down and made snoring noises. I played lullaby quality chords on the guitar. The caterpillar woke up and turned into a butterfly, happily flying around the room. Once more I reflected his play and movement on the guitar, matching his body rhythm, mood and singing.

Bill was using a powerful metaphor to send me a message about his journey. I interpreted the butterfly metaphor as a signal to start our termination process. Bill's therapeutic process had been remarkable and somewhat similar to the lifecycle of a butterfly.

We spent four more sessions terminating therapy. The team discussed Bill's progress in the classroom. His teachers reported that Bill's violent behavior had not reccurred and that he was becoming more cooperative. I discussed the termination process with the teachers and advised them how to help Bill use his coping skills. The teachers were encouraged to anticipate Bill's actions and to assist with any transitional issues that might arise during termination of therapy.

Resistance, transference and countertransference

Issues of resistance, transference and countertransference are essential to AMT and psychodynamic PT, and played key roles in the case study outlined above.

Resistance

In Bill's case, resistance was manifested as a defense against anxiety. He was in denial about his feelings of grief because he had not processed the loss of his babysitter. He was resistant to efforts made by teachers to address his behavior, because in order for him to function in his daily life he had to repress painful feelings.

It is important to anticipate and nurture healthy resistance. The therapist must find ways to externalize resistance, to address fears and to remove threats. The child is encouraged to use adaptive defenses rather than maladaptive ones by learning to understand resistance.

During Bill's chaotic and loud music making, his resistance surfaced, revealing deep emotional pain. He avoided questions and resisted accessing his emotions. Bill's violent outbursts were maladaptive defenses intended to let the world around him know that he was hurt. Our work was designed to undo the repression, to acknowledge his feelings, build up his ego and give him the necessary tools to control his feelings and actions.

Transference

Transference involves the reliving of positive or negative relationships, which the child transfers onto the therapist (Bruscia 1987). *Negative transference*, such as feeling resentful, angry or hostile, is often masked by resistance, and needs to be uncovered and worked through in order for therapy to progress. When Bill put the therapist in the role of the "bad mother", "bad teacher" or "bad sibling or peer", he repeatedly challenged limits and the therapist's ability to hold him.

The use of *positive transference* can be a powerful tool for a child in the struggle to move forward. Acting in the role of the "good mother" (Mahler, Pine and Bergman 1975), the therapist provides nurturing, understanding and love. Throughout our journey together, I tried to give Bill the hope, strength and the skills necessary to build satisfying relationships. I took on positive roles, such as Bill's father, the babysitter, siblings and teachers. He learned how to identify and articulate his feelings about these relationships. He was given the opportunity to have reparative experiences with the help of music and play, and to rehearse behavior for real situations at home and in school.

Countertransference

Countertransference occurs when, in response to the child, the therapist's own feelings, beliefs, motivations and behavioral patterns surface and affect the therapeutic process (Bruscia 1987). I used countertransference feelings that were detected through the music. These were then mirrored back to Bill musically or verbally. For example, when Bill expressed his anger, I became his sounding board, containing and absorbing his underlying feelings. Sadness, loneliness and anxiety were feelings that he communicated. During this process, I connected with my own personal feelings but always acknowledged them as mine. These connections and distinctions helped me to be authentic and empathic.

Conclusions

This case example shows how AMT is adapted to work with a young boy. AMT techniques are appropriate and effective when tailored to the developmental needs of the patient. In this case, Bill's expression was supported with chants and short improvised songs and vocalizations. Many interpretative thoughts from the therapist were carefully woven into the music and play. The organic connection between PT and AMT proved successful in many instances during Bill's therapeutic process.

My experience with Bill confirmed my belief that using different forms of symbolic expression is essential to the healing of trauma, grief and loss. To move between the very concrete therapeutic form of play and the use of music with its moments of free-flowing sound permits synthesis and a dynamic forward movement of the therapy. Creating music is a gratifying experience that allows for spontaneous responses, and helps to identify and intensify feelings. Children are amazingly resilient and often guide me along in this flow between play and music, inspiring new approaches to deal with their problems.

Transference and *countertransference* can display remarkably intense feelings in music making. One can feel overwhelmed, sad, frustrated, disappointed, angry, anxious, lost, helpless, annoyed or lonely. It is important to explore and clarify instances of transference and countertransference, because we therapists have our own inner child that needs to be taken care of outside the realm of our work.

I was privileged to take part in a child's healing and growing. I found inspiration, novel approaches and ways of synthesizing new ideas and experiences.

References

Bruscia, K.E. (1987) *Improvisational Models of Music Therapy.* Springfield, Il.: Charles C. Thomas Publisher.

Cangelosi, D. (2004) *Psychodynamic Play Therapy.* Play Therapy Training Institute, New Jersey, NY.

Kaduson, G.H. and Schaefer, C. (eds) (1997) *101 Favorite Play Therapy Techniques.* North Bergen, NJ: Jason Aronson, Inc.

Kaduson, G.H. and Schaefer, C. (eds) (2001) *101 More Favorite Play Therapy Techniques.* North Bergen, NJ: Jason Aronson, Inc.

Kaduson, G.H. (2004) *Release Play Therapy for Anxious Children.* Play Therapy Training Institute, New Jersey.

Mahler, M.S., Pine, F., and Bergman, A. (1975) *The Psychological Birth of the Human Infant.* USA: Basic Books, a division of Harper Collins Publishers.

Priestley, M. (1994) *Essays on Analytical Music Therapy.* Phoenixville, PA: Barcelona Publishers.

Winnicott, D.W. (1971) *Playing and Reality.* London: Tavistock Publications Ltd.

Further Reading

Erikon, E. (1976) 'Play and cure'. In C.E Schaefer (ed.) *Therapeutic Use of Child's Play.* Northvale, NJ: Aronson.

Erikson, E. (1963) *Child and Society* (2nd edition). New York, NY: W.W. Norton & Company.

Freud, A. (1945) *The Psychoanalytic Study of the Child.* New York, NY: International University Press.

Freud, A. (1964) *The Psychoanalytical Treatment of Children.* New York, NY: Schocken Books.

Gil, E. (1991) *The Healing Power of Play.* New York, NY: The Guilford Press.

Herman, J.L. (1992) *Trauma and Recovery.* USA: Basic Books.

James, B. (1989) *Treating Traumatized Children: New Insights and Creative Interventions.* New York, NY: The Free Press.

Kaduson, H.G., Cangelosi, D., and Schaefer, C. (eds) (1997) *The Playing Cure.* Northvale, NJ: Jason Aronson Inc.

Klein, M. (1937) *The Psychoanalysis of Children* (2nd edition). London: Hogarth Press.

Kowski, J. (2002) 'The sound of silence – the use of AMT techniques with a non-verbal client.' In T.J. Eschen (ed.) *Analytical Music Therapy.* Philadelphia, PA: Jessica Kingsley Publishers Ltd.

Kowski, J. (2003) 'Growing up alone: AMT Therapy with children of parents treated within a drug and substance abuse program.' In S. Hadley (ed.) *Psychodynamic Music Therapy: Case Studies.* Phoenixville, PA: Barcelona Publishers.

Landreth, G.L. (1991) *Play Therapy: The Art of the Relationship.* Levittown, PA: Accelerated Development.

Mills, J.C. and Crowley, R.J. (1986) *Therapeutic Metaphors for Children and the Child Within.* New York, NY: Brunner/Mazel, Inc.

Sarnoff, C.A. (2002) *Symbols in Structure and Function, Volume 2.* Symbols In Psychotherapy. USA: Xlibris Corporation.

Weber, A.M. and Haen,C. (ed.) (2005) *Clinical Applications of Drama Therapy in Child and Adolescent Treatment.* New York, NY: Brunner Routledge.

Ziegler, D. (2000) *Raising Children who Refuse to be Raised.* Phoenix, Arizona: Acacia Publishing, Inc.

CHAPTER 10

Honoring Timothy's Spirit

Mural Making to Express, Process, and Overcome Grief and Loss

Dan Summer

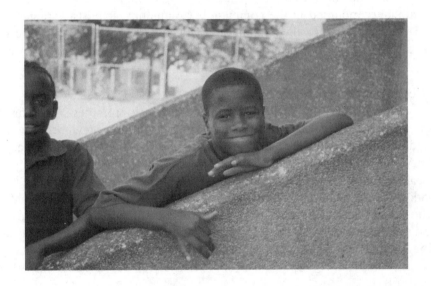

Early in 2004, a nineteen-year-old boy was shot and killed by a police officer patrolling a housing project in the Bedford-Stuyvesant neighborhood of Brooklyn, New York. This event caused repercussions in the neighborhood, ranging from protests to feelings of rage and trauma. Through a grant from Save the Children, the Wynne Center, a program affiliated with the Police Athletic League (PAL), provided art therapy for students who knew the victim, to explore feelings of loss and grief. Stages of group development, racial and religious ideology, and therapist parallel process are explored through a mural-making project.

Bedford-Stuyvesant is one of the poorest areas in Brooklyn, New York. Over 75 per cent of the residents are African-American and Hispanic. This area has one of the highest crime rates in New York City, although it has dropped over the past ten years. During 1993 there were approximately 55,000 violent crimes in Bedford-Stuyvesant and the surrounding neighborhoods. During 2002 the crime rate had decreased by over 60 per cent (Brooklyn Economic Development Corporation).

In January 2004, 19-year-old Timothy was killed by a police officer in this neighborhood. Timothy was on his way to a party in the housing development where he lived. As a short cut, Timothy and a friend walked up the stairs of a building, heading towards the roof. As the roof door opened, a police officer who was staked out on the roof pulled out his gun and shot Timothy. Timothy died shortly afterwards. He was unarmed that night. He was an invested community member, attended a local police athletic league, and was trying to raise money to go to college by working in a fast food restaurant. The police officer was White and the victim was African-American. As news spread about the event, anger mounted in the community. Community activists were enraged and the newspapers called it murder. The neighborhood became racially divided and a split began to occur between the community and the police.

The project

Save the Children, an independent organization which promotes social change for children in need, used grant funds remaining from a previous project to fund a memorial mural-making project for Timothy. The project took place at the Wynne Center, a Police Athletic League (PAL) where Timothy was once enrolled. The Wynne Center is the oldest Police Athletic League site in New York City and is housed in a converted courthouse. For $5.00 a year, children who attend are provided with literacy enrichment, homework help, martial arts, and weight training, and have access to a recording studio and a gymnasium. The students range in age from six to eighteen. All of the students are African-American or Hispanic with approximately 60 per cent boys and 40 per cent girls.

It was decided that a mural would be the best way to memorialize Timothy, and that it would be created with paint on wood. Staff and the art therapist felt that a mural would be a centerpiece that could capture and publicize emotions felt by the entire community. Because many of the senior students knew Timothy, they were chosen to create the mural, as they would most benefit from the experience. The students would be working in the gymnasium, which was a large space that did not provide much privacy, but that could provide a sense of containment.

The project lasted a few months, until the end of the school year, and was run by an art therapist (the author) and a dance/movement (DMT) therapist. High-school students worked on the mural project, and those struggling with loss received counseling and art therapy. Goals for the mural-making project included providing support to participants, and encouraging positive rather than negative feelings. A culminating community ceremony was to be held, in which members of the community, including Timothy's parents, could view the project, honor Timothy's spirit, and move on from the tragedy.

My role as art therapist

As I prepared for the project, I thought about how I could properly hold and contain the different emotions that the students would present. I needed to prepare myself for projections, while maintaining my ethical values as a therapist. I knew that I needed to be aware of the anger in the community. I was a White male entering a predominantly Black neighborhood, and I had heard about the conflict happening between a mostly White police precinct and the residents. As Acton (2001) states "Color blind therapists are not able to have a true understanding of their clients because they choose to ignore important information… harm can exist when therapists do not understand their own biases or the biases that exist…" (p.109). Many of the community members were angry about the media coverage, as well as perceived racial motives behind the shooting.

Trauma and racial tension were pervasive in this neighborhood and, being a White male, I was prepared for dealing with them openly. Waller (1993) explains "in child and family centers and schools, it can be difficult to establish a group for various reasons: timetable, group work and not being part of the 'culture' " (p. 81). As therapists, we are trained to work with people of different ages, cultures, and races. Despite these differences, similarities exist that allow us to connect as humans beings. As Ainslie and Braback (2003, p.45) say, "from the very beginning of life, every individual's psychology is simultaneously highly idiosyncratic while also deeply linked to the social and cultural realities defining the child's world."

This project to me was bigger than race. This was about healing and overcoming the grief in the community. My role was to introduce a new way for students to express themselves. By creating art together, these students would be able to process and share their past experiences and be able to make connections with each other. In keeping with a humanistic approach to art therapy, cultural biases were to be accepted while facilitating social and community change.

I considered additional areas of concern such as space, time, resistance, and attendance. The idea of deep exploration might be threatening for these students. Many, if not all, of them had been exposed to trauma in the past. I thought that an introduction to the mural-making process to honor Timothy might bring trauma-related symptoms to the surface.

Communities often unravel under the stress of the group processes that get acti-
vated by a traumatic incident...characteristics link the present traumatic incident
to prior incidents suffered by the group or community, and the emotions that are a
part of those past grievance and injustices become fused. (Ainslie and Brabeck
2003)

These emotions can be cataclysmic, and affect the community's collective
identity. For this project to be successful, it was my responsibility to hold and
contain any externalized rage or fear, and to overcome internal shame and
anxiety. The mural would be the bridge from rage and anger to calm and resolution. I understood that the students might shut down. As a therapist I would
contain this resistance and assist in transforming it into creativity.

Many of these students were emotionally unavailable or stuck. Resistance
was a defense, which they externalized through crime and violence. They had
never been allowed to process their thoughts or express themselves. In many
cases they had no voice. Students coped by not taking risks, going to school,
eating, going to bed and starting over again. Arthur Robbins states, "...some
patients will present a disbelief in anything, a lack of meaning, or a state of
emptiness and pointlessness and therefore an identification with death"
(Robbins 1996, p.22).

I saw myself as being an ally to the students during this project and a facilitator of the group process. I approached the project always remembering to
look to the artwork to obtain information. As Gonzalez-Dolginko (2003) says,
"As creative arts therapists, we can contain and organize the pain and grief that
is flowing from all this art and use its creative energy for healing and understanding."(p.106). My role was to connect with these students, and facilitate
recognition of what makes them whole.

Mural-making process

Students who were invited to participate in the project met in April 2004. The
project was announced during a community meeting at the center. The students
in the room appeared tired and exhibited low energy. As the mural project was
described, some students offered ideas while others appeared disinterested.
Many of these students had a personal connection to Timothy and were still
struggling with his loss, only three months earlier. According to staff, many of
these students had not had the opportunity to process the loss of Timothy, or
any of the multiple losses in the community prior to the murder. Before
formally starting, I reinforced to the students that this project would be an
opportunity to process loss through art. They would be provided with a safe
environment, and encouraged to verbalize their feelings if they chose to. No
other staff members would be present during the sessions, and whatever was
processed would be confidential. The students were encouraged to create
written or visual proposals for the mural. These could be about Timothy's

death or what it was like living in a neighborhood with drug activity and violence.

During the first meeting, about 15 students came in and out of the room over the course of the group. Some came in for a few minutes and others came for almost an hour. The space was a safe haven where students could interact, create, and establish a positive connection. Supplies were limited to paper, crayons, and pencils. Students began to put their ideas for the mural down on paper. One student's artwork stood out. Images that he incorporated included cemetery gates, a church and gravestones. His images were all done in pencil, and were very organized. He was careful as he created these images and stated that "This represents not only Timothy but everyone who has been killed or attacked in this neighborhood." Several other students created pictures of doves, or churches. As the students worked they connected with each other on an intimate and supportive level.

Creative arts therapists are constantly encouraging their clients to take risks. When a traumatic episode affects a community, this task becomes difficult. Owing to the trauma in the community, many of these students did not want to open themselves up, because they had been previously traumatized. The American Psychiatric Association's *Diagnostic and Statistic Manual of Mental Disorders* (1994), identifies several symptoms of post-traumatic stress disorder, which could occur if I was not careful with the mural-making process: "physiological reactivity upon exposure to internal or external cues that symbolize or resemble an aspect of the traumatic event" and "intense psychological distress at exposure to internal or external cues that symbolize or resemble an aspect of the traumatic event". It was important for me to let the students process the situation in their own way, and not to push them too hard to become involved in the project. I understood that some of the metaphors introduced in the mural content could, on an unconscious level, re-traumatize some students.

Many students in this context had never engaged in a large-scale project and most did not know what a mural was, or where to begin. When it was suggested that a large piece of wood be utilized for the mural, this further intimidated many of the students. Art therapy can be described as a problem-solving process. A client's job is to create a solution out of a blank piece of paper or canvas. Many of the students saw the big piece of wood as a problem for which a collective solution was needed. As Kaplan (2003) explains,

> A person engaged in the creative process devises or detects a problem and then goes about trying to solve it. Along the way, a certain amount of struggle is experienced that makes the eventual solution all the sweeter. (p.190)

The students were encouraged to take a risk and to explore a topic that was uncomfortable for them. This required courage. May (1975) states that

> Courage is not a virtue or value among other personal values like love or fidelity. It is the foundation that underlies and gives reality to all other virtues and personal

values. Without courage our love pales into mere dependency. Without courage our fidelity becomes conformism." (p.4)

It takes courage to create art and it takes art to recreate a community.

In subsequent meetings, the layout for the mural was developed on poster board to give the students a better idea of what the mural would look like, as well as to provide a template for the big picture. A few students began to take on leadership roles. One very quiet girl, G, created a poem related to the violence and loss in the community. The poem was shared with the group and they decided that it would be an important piece of the project. Two other students, A and L, played active roles in the process. L was an excellent student in school and attended a high school devoted to the arts. She was also on the council for programming at the PAL. She shared, "I think we should include a lot of doves in here, as well as some crosses." L conferred with the other students and decided where pictures and poems would be placed. They looked at a drawing of some cemetery plots which a fellow student had created. L stated, "I think this would be great to have somewhere in this painting, as it has so many meanings." A stated, "I think that we should create a church on here, and have praying hands come out." Meaning emerged from the images as they were displayed and arranged. Faith, loss, and moving on emerged as important components of the mural. The students felt that it was important to move on from this community tragedy but not to forget about it. They decided to include a cemetery, a church and a funeral home. Two hands would come out from the top of the church. The wooden board for the mural measured 8' x 8'. Using a small budget, paint, brushes, and primer were purchased.

Each time the group met, the number of students decreased. They were either not interested or they were not yet ready to explore intense issues in their lives.

Only four students were present when the job of painting the mural began. They were determined to make this project a success and saw it as an important step for their futures. A, L, and G assisted with applying gesso to the wood. Gesso is a primer consisting of titanium carbonate and other pigments to make the surface more flexible to paint on. It is always used on canvas, but in this case was used on wood. L commented, "I have never done anything like this before, it's kind of cool". A actively applied the gesso and G was more passive during this introductory process. These three students had known each other for the past several years. Dynamics between the three students were fluid as they continued to prime the wood. Their enthusiasm bubbled over.

Acrylic paints were introduced and the students were told that they would be permanent. A and L started working on the sky, while G started to outline different parts of the mural. The therapists contributed to the painting. As they painted, the students talked about school gossip and summer and future plans. This was a sacred time for them, and they were content to be working with each other. At this time the project was down to two students, A and L.

Slowly the mural started to take form. Color was introduced and the whole mural started to come to life. The sky was a mix of blues and pinks, with doves flying overhead. In place of a sun was a yellow opening in the sky, which the hands coming out of the top of the church were connected to. The hands created a controversy between the students. They were unsure whether to add a color to the hands. Comments included "God has no color", "We could make one hand white, one hand black", and "We could put no color in the hands." A, and L, felt that it would be best if the hands had no pigment, to symbolize purity, as well as to show equality with no racial overtones. This decision showed awareness of the larger meaning of the project. These students refused to join others as the community engaged in protests and marches. These students demonstrated art for art's sake, without allowing race, stigmas or stereotypes to impede their progress.

At the bottom of the mural, on the road leading to the church, was a gravestone painted gray. To the left side was a graveyard, with a fence and trees. In the middle was the church, which was painted in a skin tone with praying hands coming out of the steeple. To the right was a funeral home, which was also painted in a skin tone, with a brown roof. The students spent much time discussing how to place each item. Students were shown how to mix colors on the board and to sketch or erase lines. As the weeks went by, the students took more responsibility for the artwork. They took over control from the therapists and claimed ownership. The more time went on, the less talking took place, and the more ownership increased. The therapists acted as containers, and offered support, feedback, and suggestions whenever necessary.

The lettering on the gravestones was the last task to be completed on the mural. The dance therapist wrote the words with gold and silver markers. On the three gravestones, group members prepared poems that would represent individual thoughts about this experience. On the center gravestone was the poem by G which recognized all the losses in the community and how the pattern of violence created a "community trauma". The dance therapist's poem described how these students grew together and were able to properly grieve the loss of Timothy and also the loss of a part of themselves, perhaps their innocence. A's poem described losses in the community, as well as moving on with his own life, graduating from high school and going to college. L's poem talked about knowing little about Timothy, but wanting peace and minimal conflict in the community.

As the group took one last look at the mural, the student's personal growth was apparent. The mural had become theirs. They owned it. At first, a helping hand was needed to guide and lead the way. Towards the end, the therapists drew back and became observers. A and L stated that this was one of the most meaningful things they had ever done, and that they would always remember it. They were excited about presenting it at a ceremony, to honor Timothy's memory. On the last day, a small celebration for the group members was held, with pizza and soda. A and L raised their plastic glasses and congratulated themselves for working on something meaningful and everlasting.

The students wanted to know when the mural would be shown. Timothy's family was contacted, but there was little or no response. It was the end of May and the students were going to be finished with school in a few weeks. Sadly, there never was a ceremony for this project, nor was there any public acknowledgement of the students' accomplishment, due to bureaucratic complications and changes in oversight. The mural was moved to another part of the center.

The therapist's parallel process

During initial stages of the mural-making process I felt anxious, as I was unsure how the students would respond to the idea. The anxiety stemmed from fear of the unknown. Owing to the conflicts in the neighborhood, I wasn't sure whether a White therapist would be perceived as an enemy or friend. As an art therapist for the past seven years, I have always wanted to be accepted by the individuals I encounter. This need to be accepted stems from youthful experiences in which I was not accepted. A strong willingness to connect with people from different backgrounds brought me to the field of art therapy.

As I approached this project I was concerned that if I were not accepted, more fears would surface within me. Questions would arise, such as "was I good enough?" and "would I be harmed?" I realize, now, that I harbored some of the fears that the people in the community were projecting. I intellectualized that these projections were about race and surmised that those around me were thinking, "If one White man is going to kill, why won't this one? He's like every other White male." These thoughts were not rational, and they created anxiety and fear in me. On some level I was fearing for my life.

Many times during the process I felt like an outside observer, watching the process unfold. This was uncomfortable at first. It seemed that six hours a week was not enough to develop significant relationships with the students. As an outsider, I wanted to fit in. During art-making I engaged in conversations with the students, asking them what their connection to Timothy was, or trying to find out a little more about them. Many of the students were guarded and did not offer much, but remained engaged in the art-making.

During art therapy the role of the therapist is to provide a safe space, as well as to contain projections and introjections. These students were in the process of becoming more cohesive as a group. Yalom (1995) describes group cohesiveness and acceptance of each other, as well as therapist.

> The group will accept an individual, provided that the individual adheres to the group's procedural norms, regardless of his or her past life experiences, transgressions, or social failings…all can be accepted by the therapy group, so long as norms of nonjudgmental acceptance and inclusiveness are established early in the group. (p.49)

My fears that I would be judged or threatened soon morphed into an easy comfort level.

I began the project with many expectations. I thought that the students would open up and connect freely with me. I learned that as lead therapist my role was to contain, and not necessarily be accepted by the members of the group. My being physically present was enough for them. Their investment and ownership of the project demonstrated to me that they were capable of handling themselves after the mural was finished. In many cases they did heal, by working together. Students spoke to me when they needed to. I listened and provided feedback when I felt they needed it. The therapeutic safe space was created, and the participants felt it.

My comfort level as facilitator changed over time. It went from a state of fear and anxiety to a state of being calm and at peace. As Schwartz (1996) says,

> When art is produced in a therapeutic situation, the therapist responds as both a facilitator of the artwork as well as an observer…the response to the product must be therapeutically motivated, involving awareness of one's reaction to what one sees and perceives and using that self-awareness to relate to the needs of the clients and the work at hand. (p.244)

As the process unfolded, I grew more aware of the greater meaning of the mural. It was a representation of mourning, remembering and moving forward.

Both the students and myself needed to muster up the courage to embark on this collaborative art-making experience together. Simultaneous growth needed to occur. As Moon (1999) writes,

> Art is the anchor, the heart, the taproot of the work with teenagers. A logical out-growth of this is that we art therapists must make art in the company of our patients… Artists-therapists who work with suffering adolescents should have a profound belief in the power and the goodness of art-making. (p.78)

Shortly after the proposals were submitted, it was difficult for me to decide whether to join the students in the art-making process or to let them do it them-selves. My joining in after a few sessions created a therapeutic alliance with the students. At the same time, I was allowing myself to be vulnerable, just as the students were, in sharing a piece of myself. It was an empowering experience for me. Moon (1995) states,

> The creative arts provide opportunities to make concrete objects which symbol-ized feelings and thoughts that are evasive, obscure and mysterious. This offers both the therapist and the patient a thing to talk with and about. Many people experience talking about the characters in their images as less threatening than discussing their emotions or relationship difficulties directly. (p.81)

For the students, the streets, drugs, murder and violence were their reality. The mural was an extension of their experiences. As facilitator, my experience was one of growth. I learned how to trust the process, and was able to see the mural as a piece of art as well as a healing symbol. Being involved with a project of this magnitude helped me to focus on the needs of the students and staff, and to remain open to issues of countertransference.

Although only a few would be able to see the finished product, it was hoped that those who directly knew Timothy would have the opportunity to view it. A larger goal was to have local community activists view the mural and to use it for political implications. Because this incident received much coverage in the press and occurred in a neighborhood with a history of violence, the mural project became a societal one. This project was designed to memorialize the loss not only of Timothy, but of others who were victims of violence in the neighborhood. Although this would not completely alter the fear and racial tension in the community, it would be a step in the right direction. Warner (2001) describes how the arts play a role in social activism and states that

> Artists who contribute to social issues may be part of a movement known as either issue art, activist art, socially conscious or socially relevant art… The talents of the socially conscious artist are used to bridge the past and present and to provide a future view. (pp.17–18)

My new role as art therapist and social activist soon emerged.

When it became clear that a community ceremony would not occur, I was heartbroken for the students and sad that the community could not share in such a moving tribute to Timothy. I thought that a ceremony would provide necessary closure for the students. I soon realized, however, that these students did in fact get their needs met and achieved a sense of closure. To be able to connect and to watch the development of the mural and the students was a gift for me. As McNiff (1998) says,

> We do not have to know where we are going at the beginning of the creative act. People who control the work in advance are pushing against the grain of creation, so no wonder there are feelings of inhibition and emptiness. Creators learn how to cooperate with the forces around them. (p.60)

As the students became able to channel their emotions, achieve a sense of ownership and begin to move on, my role in the process became clear. I realized that I was a container for these students, provided a safe space for them, guided them into previously unexplored territory, showed them how to have the courage to be creative, and encouraged them to take risks. I learned to just be, and to stay in the moment. These were important lessons for me.

Conclusions

The people at the Wynne Center needed a large-scale project to externalize their inner trauma and to express what it was like to live in a difficult environment. Murals promote working together, conflict resolution, and communication. The process of honoring Timothy's spirit through mural-making became a catharic one, promoting growth, empowerment and independence.

Investment in the process was attained as the students slowly became more engaged in the mural-making process. Many of the students had previously been involved in art at school but had never engaged in a group art-making process with a targeted purpose. This was an opportunity for the students to learn about art therapy, to experience the art-making process, and to reach a common product.

During this art-making process I realized that the project allowed me to heal as well. Many of my fears and anxieties were alleviated while creating the mural. As facilitator I was able to develop a therapeutic alliance with these students while allowing freedom and ownership. This project enabled me to shed some of my rigidity as a therapist. The experience of being vulnerable enabled me to have more empathy for the students, and allowed me to be more present.

This past year, I have been making efforts to have the mural displayed outside of the Wynne Center or somewhere in the community. However, when I went to Wynne, the mural had been moved and was not accessible to students. Symbolically this represented forgetting about what had happened and put the violence issue on hold. Recently I went to the Wynne Center, only to find the program closed. No children, no staff, no mural. To me this epitomized the neighborhood and the cycle of ongoing neglect and violence. It saddened me that these students never received public recognition for this project. However, to these students it wasn't about praise for the product but about the process. Exposure to art therapy, working collectively, and creating memories was something that would linger with the students and myself.

Afterthought

This past month in New York, there was a screening of a film created by two young filmmakers from Bedford-Stuyvesant. The film was called "Bullets in the Hood: a Bed Stuy Story". The director of the documentary was a close friend of Timothy's, and was standing behind him when the officer shot him. It is an excellent portrait of a community saddened by loss, but at the same time shows how a community can come together in a non-violent way to identify how gun violence and race can disrupt it. I had a strong connection with this film and spoke to Timothy's mother afterwards. I introduced myself and explained the mural project. She was aware of it, and was appreciative. I promised that I would do what I could to get the mural displayed. This is a promise I will keep.

Acknowledgements

I want to personally thank all the students for allowing me to come into their program and provide a service that was meaningful and moving. This one is for you, Timothy…

References

Acton, D. (2001) 'The "color blind" therapist.' *Art Therapy Journal of the American Art Therapy Association 18*, 2, 109–112.

Ainsley, R & Brabeck, K. (2003) 'Race murder and community trauma: Psychoanalysis and Ethnography in exploring the impact of the killing of James Byrd in Jasper, Texas.' *Journal for the Psychoanalysis of Culture and Society 8*, 1, 42–50.

American Psychiatric Association (1994) *Diagnostic and Statistical Manual of Mental Disorder, Fourth Edition.* Washington, DC: American Psychiatric Association.

Brooklyn Economic Development Corporation (Undated). Accessed October 2003 at www.bedc.org. Accessed

Gonzalez-Dolginko, B. (2003) 'Art therapists are increasingly dealing with trauma: let's make sure we're all prepared.' *Art Therapy Journal of the American Art Therapy Association 20*, 2, 106–109.

Kaplan, F. (2003) 'Picture peace.' *Art Therapy Journal of the American Art Therapy Association 20*, 4, 190.

May, R. (1975) *The Courage to Create.* New York: Bantam Books.

McNiff, S. (1998) *Trust the Process: An Artist's Guide to Letting Go.* Boston: Shambhala.

Moon, B. (1995) *Existential Art Therapy: The Canvas Mirror.* Springfield Illinois: Charles C Thomas.

Moon, B. (1999) 'The tears make me paint: The role of responsive artmaking in adolescent art therapy.' *Art Therapy Journal of the American Art Therapy Association 16*, 2, 78–82.

Robbins, A. (ed.) (1997) *Therapeutic Presence: Bridging Expression and Form.* London: Jessica Kingsley Publishers.

Schwartz, N. (1996) 'Observer, process, and product.' *Art Therapy Journal of the American Art Therapy Association 13*, 4, 244–251.

Waller, D. (1993) *Group Interactive Art Therapy.* London: Routledge.

Warner, D. (2001) 'The lantern-floating ritual: Linking a community together.' *Art Therapy Journal of the American Art Therapy Association 18*, 1, 14–19.

Yalom, (1995) *The Theory and Practice of Group Psychotherapy.* (Fourth edition.) New York: Basic Books.

CHAPTER 11

The Architecture of Self-expression

Creating Community through Art
with Children on Chicago's South Side

Dorothy C. McGuire

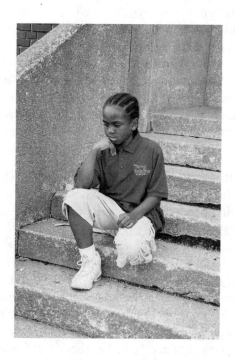

This chapter illustrates the use of art therapy with children from one of Chicago's low-income and predominantly African-American neighborhoods. The art work presented serves as visual documentation chronicling the psychological and behavioral impact of a large-scale public housing demolition / reconstruction initiative. Over a three-year period, children aged 6–14 identified feelings, needs and hopes regarding the violence, poverty and trauma in their community. As "architects" of their own miniature "community", children gained empowerment through art-making, while voicing their valuable experiences as witnesses to social change.

Introduction

Community can be defined in many ways. In its most literal sense, it is "a group of people living together in one place, considered collectively; a society" (*Concise Oxford English Dictionary* 2004, p.289). Though geographic proximity can indicate commonalities among people, the term "community" seems to suggest something larger. Its meaning can be as diverse as the society it describes or as personal as any one individual. In its broader context, "community" can be defined as "kinship" or "family", or by those relationships in which ideals are shared through the "convergence of a cooperative spirit". How we define the word "community" is a semantic task. How we create community requires action – the action of living subjectively day to day, finding connection through similarities and enrichment through differences.

Communities are living organisms, constantly in flux, susceptible to injury (internal and external), and permeable to change. How we adapt to our community depends on our ability to take meaning from its fluctuations, accommodate ourselves to its contradictions and act purposefully on its behalf or against it. Ultimately, it is a result of our openness and our capacity to integrate its injuries as well as celebrate its successes.

This chapter describes the creation of community through a series of lenses (racial, economic, and political) and their interplay with the therapeutic and creative cultures of children on Chicago's south side. Unique solutions for physical and emotional changes are explored and created by young, inner city "architects" using art therapy initiatives as a blueprint for change.

Community Counseling Centers of Chicago (C4)

Community Counseling Centers of Chicago (C4) is a non-profit organization that has been providing supportive psychiatric and behavioral healthcare services to consumers in and around the Chicago area since 1972. Comprehensive psychiatric and behavioral health care services are provided at nine different sites across the Chicago area and are funded through grants from the state of Illinois, the city of Chicago, and other corporate and foundation sources. As one of the larger social service agencies in the state, it serves nearly 7,000 consumers with the following demographics: 46 per cent African-American, 30 per cent Caucasian, 18 per cent Latino and 6 per cent other races or unknown. Additional statistics show that nearly 51 per cent of all C4 consumers have no income, and that 80 per cent live below poverty level (Community Counseling Centers of Chicago 2003).

C4 serves the community by providing acute or ongoing outpatient, linkage and supportive services to children and adults with needs ranging from chronic mental illness, to substance abuse, trauma, and untreated sexual abuse/assault. The treatment provided is considered a collaborative effort between the C4 consumer, its staff and other local support networks. Services are provided with a focus on identifying and implementing the highest possible care in a culturally competent, client-centered and community-based manner.

The ABLA program

Within the C4 network, support services for child and adolescent programs operate with the primary goals of identifying, reducing and preventing psychiatric and behavioral problems, while promoting successful family and community integration. Located on Chicago's south side, C4's ABLA program is a grant-funded initiative that was designated specifically to identify, assess and link at-risk children and families to existing psychiatric and social services in the area. The name "ABLA" is an acronym representing four major housing developments in the area just west of the city and bordered by Cabrini Street (North) and 14th Street (South). These are the Jane Addams House, Brooks Homes, Loomis Courts and the Grace Apartments.

As a primarily (80–90 per cent) African-American neighborhood and one which has been chronically neglected and underserved, the area has a history of high crime and gang activity, incarceration, chronic poverty, adolescent truancy and poor academic performance. Many of the staff at ABLA reside in, or are personally connected to, the surrounding community, and as such possess an immediate investment in their work. Despite what often feels like overwhelming odds, the staff consistently identify the particular needs of children and families in order to link them with appropriate supports such as outreach schools, community organizations, local social service agencies, and neighborhood groups. Services can include individual and group therapy, medication evaluation and maintenance, parent education, psychiatric assessment and support, as well as family-based therapy.

A complex therapeutic culture

Though many of these services are highly warranted and intensively needed in many of Chicago's south side communities, implementation has been inherently challenging for a number of complex reasons. One primary obstacle to the intended goal is that, traditionally, the provision of therapeutic services among minority populations has proven difficult. Owing to a high incidence of mistrust in "self-disclosing" situations, African-American individuals may perceive the conventionally accepted idea of "therapy" itself as one entailing an increased level of social and cultural vulnerability (Sue and Sue 1990). Historically, African-American people have experienced racism, discrimination and oppression, creating pervasive mistrust that may be culturally embedded. As a result, institutions intending to provide support (such as the mental health system) have often been met with psychological and social barriers that interfere with the counseling process and its intended benefits.

A further complexity exists when one considers communication styles among minority populations. Within African-American communities, nonverbal communication has been found to be a core component of interpersonal exchanges and is often considered a more accurate barometer of true feelings and beliefs (Hall 1976; Weber 1985). As a result, the primarily "verbal" approach of contemporary therapy that places high value on intellectual and verbal expression may fail to provide an accurate measure of feelings and needs for certain populations. Therapy, then, can be met with resistance and suspicion when imposed upon a cultural group that relies on the interplay between both verbal and nonverbal cues for effective self-expression. Taking this into consideration, the integration of non-traditional therapeutic ideals (such as those inherent in art therapy) with more traditional forms of therapy can effectively utilize the cultural strengths of the community, improve receptivity to outside intervention, and act as a catalyst for internal motivation toward change.

The art therapy program

The art therapy component of C4's ABLA program was introduced in the spring of 2002 with the primary focus on providing after-school arts programming to a largely underserved community with little or no access to the arts. The art therapy program contributed multifaceted benefits to the inherent goal of the ABLA program by acting as a non-threatening catalyst for engaging and linking families to supportive services, while simultaneously building a greater understanding of the benefits of therapeutic intervention with children chronically exposed to violence, poverty and loss. In the informal and creative context of an after-school art studio, art therapists were able to assess those children demonstrating a greater need for psychiatric or behavioral assistance, while creating constructive opportunities for all participants to develop strengths and build positive adaptive skills in a safe social environment.

While children from at-risk communities experience the same developmental struggles as other children, in order to survive they must also learn to cope with additional stressors that accompany low socio-economic status and diminished support systems. Since many school systems are unable to offer inner city youth appropriate opportunities to learn creative problem-solving skills or to develop alternative kinds of intelligence (creativity, spatial and visual skills, relational sensitivities), students are often forced to cope with the demands of their overwhelming environments with over-extended and ill-equipped coping strategies (Linesch 1998). It is imperative that inner city children and adolescents are given greater opportunities to learn and utilize creative thinking and to release emotions residual to their traumatic life experience. Without these outlets, they may find alternative ways of achieving these goals through negative and maladaptive means such as violence, substance abuse, and other self-destructive behaviors.

The ABLA art program participants were targeted by area schools and community outreach by ABLA staff. Identified participants experienced one or more of the following therapeutic issues: academic difficulties, stressed and disorganized family relationships, low self-esteem, poor communication skills, history of abuse and/or neglect, witness to, or participation in, social violence, and other behavioral issues. All were identified as needing alternative outlets for recreation and positive social interaction. During their participation in the art program, nearly all of the children demonstrated symptoms of post-traumatic stress, including social withdrawal or dysfunction, acting out behaviors, feelings of depression and anxiety, hyper-vigilance, and difficulty with self-soothing.

The children of ABLA

Children participated in art therapy once a week after school for two hours in a makeshift art studio housed in a rented schoolroom central to the neighborhood's families. Each week participants ranged in number from six to twenty and varied in age from 6–14 years. Often the children were siblings or close neighbors, indicating the value of community ideals despite everyday obstacles. Week after week the children would show up like clockwork, often trickling into the studio early, depositing schoolbooks and sweaters onto the red sofa in the corner of the room, promptly asking what was planned for the day. Often as this question was posed, wide eyes and small arms would wrap enthusiastically around the addressee in a gesture both of greeting and of purposeful intent, simultaneously stating "I'm here" and "What can I create today?".

What was immediately obvious in such moments was the children's unrelenting desire to be seen and to create and own something that expressed their value in the world. Their ability to risk making meaningful connections, despite pervasive evidence of the potential losses and betrayals in their personal and cultural histories, was evident both in their willingness to trust and in their unfailing capacity for resilience from week to week. Despite the regular indications of behavioral deficits, poverty, and neglect, the art studio brought out strengths, accessed meaningful and creative expression, and allowed students to witness their own visible successes. By addressing and encouraging strengths rather than deficits, the ABLA art studio and the art therapy process offered these young artists the opportunity to identify and build upon what makes them "able", while simultaneously providing situations in which alternative and creative strategies for solving problems and coping with change were explored.

Chicago Housing Authority and urban renewal on the south side

Over time, visual changes to the neighborhood surrounding the art studio became tangible. Interspersed between the fixed landmarks of Ladder 19, the oldest fire house in the city, and St Ignatius Church, and occupying the area just west of the University of Illinois at Chicago and south of downtown Chicago, were many of the city's oldest and most notorious housing projects. These same high-rise buildings, comprised of layer upon layer of red brick and grey cement, aesthetically sterile and devoid of anything "natural" beyond the rare untended tree, housed many of the children and families that participated in ABLA and the art therapy program. These buildings had been an earlier solution to urban overcrowding and an inadequate attempt at providing low-income housing for Chicago's resident poor. Years later, the dilapidated buildings themselves became the physical manifestation of a neighborhood's chronic social neglect and lack of opportunity.

Over the next decade and with financial and political impetus in place, the Chicago Housing Authority (CHA), in partnership with mayor Richard M. Daley and the US Department of Housing and Urban Development, initiated a large-scale public housing plan called "The plan for transformation" to redevelop and rehabilitate some 25,000 existing CHA apartments (Chicago Housing Authority 2003). The idea itself was welcomed by many who lived there, as violence and crime rates had skyrocketed among low-income areas on Chicago's south side, rendering them increasingly dangerous for its inhabitants. At the same time, it had become increasingly difficult for families residing there to find affordable housing outside of the area owing to rising costs of living and insufficient incomes to support a viable move. The plan was intended to renew or replace the structures themselves while attempting to reduce the isolation of public housing residents by integrating them into more mixed income communities. Additionally, the city's initiative represented a unique opportunity to assist local residents and businesses in beautifying their living and working communities while raising the standard of living.

"Tearing down and building up"

Though from its inception the new housing initiative was largely viewed as a positive change, the psychological impact on its residents was significant. The plan for transformation mandated both temporary and permanent relocation of large numbers of children and families to accommodate the renewal process. Each week more and more buildings were demolished, leaving vast, empty lots full of dust, rubble and contorted steel beams. The effect was one of progressive devastation, infusing the physical landscape with the surreal impression of a city under siege; one in which the daily life of its occupants continued unflinchingly around the destruction of space. As the ongoing physical transition provoked intense visual changes in the urban landscape, so did the psychological impact of the initiative affect the children and their families. Though many living and/or working in the area were hopeful that the structural changes would eventually bring positive change to the greater community, the immediate magnitude and meaning of such integral shifts were profound.

Of primary consideration was the cultural idea and psychological meaning of "home". Even an imperfect home meets certain psychological and physical human needs, among them the need for safety, identity, comfort, nurturance and love. In African-American communities, the notion of "home" is related to the concept of "family", which can include cultural identification with the broader social network. According to Thomas and Dansby (1985), African-American family structures often exist as extended social networks which include relatives, older children, and close family friends, many of whom share responsibilities for emotional and economic support. The impact of change and the relocation of families upon one individual can expand exponentially among others in the community system, in much the same way as a drop of water creating ripples in a pond. The effect of tearing down large numbers of homes and constantly relocating families and social resources produces intensified and unabating emotional effects on the community, particularly for its youngest members.

The impact of a changing landscape on resident children

As the CHA initiative continued to move forward, many of the neighborhood children, already suffering from untreated trauma and chronic social stressors, inadvertently expressed feelings and thoughts about their changing environment through art and play in the safety of the art studio.

An illustration

James, a quiet nine-year-old waiting for a ride home after art group, occupied his spare time with two small figurines (Ronald McDonald and Big Bird) retrieved from a collection near the "quiet space" on the rug in the far corner of the art room. From all outward appearances, Ronald and Big Bird appeared to be talking happily as James played, intermittently leaning towards one another in response to an involved conversation. As the therapist approached, James readily stopped his play and looked up unremarkably to see if his ride had come. When asked what the two had been talking about, James simply replied, "Ronald McDonald is crying because his house is being torn down."

Though the children frequently entered the studio with updates on the physical changes around them, they seemed to have great difficulty identifying their own feelings, even when questioned directly. Generally, feelings were expressed as behaviors and through body language such as aggressive anger directed loudly at a peer, or distressed silence manifesting clearly in tearful disappearances under tables, or in the solace of the owner's thumb. For most of the children there simply were not adequate words to express the source of their emotional impulses, and as a result the range of direct emotional discourse proved limited. In response to this discrepancy, art projects were designed to integrate the identification and expression of feelings nonverbally through the children's natural capacity for physical expression and their love of storytelling and narrative play. The children were readily able to act out scenarios based on daily events, or to create emotionally complex characters that mirrored what they were often unable to say.

The "Create Community" project

The "Create Community" project was the natural derivation from the need to find creative and meaningful ways for the children to gain ownership in the rebuilding of their own community. The project supported their unique voices and allowed them to identify and express the hopes, fears and anxieties that paralleled the changing landscape they observed each day. At its inception, the focus of the project proved twofold: first, to find appropriate and meaningful outlets for children to identify, express, and gain greater awareness of their feelings as they emerged, and second, to rebuild the children's sense of empowerment and control by engaging their imaginations in the task of actively contributing to the changes at hand. Abstract goals evolved into simple art ideas, which quickly became the blueprints for creative city planning. The children were no longer passive bystanders to social change, but architects of their own design.

Art and play as an emotional mirror

The initial task was to find creative ways to help the children name and describe their emotions. Because children who experience chronic trauma or neglect often develop emotional numbing and do not often have recourse outside of the traumatic environment to mirror their experiences, the simple task of identifying basic feeling states can be paramount in recovery (Herman 1992). To this end, a game called "Act out" was created, which allowed the children to re-enact their feelings and experiences in a fun and permissive, charade-like atmosphere. One at a time, children were asked to choose simple "feeling" words and to act them out for the group, using only facial expressions, body language and movement. In this way, children began to notice and identify their own and others' body language and expressions as a resource for distinguishing one feeling from another. Photographs were taken as an additional and tangible reference point for the children to create life-size, three-dimensional sculptures or "feeling portraits" depicting the feeling they most wanted to convey. (See Figure 11.1).

Children began this phase of the project by constructing the head of their figure with a balloon form using plaster gauze. Once the form hardened, detailed facial features were added, using air-dry clay. Notably, many of the children chose emotions which they identified as "feeling a lot", which were also those which they had the most difficulty expressing with words. The

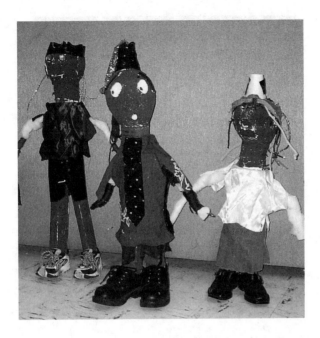

Figure 11.1 A 3D "feeling portrait"

emotions most frequently depicted were "worried", "angry", "frustrated", "confused", and "shocked", with a solitary "happy" figure among the group and a few "sad" and "lonely" sculptures rounding out the expressive assemblage. Once the head of the sculpture was complete, therapists assisted the children in building bodies out of cardboard, oatmeal containers, wire, and other found objects to mimic the exact physical representation of the emotion they were trying to convey.

The children then dressed and styled their figures, including personal details such as complex braids and hairstyles, earrings, hats, purses, and designer outfits, all made up of creatively juxtaposed pieces of fabric, ribbon and glue. Real shoes anchored the figures to the floor and also held the weight of the personified emotions upright. Quite appropriately and symbolically, the now expressive bodies were placed firmly in the children's shoes.

The "rebuilding" of a community

As the children continued to develop awareness of, and ability to manage, their feelings about the changing environment, they began the task of creating their own unique miniature community structures, using mixed media on simple cardboard frames (see Figure 11.2). Children searched for and collected a myriad of raw materials beyond the art room doors to use for their constructions. Most buildings were designed and constructed by groups of three or four under the supervision of art therapists. With the same enthusiasm that inspired the creation of their "feelings", they began with the most immediate need, a

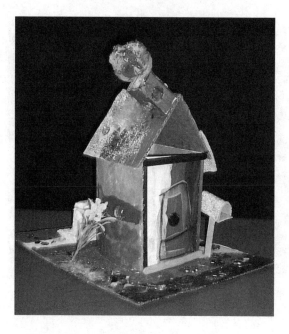

Figure 11.2 Sculpture of a home in a miniature community

home. Young "architects" were asked to imagine and build homes for themselves and their families, incorporating both "wishes" and "needs" in the design.

Some created simple structures with elaborate facades such as rainbow-painted houses with glittered roofs and jeweled windows, while others preferred more open family compounds where both family and friends resided together. Still others built high-rises and condominiums with built-in night-clubs and grocery stores, ample parking and elaborate landscaping. With the number of structures expanding as friends and acquaintances were considered, it became necessary for the project to grow as well. Individual houses were placed on masonite city "blocks" (see Figure 11.3) and neighborhoods were suddenly established.

As the primary need for a home was now a reality, the "architects" became "city planners", moving on to developing other communal structures that might be needed by its residents. The group decided collectively upon a lengthy list of possibilities, and in this they were unusually mindful of communal needs as well as personal ones. Education, health and spirituality were of primary concern and gave rise to the construction of a church (see Figure 11.4), a school, and a library as well as a homeless shelter, "old folks" home, and animal sanctuary for lost and abandoned pets.

Communal areas that focused on culture and leisure activities followed and included a movie theater, a neighborhood park complete with sculptured gardens, swing sets and sand boxes, and a rather extensive city zoo. Sand was collected for zoo animals' habitats, broken twigs were gathered and trans-

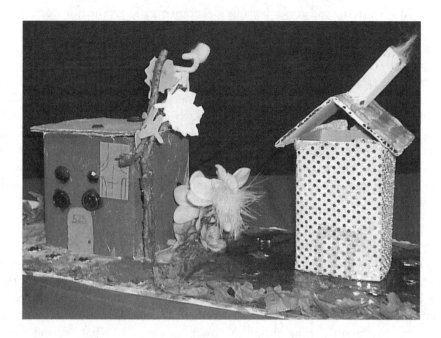

Figure 11.3 House sculptures on a "city block"

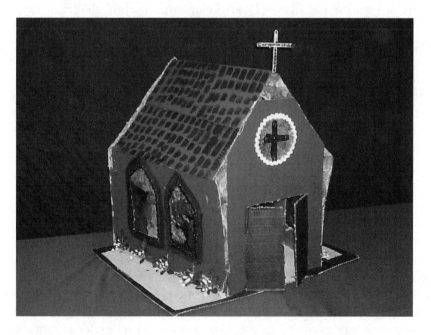

Figure 11.4 Church sculpture

formed into trees, and rocks became decorative pathways in the park. Each child, according to their own ability and inspiration, was supported in contributing to the expanding effort.

As the imaginative structures began overflowing into the hallways and offices, the fact emerged that as the children became more secure in their ability to create their own community, the limits of their miniature landscape expanded. The colorful and imaginative additions which came about over time did not suggest the meager requirements of a neglected community attending merely to the survival of its residents, but were inspirations that grew in an atmosphere in which primary needs were symbolically met. The inherent knowledge that shelter, safety, and meaningful connection to others existed, and were self-created, provided soil for other hopes to take root.

Putting 'community' into words

As the space to store the projects became limited despite the continual flow of ideas, the children were asked to further document their ideas, thoughts and feelings about both their existing community and the changes they hoped to see as a result of the ongoing reconstruction. Individual journals with questions such as "My favorite thing about my community is…", "What I wish I could change about my community is…" or "What makes me frightened about living in my community is…" were created, and each week the art studio participants chose one question to answer. Overwhelmingly, the children identified " gang violence", "people getting shot", and "not having what I need" as those things they would change about their community if they could, while "playing with friends", "my family", and "being outside" were the things they valued most. Through this exercise, the children were better able to put words to their experience of "community" by looking at and evaluating the meaning of what they had created. With this as counterpoint, they became increasingly equipped to identify the changes they had witnessed and to convey their hopes for the community that continued to transform around them.

Creating communities through art

In conclusion, the outcomes and benefits of the "Create Community" project proved valuable both to the children and their community on many levels.

The initial and most primary goal was to assist children to develop more effective and productive ways of identifying and naming feelings. As children suffering from the effects of sustained trauma have minimal outlets for self-expression, art as a therapeutic modality provided a non-threatening and nonverbal outlet for practicing these skills productively. Through games and dimensional art directives, children were assisted with simple identification of their emotional states and were encouraged through positive reinforcement to practice greater awareness and expression of their feelings.

Additionally, the art experience itself acted as a catalyst for reducing the helplessness and isolation felt by children who were frequently unable to express feelings verbally, if at all. Over time, behaviors changed from outward aggression and regressive distress to purposeful activity and meaningful self-expression. Children who had previously entered the studio with no purpose but distraction entered with creative ideas and collaborative plans for achieving them. As children created larger and more intricate designs, collaboration and creativity were primary outcomes.

As an additional benefit, more positive coping strategies were developed through the problem-solving, decision-making and interpersonal interactions inherent in the art process. One child's idea would inspire the creativity and support of several others towards a common and creative goal. In an atmosphere in which "belonging" often involves negative peer pressure and violent outcomes, an opportunity to work together to create rather than destroy proved valuable to children often distinguished by behavioral deficits rather than abilities.

Ultimately, through the symbolic "community" that the young artists of the ABLA program created, their larger community grew unknowingly. In ways not quantified by blueprints or a changing landscape, the children, who were offered a unique outlet to find identity and meaning in the changes around them, embraced their creativity and were empowered to act in an environment that often allowed them merely to survive. Through art, this act of surviving was transformed into an opportunity to thrive, creating what was needed and what was hoped for. Silently, and in ways more subtle than the raising of a building, a community based on potential, resilience and hope was built.

Postscript, 2005

Ironically, even as this chapter is written and the value of "community" and "belonging" is discussed, the art program at ABLA finds itself unexpectedly homeless. Feelings evoked as the children's artwork was packed up (and much of it damaged by careless movers) were similar to those expressed as real homes were torn down one by one. "Worry", "sadness", and "anger" all came to mind as bits of a popsicle-stick fence were restored to the park where it had been carefully built, or as the pom-pom kangaroo with its felt pouch and baby was rescued from the floor. Most of the work now finds itself stored in boxes and bags, waiting to see if the community in which it was created will conspire to find it a new home.

Though the intent of this project was to witness the process of urban change as seen through the eyes of the children residing there, the reality seems to remain that certain "communities" still fail to see what is ultimately valuable. A new facade does not simply eliminate the residue of poverty, neglect and violence at the core. If there is a lesson to be learned here, it is that the value of a community is defined not merely by the beauty and newness of its visible structures, but by the inherent value and potential of the people who belong to and create it. Community exists in connection and collaboration, in the willingness to support and provide for what is imperfect as well as that which is whole, and in the knowledge that a home represents more than simply a building of residence. Only at that point can we look beyond the basic needs of a community and consider all that may be possible.

References

Chicago Housing Authority (2003) *Plan for Transformation.* Retrieved 22 July 2005 from http://thecha.org

Community Counseling Centers of Chicago (undated) *About C4.* Retrieved 24 June 2005 from http://c4chicago.org

Concise Oxford English Dictionary (11th edition) (2004). *Oxford: Oxford University Press.*

Hall, E.T. (1976) *Beyond Culture.* New York: Anchor Press.

Herman, J.L. (1992) *Trauma and Recovery.* New York: Basic Books.

Linesch, D.G. (1998) *Adolescent Art Therapy.* New York: Brunner/Mazel.

Sue, D.W. and Sue, D. (1990) *Counseling the Culturally Different: Theory and Practice.* New York: John Wiley & Sons.

Thomas, M.B. and Dansby, P.G. (1985) 'Black clients: family structures, therapeutic issues, and strengths.' *Psychotherapy 22*, 398–407.

Weber, S.N. (1985) 'The need to be: The socio-cultural significance of black language.' In L.A. Samovar and R.E. Porter (eds) *Intercultural Communication: A Reader.* Belmont, CA: Wadsworth.

Further reading

Benard, B. (1997) 'Tapping resilience through the arts.' In D. Magie and C.E. Miller (eds) *Art Works! Prevention Programs for Youth and Communities.* Rockville, MD: National Endowments of the Arts.

CHAPTER 12

SOHO – Space of Her Own

An Art-based Mentoring Program for Girls

Linda K. Odell

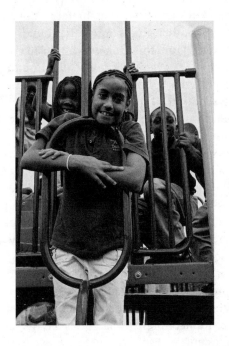

SOHO, Space of Her Own, is an art-based mentoring program serving low-income, at-risk middle-school-aged girls in Alexandria, Virginia. Girls and mentors participate in a 16-week arts and life skills program, culminating in the redecoration of girls' bedrooms,in the manner of "Trading Spaces" (a room makeover series on American TV). A creative partnership between the non-profit Art League and the 18th District Juvenile and Domestic Relations Court Service Unit has worked to target key areas of need identified in a recent city-wide survey of Alexandria's teens

and parents – for example, promoting positive inter-generational relationships, engaging in creative art activities, and participating in meaningful community service projects. The ultimate goals of the program are to prevent juvenile crime and misuse of drugs and alcohol, improve social skills and self-esteem, promote engagement in and appreciation of the arts, and foster long-term mentoring relationships. SOHO has served 42 girls to date, all of whom have displayed improvements in targeted areas in post-project surveys.

Working towards home improvement and relationship building

On alternating school nights inside the walls of a large, unassuming warehouse off the Potomac River in Old Town, Alexandria, Virginia, a bit of magic is occurring. Soothing jazz churns out of an old CD player as some 15 girls work diligently with their mentors to create masterpieces that will be used to morph their currently dismal bedrooms into fresh new spaces, personifications of their burgeoning youthful identities. A buzz of chatter resounds about which colors of paint to mix, where another glue-gun can be found, or who is available to assist. Comments such as "Does this look good?", "Can you help me?", "Do you think I should redo this?", "Where is a ruler?" fly around the room.

She may have received a failing grade on a test or been to the principal's office at her middle school for fighting, but tonight she is a winner, an *artist*, warmly welcomed and valued just for showing up. These SOHO participants, who live in low-income housing, have a commonality as they struggle to find their identity. Each one lacks a sense of place or organized living space. She may have to share a makeshift bedroom with multiple family members. Her room may lack adequate lighting, storage, or study space. She may not have a bed, or her mattress is on the floor, worn and stained. She might lack a chest of drawers, or hangers in the closet, forcing her to store her clothes in trash bags – one for clean clothes, the other for dirty. Her family may be frequently uprooted, forcing her to gather up her few belongings and move from one not-so-safe neighborhood to another. The instability of this lifestyle increases the risk of family problems and mental health issues. At home there may be chaos, needy younger siblings, addicted parents, unkempt and unsanitary sur-roundings, or an untrained puppy that bites at the ankles and defecates throughout the apartment.

At SOHO the energy is positive, a creative chaos and a wealth of arms all wanting to embrace these girls and provide a nurturing web of guidance and support. The physical quality of girls' spaces in their homes is improved. Each girl is provided with her own adult female mentor and together they learn creative art and design techniques. Instruction in social skills and positive conflict-resolution techniques is infused throughout the program. SOHO is working to enact a positive influence in the lives of girls who want to make a change, and also in the lives of those who do not yet realize that they are capable of change.

Community-wide developmental assets survey fosters plan and partnership

In the year 2000, the City of Alexandria completed a community-wide assessment of teens and parents, identifying the following key problem areas: lack of positive inter-generational relationships, lack of engagement in creative art activities, and lack of participation in meaningful community service (Search Institute 2001). The following six areas of need for teens were identified:

- a feeling of control over personal events
- the ability to resolve conflict non-violently
- a sense of value and useful roles in the community
- active engagement in school and after-school activities
- more time engaged in art activities
- adults who model positive, responsible behavior.

Alexandria's City Council established a Youth Fund to support grassroots efforts to address these target areas. The Youth Policy Commission, made up of adult and youth community members, selected SOHO for three consecutive years of funding. This program runs on an annual budget of just $12,000 and relies on community-wide support in the form of volunteers and in-kind contributions.

The concept for SOHO is based on key target areas for fostering developmental assets in youth. The program was designed specifically for girls because of a lack of programming for at-risk and court-involved females in the community. Bilchick, Butts and Poe-Yamagata (1996) of the Office of Juvenile Justice and Delinquency Prevention (OJJDP) identified the need for gender-specific programming. Throughout the past decade crimes committed by females have been on the rise, but traditional community-based programs have been primarily designed to serve the needs of male offenders. As a result of a lack of alternative programs, juvenile female offenders have been incarcerated in detention centers at a disproportionately higher rate than their male counterparts. SOHO targets girls in order to provide an array of services designed to meet gender-specific needs in the least restrictive environment and to prevent future criminal involvement. Best program practices for females, as outlined by OJJDP, include the promotion of social competence and positive self-esteem, participation in extracurricular art activities, life skills instruction in problem-solving and anger management, and interventions that help girls to make positive decisions and life changes. SOHO aspires to meet these needs.

Long-term relationships with adult mentors trained in the issues faced by at-risk girls promote healthy decision-making. A study of the nationally respected Big Brothers Big Sisters of America mentoring programs reveals that mentor relationships are effective in reducing criminal activity and drug and alcohol abuse and in promoting school success, when meetings are frequent and ongoing (several times per month over one year's duration) with mentors who have been screened, trained, supervised, and monitored (Tierney, Grossman and Resch 2000). SOHO works to match girls with mentors and to encourage bonding between mentors and girls to promote healthy long-term relationships.

The "hook"

Initial focus groups with women and court-involved girls helped to shape the concept and ensured enthusiastic participation. The aim was to provide positive influences in the lives of girls who wanted to make constructive changes for themselves and others, by improving the physical quality of girls' spaces in their homes. One SOHO program graduate, Stephanie, summed up the "hook" at the 2005 All American City Awards Competition in Atlanta, where the SOHO program was featured as an example of creative programming: "Why do you think *every* girl in Alexandria wants to participate in SOHO? Well, at the end of the program, each girl gets her bedroom remodeled beautifully."

The most common delinquent behaviors among young females in Alexandria are truancy, substance abuse, running away from home, shoplifting and fighting. Offenders tend to come from ethnically diverse, low-income and single-family households. Designing a needs-based learning environment so compelling that girls would be motivated to participate and attend on a regular basis proved challenging. Program creators wanted to find a hook. They noticed that the recent onset of a multitude of remodeling programs on television had created a national buzz. Most projects on these television programs targeted middle- to high-income families, neglecting families and individuals living in low-income housing. By developing a program that would result in newly remodeled bedrooms for low-income, at-risk youth, both adult females and teenage girls might be motivated to attend bi-weekly classes, work together and create long-term relationships. Adults volunteered for altruistic reasons; many had untapped interest and potential for interior design. Girls liked the fact that the program resulted in redecorating their own personal spaces and met specific individual needs.

SOHO participants are teen females who live in low-income housing and appear to have a commonality in their struggle to find their identity. In giving them a sense of place, an organized living space (including the basics such as adequate lighting, storage or study space), and an outlet for artistic expression and creativity, the hope is to improve their outlook. This program begins to positively counteract the many challenges faced by these girls.

Partnership

What has worked to make SOHO a success has been the partnership between the Court Service Unit (CSU) and the Art League. While the CSU has a long history of providing services and developing community-based programs for court-involved youth, this type of program could not have been realized without the partnership of our community's most respected art center. The Art League has written grant proposals, managed the SOHO budget, recruited "teen-friendly" art instructors of the highest caliber, provided rent-free program and storage space, and secured free parking for mentors.

Alice Merrill (BFA, MA Fine Arts and Art History), director of the Art League School for six years and current Director of Development for the Art League, Inc., brought a wealth of knowledge and art program experience to SOHO as its co-creator and co-director. Ms Merrill embraced the program plan as a way of "expanding League outreach by reaching underserved and challenged constituents with the creative process." According to Ms Merrill, who has volunteered literally thousands of hours of her time to SOHO over the past three years,

> The League's mission reads, 'By nurturing the artist, we enrich the community.' The League works to develop the artist through education, exhibition and a stimulating, supporting environment, while sharing the experience of visual arts with the community. (Merrill 2005)

The Art League provides the classroom and work space for the program and handles all aspects of art curriculum, materials and course instruction. Additionally, Ms Merrill has volunteered to provide nutritious dinners for all participants and has assisted with mentor recruitment, donations, and assistance during remodeling weekends.

The role of the Court Service Unit is to recruit at-risk youth through the courts and schools, recruit and train mentors, conduct required background investigations for instructors, mentors and other volunteers, schedule remodeling weekends, solicit donations, and provide life-skills curricula and behavior management.

SOHO – an overview

Participants begin to arrive at 4.00pm and immediately begin working on homework. Mentors who are able to arrive early are on hand to provide tutoring and organizational assistance. At 5.00pm girls participate in life skills and team-building activities. Through mini-lessons and role-play, they learn everything from table manners, to phone etiquette, to anger management, to ways of resisting negative peer pressure. Teen pregnancy has been on the rise in Alexandria. To address this need, community agencies have provided sex education through SOHO and have worked with girls to practice refusal skills. By 5.30pm, most mentors have arrived and the group shares a healthy dinner buffet that includes a medley of meat, fruit, vegetable, nut, cheese and whole-grain options. Art instruction takes place between 6.00pm and 7.30pm. Artists present lessons to the group and then circulate among small groups to reinforce skills.

On most evenings, participants have a variety of projects to choose from, depending on interests and needs. One girl may work with her mentor to sand and prime a donated dresser, another may make a mask replica of her face, and yet another may mix colors to repaint her hope chest or sketch a design for her chair. If a girl has had a particularly bad day at school or is having a conflict with another program participant, she may take a walk with her mentor or receive mediation support. At 7.30pm, the clean-up call is made, usually met with a loud group sigh and comments like, "Already?", "Just a few more minutes," or "Why can't we stay later?" Art supplies are cleaned and stored with utmost respect for the environment, with paintbrushes blotted with old paper prior to rinsing, and leftover paint sealed for future use. During the final half-hour of the evening, girls and mentors participate in a team-building activity and then share insights in a closing circle that ends with a SOHO cheer. Mentors provide transportation home from the program, which offers the opportunity to touch base with parents and guardians and to problem-solve family issues as they arise.

One key to the success of SOHO and retention of participants has been the ability of staff and mentors to meet the diverse and ever-changing needs of SOHO girls. One girl reported that her family was being evicted from their home. The girl's mentor contacted her mother to ask how she could help; the room was designed so that it could be mobile. Another girl shared about an instance of sexual abuse. In response, the mentor contacted authorities and provided assistance for the guardian to obtain counseling services for the child.

SOHO participants

Alexandria Public School truancy outreach specialists, guidance counselors, and juvenile probation officers recruit middle-school girls to participate in the SOHO program. A girl must meet two or more of the following criteria to be eligible for participation in the program: she is either on probation or the younger sibling of a young person on probation; she has committed status offenses such as skipping school or running away from home; she is struggling to get along with others at school, at home or in the community; she is the child of an incarcerated parent. The girls must express a desire to have a mentor and an interest in learning art. Participation in SOHO is voluntary. Girls attend an informational meeting and discuss the value of having a mentor, then watch a four-minute promotional video that shows art classes, friendly mentor/mentee relations and "before" and "after" bedroom scenes. When the video ends and the question is posed, "Are any of you interested in participating in SOHO?" a multitude of hands fly up.

The next phase of the recruitment process is a mandatory orientation session with the girls and a parent or guardian. Both must express a desire for an adult female mentor and commit to a relationship that will span at least one year. Mentors and volunteers need frequent access to girls' homes, which may be perceived by adults as an invasion of privacy. Parents are expected to provide a welcoming environment for mentors to work with the girls to plan and remodel, and are expected to assist with remodeling projects by being at home throughout all phases of the process. They must also provide supervision for younger siblings, and assist with tasks and provide meals as needed. At times these expectations have been too great and parents, wanting to maintain a right to privacy, have denied permission for their daughters' participation with SOHO. For the most part, however, parents and guardians welcome the opportunity for their children to be involved in such a positive experience. All parents are invited to participate in SOHO nightly art classes and to join the group for dinner.

Merely showing up to the SOHO program is not enough. Participants may not miss more than one session, and are required to maintain a cooperative work ethic and positive communication with peers and adults. Over the past three years approximately one third of the girls did not meet these expectations, were referred to other services and invited to try again the following year. Girls are not matched with mentors until week four of the program, after demonstrating the motivation and enthusiasm needed to promote, long-term participation and mentoring relationships.

Mentors and volunteers

From the onset, community response to the SOHO program has been outstanding, with an abundance of volunteers offering support. Responding to word of mouth and media attention, volunteers seek out SOHO, making the mentor recruitment process a simple one. A video presentation at a youth violence prevention conference last year resulted in 14 volunteers and an unsolicited check for $5,000.

Women choose to volunteer with SOHO for a multitude of reasons. Businesswomen join because they yearn for participation in the creative artistic process and have the desire to make a difference in a child's life; aspiring interior designers and art therapists come from local universities to get hands-on experience; teachers and social workers are motivated to participate because, while regularly working with large numbers of students, they want to have a long-term impact on one particular child; photographers have come forward to document the program because of its beautiful subject matter; women have offered to teach classes or assist with logistics and donations because they don't have the time to devote to a mentor relationship but want to contribute to SOHO and its girls.

Each mentor receives training, using a national best practice mentor-training curriculum from the National Mentoring Partnership (2005) and specific training to address needs of at-risk girls in Alexandria. The one-year mentoring commitment is tracked with support such as quarterly follow-up group activities that range from camping trips, to bowling, to dinners. Amy Cable, a middle-school teacher and mentor to Juju, shares her insights:

> The most amazing part about the program is that it does such a complete job at meeting the social and emotional needs of these girls. I joined SOHO because I wanted to build lifelong relationships and experiences as a mentor. Juju started off as a girl with a major attitude, not just at school but also at SOHO. I agreed to work with her because I knew no other mentor wanted to work with her. Yet part of me was not thrilled with the idea of working with this girl who had a major attitude. Once SOHO started, I realized that underneath the attitude was a truly artistic girl who just needed to be provided with an outlet before she could start blossoming. The art allowed her to open up and express her feelings. As her artwork progressed, she started to believe in herself and her talents. Her nasty attitude was gone, in part because she started to believe in the power of herself through her artwork versus getting power through being nasty. Her teachers at school confided in me that they could not stand Juju because she was so nasty. Yet during and after SOHO, teachers all noted a change in her attitude. Juju was actually smiling and making jokes with teachers, and more importantly, she was listening to teachers, unlike her pre-SOHO days when she would just stare off into space with a scowl on her face. Juju learned so much about herself and her abilities through her experience at SOHO. What she learned are things that you just can't teach during school hours.

Juju describes her mentor, Amy as "very nice and helpful" and says she enjoys hanging out with her, going to her house and cooking together. SOHO "made me be creative and helped us (girls) to think positive things about ourselves." Working on art projects makes her feel "peaceful and calm." At home, when the house is hectic and Juju finds herself in a bad mood, she now retreats to her gorgeous new bedroom and draws.

The SOHO Art Curriculum (Merrill 2005)

SOHO co-creators and instructors developed the initial comprehensive 16-week art curriculum, which has been refined over the years to include input from program participants. According to co-creator Alice Merrill, "It is designed to engage the girls at any level of artistic proficiency and to build upon and encourage that proficiency," with the following goals:

- opening and/or expanding avenues of self-expression
- building technical expertise in art processes and handling of materials

- demonstrating that expressive and personalized artworks can be created by using often inexpensive materials
- becoming acquainted with outstanding artists who make their living producing works of art
- experiencing the natural high and empowerment that hands-on participation in the creative process can bring.

Space designing

Beginning at an initial mentors' orientation, professional space designer Sheila Kaplan speaks about the psychology of color, room layouts, traffic flow, cost cutting (yard sales, thrift shops, dumpster diving, contributions), clutter control and other space design concepts. This lesson was initially presented to mentors and girls together. Many of the girls lost focus, so the lesson is now given to mentors only.

Dream chests

During their first art lesson, girls and mentors assemble "dream chests" – small, wooden chests measuring approximately 2' x 3' x 1.5', which are used to house smaller art projects, supplies, materials, and work clothes. During early sessions, the box tends to serve as a test template for developing painting, decoupage, and other skills. We've watched many boxes change colors and designs several times. Ultimately, however, they are designed as art projects and become part of the personalized expressions of the participants. The box is taken home at the end of the 16 weeks, where it is a true "space of her own".

Journals

At the second art lesson, each girl is given a pencil, pen, and sketchbook to be used as a journal for recording her artistic ideas, hopes and dreams, and notes, and for pasting color swatches, room layouts, themes and subjects of interest. Girls make color wheels and are taught how to mix paint, use a paintbrush, properly clean up, and other studio protocol. Frugality, conservation, and cleanliness are strongly stressed.

Floor cloths

Patrick Kirwin is a renowned *trompe l'oeil* professional artist who begins his instruction by showing examples of his huge murals and extraordinarily realistic paintings. He teaches the girls painting techniques, beginning with faux finishing (a painting technique that involves using paint to make textures that look like brick, stone wallpaper and other materials). He also offers instruction on cutting and using stencils, usually of calligraphy, floral, animal and other motifs. His lessons culminate in the girls producing floor cloths, a sort of poor man's carpet made by America's first settlers, using cloth from ship sails. By the end of this project, most of the girls have developed individual themes and/or characteristic aesthetics for the artwork they are creating.

Plaster molds

As a team-building exercise as well as an art technique, plaster molds are made of each girl's face. Multiple paper castings are produced, which can be incorporated as papier-mâché sculptural components for other projects.

Personalized chairs

At the third class, the core art projects begin. Steve Prince, an outstanding and charismatic professional artist in printmaking and sculpture and League instructor for over ten years, starts with the project "Sit down to rise up," involving the creation of a personalized chair or throne by "taking an existing chair and inscribing it with the personality of the student through various concepts and techniques" including chair reconstruction and design, sculpture, symbolism, patterns, transfer, calligraphy, decoupage, and poetry (see Figure 12.1). He engagingly discusses aesthetics, symbolism, composition, and structure. The project theme is reflective of Steve's philosophy that "in order for us to excel in life, we must first humble ourselves and not get caught up in the superficial, materialistic aspects of the world."

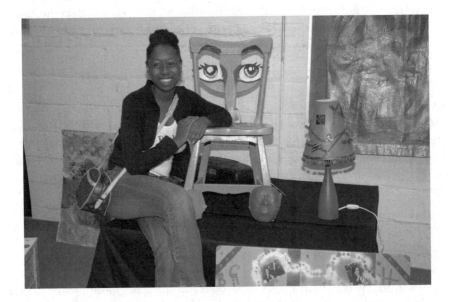

Figure 12.1 Shae's work. (Photograph by Dana Howe)

Art projects continue, including a lamp design project similar to the chair project. Design options and incorporation of varying textures, patterns and colors are further explored. At this point, many of the young participants are beginning to develop an aesthetic theme through coordinated colors, patterns, symbols, and subject matter. Other classes (including knitting, paper collage, and sculpted papier-mâché mirror frames) have been offered successfully, but the chest, chair, lamp, and floorcloth projects continue as the core of the art instruction.

Remodeling work

The remodeling weekend is the culmination of a long process in which the process is just as important as the product. Girls and mentors communicate and negotiate a plan for each room. One girl wants a black ceiling and red and black walls in her room; the mentor works with an art instructor to provide a visual image of what that space would look like and persuades the girl to select a more subdued color scheme to enhance the display of her artwork. In another room, Barbie doll heads are separated from Dorito crumbs and an incomplete deck of playing cards; this girl works with her mentor to decide which items to keep, which to discard, and which to donate to charity. A mother demands that her daughter's mentor use her budget to put a down payment on a new bedroom set; the mentor carefully persuades the mother that this is not in line with the purpose of SOHO. Girls now have a multitude of artistic creations to spruce up their spaces, and look forward to the surprise that will be revealed.

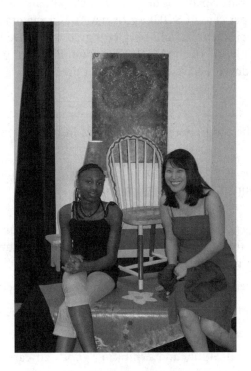

Figure 12.2 Juju and her mentor, Amy, show off work at a SOHO gala. (Photograph by Dana Howe)

Remodeling weekends are coordinated completely by the mentors, who, after weeks of planning, have acquired the goods (beds, dressers, hangers, bedding, lamps, desks, curtains, etc.) and services (often provided by a small army of friends and family members) that they need. Each mentor is given a budget of $250 for each room renovation, an additional $50 for paint, and another $50 for meals on remodeling weekends.

A girl and her mentor form a dyad with another mentor/mentee pair to plan for remodeling weekends. The mentors coordinate dates with the girls' mothers for home visits. The first visits are to assess the space and determine needs and wants. Subsequent visits are for cleaning, clutter control, and minor home repairs. On remodeling weekends, Saturdays are used to paint the room and clean the floors. On Sundays, the girls "trade spaces" and work with each other's mentors to do a good deed for one another by completing remodeling work. At the end of the day, girls return home for surprise unveilings. Smiles, hugs, and shrieks of joy tend to top off the day. The final product is a lasting memory that can have long-term effects. Each girl now has her own study space, adequate lighting, organized storage space, and some form of privacy, created from trendy and hip designs that are ideal for showing off to friends and hosting sleepovers (see Figures 12.3 and 12.4).

Outcomes

By the end, every participant has developed social and life skills and art appreciation. Eighty-six per cent of SOHO girls have so far maintained ongoing relationships with their mentors, and only two graduates have been convicted of crimes since completion of the SOHO program. Program goals and measurement tools were developed to assess program outcomes.

Program goals

SOHO expects the program to foster changes in behavior, skills, and competencies, so that:

- Eighty per cent of mentoring relationships continue for one year after completing the program (positive inter-generational relationships, and valued by the community)

- Eighty per cent of girls do not take drugs or alcohol or use physical violence for one year after completing the program (service to the community – crime prevention)

- Eighty per cent of girls report increased in competence in:

    ◦ communicating with confidence

    ◦ etiquette and social skills

    ◦ eating healthily and exhibiting good self-care

- ◦ creating a beautiful bedroom living environment
- ◦ making new friends easily.

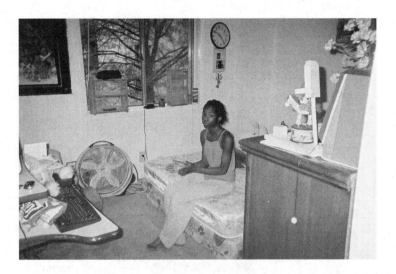

Figure 12.3 Rashawn's room before

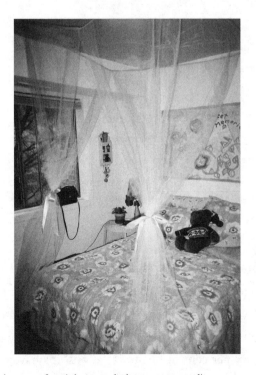

Figure 12.4 Rashawn's room after. (Photographs by Jenna Fournel)

Measurement tools and outcomes

Program outcomes were evaluated according to the three areas shown in Figure 12.5.

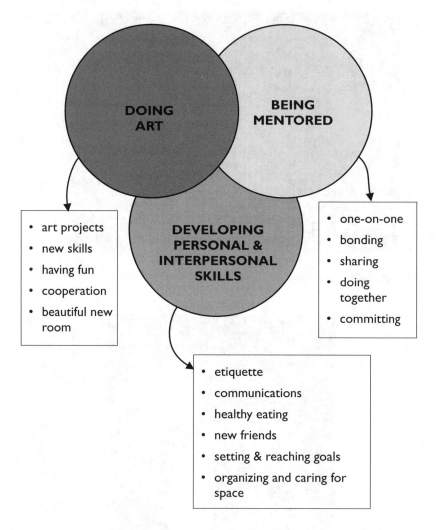

Figure 12.5 SOHO project outcomes

1.   *Mentor relationship* supported by mentor contract was measured by:

     ◦   logs to document contacts between mentors and girls

     ◦   mid-year formative evaluation by mentor, and changes made

     ◦   year-end summative evaluation of program by mentor.

Outcome: Eighty-six per cent of mentor relationships have continued beyond the completion of the group component of SOHO.

2.   *Art skills and accomplishments* were supported by Art League training and were measured by:

   ◦ list of art projects and skill development (painting/drawing/theory)

   ◦ "before and after" photos of room.

Outcome: One hundred per cent of SOHO graduates have completed art projects, demonstrated improved skill development, and expressed pride in their remodeled bedrooms.

3.   *Self-esteem and social skills* were supported by programs and rite-of-passage event and were measured by:

   ◦ pre- and post-test of girl's report of experience

   ◦ personal interview with each girl and family at start of program

   ◦ personal interview with each girl at end of program.

Outcome: One hundred per cent of SOHO graduates have expressed satisfaction with the SOHO program, acquisition of social skills, and improved perceptions of key target areas. Eighty-five per cent of parents/guardians have noted an improvement in behaviors (attendance, anger management, cooperation, friendliness, etc.) either at home or in school.

Overall changes in behavior are measured by a review of crime rates one year after a girl completes the program. The results show that 40 of the 42 girls who have graduated from SOHO to date have had no court involvement for criminal activity. One girl has been arrested for shoplifting, another for assault; both of these participants had prior delinquency charges.

The program has been particularly gratifying to the Art League as it has enabled young girls to discover that they have creative abilities, can produce unique and expressive objects of personal and marketable value, can change the space where they live for the better, and can enhance that space with objects they have created. The extraordinary combination of mentoring and use of the creative process can be, in the words of a volunteer, "transformational" for all involved. The powerful impact of this project for mentors was perhaps best expressed in a poem written this year by volunteer Tara Cristian:

SOHO Spring 2005

To have the opportunity to receive true self-expression
That late night and early morning telephone calls are a
Welcomed surprise regardless of the conversation

To care for without reservation or judgment
Like new parents with a newborn infant where their greatest
Wish is for the child's happiness
To be thought of and treated as additions to her family,
An extension of her heart
A strong sisterly bond consisting of love and friendship
Oh, to be mentors of (SOHO) young women
To share in the lives of aspiring, creative, and powerful
Female spirits
What an amazing gift!

The unexpected

The greatest unexpected impact of SOHO has been on the families of participants. One drug-addicted mother, who had virtually ignored her daughter's mentor and other remodeling crew members all day Saturday, borrowed SOHO cleaning supplies and scrubbed her entire house. The following day, she asked, "Is there anything I can do to help?" and assisted the crew throughout the day. This mother had denied years of court-ordered services of home-based counseling, only to let SOHO volunteers into her home. By the end of the weekend, the mother was implementing advice on behavior management strategies and seeking sex-abuse treatment for one of her children. One mother had been using bleach in the dehumidifier in order to "clean the air" and relieve her daughter's asthma symptoms. The mentor was able to guide the parent to use scientifically proven methods to treat the illness. Mothers have received assistance from SOHO volunteers for finding jobs, seeking drug and alcohol treatment, and accessing mental health services, childcare, and special education services for children.

Sadly, another unexpected discovery at SOHO was the high number of pre-teen participants who had already been sexually active, were failing at school, and had an extremely low self-image. These disclosures emerged thanks to the trusting relationships developed between girls and their mentors. The SOHO curricula and mentor training continues to evolve to address expressed needs.

Community-wide collaboration

Media attention from *The Washington Post,* WAMU Radio, *The Alexandria Gazette Packet, Alexandria Journal,* and *The Chronicle of Philanthropy* has worked to promote knowledge about SOHO, yielding dozens of volunteers, financial contributions, discounts from local restaurants and paint companies, and donations of dressers, beds, hangers and pillows. In response to a copy of a newspaper article and a plea for support posted on the Alexandria link at

Freecycle.com, literally thousands of dollars' worth of furniture, futon frames, loft beds, dressers, nightstands, bookshelves, desks, and other items have been donated.

In her own words

"I've learned that you can mess round with art, and you have to keep trying different ways and see what you like." (Lauren, age 12)

"Art is important because it makes me feel great. My mentor picks me up in her car – a jeep – I just like to ride here." (Dominique, age 11)

"My dad came to visit and spent the night in my extra bunk, and I told him to try the bed, and he tried it out and said, 'I'm going to melt'; I told him to try the pillow; he tried the pillow – he sank into it until he couldn't even see; he said 'I've melted in comfort.'" (Alicia, age 10)

"Before, I felt bored in my room, now it's fun– when my mom tells me to go to my room, I have no problem with it! [At SOHO] you learn how to repair broken things in your room – my mom even asked me if I would help her remodel her room." (Tasha, age 12)

"My room is sputnik! I just made that word up. It has a study place and a buncha lights, so I never have to run out of light or be in the dark. Now I sleep in my room every night; before I was never in my room; it was dark; it didn't have light. My mentor is my best friend now." (Tiara, age 12)

"I was afraid because I didn't know how to draw – And I still don't know how. But I'm not scared any more." (Brittany, age 12)

"The most helpful thing I learned from SOHO was how to cope with problems between girls." (Stephanie, age 13)

Still to do...

SOHO hopes to attract year-round funding for a program coordinator position, so that all interested girls and volunteers are able to participate. A scientifically based social skills curriculum will be adopted in order to standardize pre- and post-tests. In 2006 SOHO plans to pilot a program with fourth and fifth graders, particularly Latina girls, in an effort to prevent sexual activity at an early age, prevent school failure, address plummeting self-esteem and reduce gang involvement.

What about boys? As a result of multiple focus groups with boys, should funding be secured, Alexandria will launch "COHO", Crib of his Own, where boys will build dressers and loft beds and create new bedrooms with the support of male carpenter mentors. Another popular idea is to steal the concept from television's "Pimp my Ride" to create a fun automotive program for boys.

Closing

Steve A. Prince's poem, which he wrote in 2005 to celebrate the SOHO girls, was reproduced, framed with an original wood block print, and given to each girl at the ending gala celebration:

It was not by accident

It was not by accident
That I was there the day you were born.
It was on a Tuesday…
Lilies from the field
Sprung from the concrete
And recycled wood.
You are an ancestral
Blend of blood
Of love, of tears, of eyes
Of butterflies fluttering in the wind
Of change. Your life
A cornucopia of hand
Shaped dreams.
Your splendid mind shines
Bright in the shadowed night.
It was not by accident you were
Born beautiful

Especial

And free
You were meant
To be!

Note

SOHO creators Alice Merrill and Linda Odell were the recipients of the 2005 Northern Virginia Leadership Award for Community Partnership.

Acknowledgements

I thank the following individuals and businesses for their extraordinary contributions to SOHO: Alice Merrill for her thousands of hours volunteering to fundraise, plan curricula, hire instructors, purchase supplies, prepare healthy meals and provide an overall positive and nurturing atmosphere for girls and mentors alike; Kris Rosenblatt for her support in the creation of SOHO and three consecutive years of volunteer work as mentor, instructor, and supply manager; Gwen Mathews for her work in the initial development of SOHO, recruiting mentors and providing technical assistance in program promotion and mentor training; Steve Prince for his dedication to SOHO, his first-rate art instruction and service as inspiration to all SOHO participants; and Karen Vigmostad for her assistance with the development of evaluation measures and charts. I also thank other major contributors, including the Alexandria Youth Fund, the Otto-Whalley Family Foundation, Alexandria City Public School social workers and teachers, the Art League, 18th District Court Service Unit, Bugsy's Restaurant, Duron Paints, Golden Paints, Home Depot, Freecycle.com, and the Alexandria Seaport Foundation.

References

Bilchick, Butts and Poe-Yamagata (1996) *Female Offenders in the Juvenile Justice System.* Washington, DC: Office of Juvenile Justice and Delinquency Prevention.

Merrill, Alice (2005) *SOHO Art Curriculum.* Inc. Alexandria, VA: The Art League.

National Mentoring Partnership (2005) *The Learn to Mentor Toolkit.* Accessed 5 October 2005 at www.mentoring.org. Washington, DC.

Search Institute (2001) *Developmental Assets: A Profile of Your Youth.* Report Number 80223. Alexandria, VA.

Tierney, J. P., Grossman, J. B., and Resch, N. L. (2000) *Making a Difference: An Impact Study of Big Brothers Big Sisters.* Philadelphia: Public/Private Ventures.

CHAPTER 13

Collaboration and Creativity

Art Therapy Groups in a School Suspension Program

Ashley R. Dorr

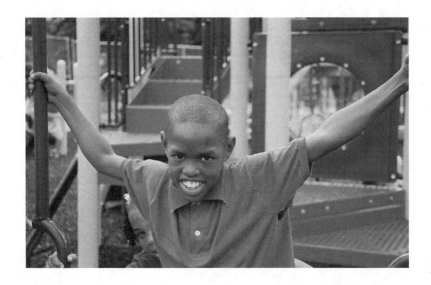

This chapter will focus on art therapy groups in a school suspension program in New York City. Adolescents who get suspended from school naturally carry with them unresolved conflict, feelings of anger, and low self-esteem. This chapter will describe the efficacy of art therapy groups in addressing these issues as illustrated by two components of the art therapy process: the collaborative group process, and the creative art-making process.

Background

During the 2004–2005 school year an estimated 44,000 school suspensions took place in the New York City Public School system (Lovett 2005). These suspensions ranged from week-long, to 30, 60, or 90 days or year-long. A year-long suspension is called a superintendent suspension. An estimated 576 high school and junior high school students in the New York City Public Schools received superintendent suspensions in the 2004–2005 school year (C. Burnet, in unpublished personal communication, August 2005).

Suspensions are often necessary to keep a school safe, ensure consistency, and follow through with rules and consequences, but, though necessary and warranted, these suspensions can result in stressful and damaging experiences for the youth who receive them. For some, school may be their only safe and consistent environment and their primary social network. To be ousted from that context is a major interruption in an adolescent's world. Their entire social system, daily routine, commute, environment, and school structure is changed abruptly. Waller states, "A growing field of research supports the belief that suspensions weaken a student's bond to his or her school, increasing the likelihood that a child will drop out" (Waller 2004, p.1).

In New York City, suspensions are on the rise and the number of youth out of school on a daily basis is escalating into a crisis in the educational system. The suspension school program described here was created in response to this crisis. It is held in a youth development agency and serves students who have received year-long superintendent suspensions. The goal is to help these students develop the necessary skills for school and to assist them in transitioning back into the regular school system.

The students in this suspension school include junior high and high school students aged 12–19. They are referred for a high-end suspension (which means that the suspension usually occurred because of a serious offense such as physical violence involving peers, teachers, security officers, or principals, or possession of weapons, or possession of drugs). These students have been unsuccessful in the standard public-school classrooms in New York City. Some have a history of minor suspensions, while others have shown pervasive truancy, behavioral problems and academic problems. Because these students are often considered oppositional, truant, and hyperactive, their educational needs are often overlooked. While some students have had experience in counseling or therapy, many of them have not experienced counseling before. Some students are naturally defensive upon entry to the school. Their defensiveness is expressed in acting out, guarded affect, and resistance to therapeutic services or to staff members in general. In addition, there has often been a gap of one week to six months since they left their previous school setting. This could mean that they have spent time in a detention center, at a temporary educational site, or at home, awaiting answers and information from school personnel.

While some take responsibility for being suspended, others report feeling unfairly or unjustly treated. Some students feel that many cards have been stacked against them. Taking responsibility is difficult because students are often unable to identify or acknowledge underlying feelings, issues, and events that led to the suspension. Those students who do take responsibility may experience feelings of guilt, failure, and lowered self-esteem. Students react differently to being in the suspension school. One common factor, however, is that all of them have left their previous school with unresolved conflicts and feelings. These students are in need of a reparative and holding experience. When given a place to be safe and creative, adolescents can take advantage of the opportunity to make art and express themselves (Riley 1999).

Art therapy groups

The challenge of using creative arts therapies in a school setting is that there are often differences between therapeutic and educational goals, methods, and evaluation techniques. Communication and understanding between the therapeutic and educational staff are essential.

The suspension school program presented in this chapter is designed to provide academic classes and therapeutic services. The therapeutic component is designed with a strong creative-arts-therapies approach. The students each have an individual counselor and are seen in individual art, dance, music, or verbal therapy sessions as well as in groups. Each group focuses on a specific issue such as anger management, self-esteem, or conflict resolution, all of which have been identified as major issues for this population. Notwithstanding these specific group focuses, therapists usually address all of these issues simultaneously, since they are inter-connected.

The first step in setting up groups at the suspension school is for the therapists to have individual conversations with each student before the group begins. This provides an opportunity for the therapist to explain the purpose of the group, and for the therapist and student to get to know each other. Students want to be seen as a whole person, and not just as the part that is referred for treatment. It is important that a therapist gets to know that whole person and not just the part that needs "anger management," or "conflict resolution" (Malekoff 2004).

A group structure that creates the safe environment necessary to handle conflict as it arises is developed by establishing a shared purpose, exploring what art therapy is, exploring the topic at hand (anger management, conflict resolution, or self-esteem), and explaining rules (especially discussing respect and confidentiality). Group members can contribute their own rules in their own words. Allowing group members to establish their own rules empowers them and shows respect for them as stakeholders in the group. The students are mandated to attend the suspension school and mandated to attend the art therapy group, so any amount of control given to them goes a long way. The process of establishing rules can be arduous, humorous, empowering, and challenging but essential. Students need to know that there are rules, in order to feel safe. This is also a time when students may "test" the therapist. When tested, it is important for the therapist to set limits, but at the same time accept the expression that is shared. For example, one student smugly shared his rule to "Smoke weed everyday in group." The group laughed and he smiled. The therapist handled this by stating that surely we would not be *smoking* weed, but that we could indeed *talk* about it, and would do so confidentially. This allowed the student to feel heard and validated, while showing him that his expressions would be kept confidential.

Building trust is essential in the beginning phases of groups. Malekoff (2004) describes the beginning of group as being "particularly difficult for adolescents who come from unstable environments characterized by inconsistent comings and goings" (p.53). He goes on to say "When a lack of trust pervades one's life experience one can expect that experience to be carried into the group" (Malekoff 2004, p.53). As the group structure is set and trust is built, cohesion and collaboration emerge, allowing the group to move forward.

Conflict, anger, self-esteem

Inner city adolescents not only live in a world full of conflict, but must do so while "growing up." They are in transition from being children who are unable to fully understand conflict, to being adults who should have this capacity, as well as the coping skills necessary to resolve conflict. Adolescents face conflicts with peers, family members, authority figures, and most of all, within themselves. In addition many inner city youngsters must survive in neighborhoods where conflict and violence permeate streets and families. Exposure to and involvement in conflict not only affects mental, emotional, and cognitive well-being (Lorion 1998), but makes negotiating normal developmental changes a challenging endeavor (McManus 1993).

Conflict can cause a young person to feel angry, disempowered, and "out of control." Research by Rosenthal (2000) found that exposure to community violence during adolescence often resulted in psychological trauma manifesting in anger, anxiety, and depression. Lacking alternative modes of expression, "holding it in" or "acting it out" become modes of expression, and the cycle of negative events repeats.

Yalom (1995) indicates that groups resemble the primary family setting. The way an individual interacts in groups is related to experiences in his or her primary family. It is no surprise that many young people who have grown up surrounded by conflict have difficulty succeeding in school. They act in school as they would at home or in their neighborhoods.

When adolescents act out their conflicts in school it can result in feelings of anger, rage, revenge, injustice, confusion, guilt, and sadness. These overwhelming feelings are often difficult to modulate, resulting in low self-esteem. During adolescence, the individual develops his or her identity. As the identity develops, adolescents are in a constant state of self-exploration (Blos 1962). This time is filled with questioning, ambivalence, and a fragile sense of self. Getting suspended from school as an adolescent is equivalent to being fired from a job as an adult. A blow to the ego is hard for anyone to take, and so much the more if it occurs during adolescence, when ego-strength may already be fragile.

Conflict resolution

Students at the suspension school have all experienced the unresolved conflict of being suspended. Conflict is therefore expected to arise during the therapeutic process. Conflict presents itself in many ways: between group members, towards the leader, through resistance to group rules, or as conflict with the art materials. These conflicts can be used as opportunities to teach how resolution can occur, if a safe climate is established. If group members have concrete experiences of collaborating and resolving conflict they can then begin to internalize and use these skills in other situations. Kaplan (1994a) defines conflict resolution as "a nonviolent, non-adversarial, cooperative problem-solving approach."

Students who come to the suspension school have lost their support system at school as a result of a conflict. If a support system is lost in an early stage of development, the adolescent will unconsciously search for an environmental support system (McManus 1993). Art therapy groups can serve this purpose, and provide an opportunity for group members to look at their own conflicts as well as explore group conflicts. Liebmann (1996b) states that "people in conflict with themselves or others do not have the communication skills to resolve situations verbally and therefore arts approaches are extremely helpful" (p.3). Words can escalate conflicts, whereas art-making can respond to conflict with more distance and safety (Liebmann 1996a).

Conflict resolution Case Study 1: Conflict and non-conflict images

During one session in an all-female art therapy group, the topic of conflict was explored. This group had been through many trust-building steps and had formed a very cohesive group. The women brainstormed about different types of conflict and shared examples, such as conflict with self, teachers, peers, and parents. They discussed how a conflict looks and feels depending on where you are standing: whether you are in the conflict, watching the conflict, or completely outside the conflict and conflict-free. They discussed how, when a conflict happens in schools, bystanders experience the conflict as well, which can perpetrate it. A conflict can go on longer because the students fighting often gain an audience, and because the people witnessing the conflict experience feelings of fear – which disturbs their sense of safety, perhaps even leading them to joining in with the conflict.

The young women were asked to create two images depicting what it feels like when they are involved in conflict, and what it feels like when they are not involved in conflict. They were encouraged to use lines, colors, and shapes to

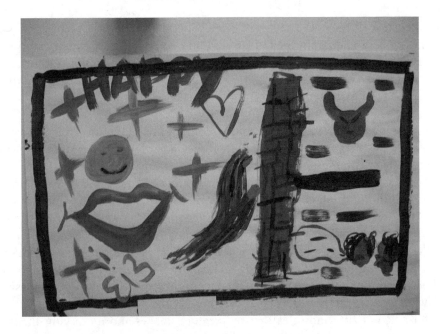

Figure 13.1 One young woman's conflict image

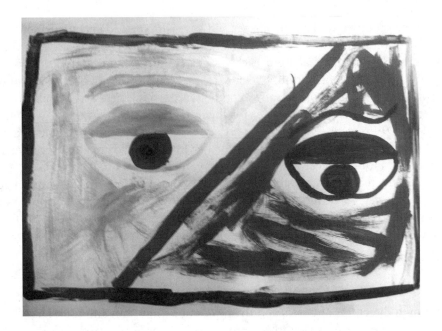

Figure 13.2 A young woman's conflict image representing two sides of her personality

illustrate the difference. They were given paper with a black border as a way to frame, hold, and contain their creations and expressions of difficult emotions. They were invited to create the two images in any order that felt comfortable. Most of them chose to create the image of themselves in conflict first, and then created the one of themselves out of conflict.

The majority of the non-conflict images still indicated a sense of conflict. For example, one young woman's non-conflict image (Figure 13.1) included her hand pushing against a wall, on the other side of which was a devil's head, which she said represented girls gossiping about her.

She said, "Even when I am out of conflict, it's still there and I have to try so hard just to not think about it or get involved in it." The young women talked about how their guards are always up, meaning that they have to portray a tough exterior and be ready for conflict at any time. Another young woman talked about her non-conflict image (Figure 13.2) as representing two sides of her personality. The difficulty in distinguishing between in and out of conflict illustrations could be due to the fact that conflict in their lives is so pervasive. The art process led to a deeper discussion of what actually causes conflict.

Kaplan (1996) indicates that by creating images and modifying them, a person can own and begin to take charge of their emotions. Her research also shows that specific changes in the way someone expresses their emotions can occur when they are enabled to modify and work through emotions using the art process.

The group viewed all the images and gave support and encouragement for each person's creation. In witnessing and supporting each other's artwork they were able to accept and hold each other's feelings about conflicts. Yalom's (1995) theory of universality relates to this experience, in that the young women were able to universalize conflict and see that it exists for all group members, and this made it easier for them to accept it within their own lives. Yalom (1995) states, "As patients perceive their similarity to others and share their deepest concerns they benefit further from the accompanying catharsis and from ultimate acceptance by other members".

This activity was possible because the young women in the group had gotten to a stage in the group process where they shared a sense of trust and safety. The collaboration that occurred in the early stages of group formation developed a safe space for them to explore conflict. Group cohesiveness is necessary before any deep work can begin (Yalom 1995).

Conflict resolution Case Study 2: Clay

Though direct use of topics and themes can be important and useful, as illustrated in the previous example, many times metaphor is a safer way to work. The use of metaphor provides a way to use symbols and representations as an indirect exploration of themes. The material will surface within the metaphor and can be worked out in a non-threatening way.

All students in the art therapy group described here were male and ranged in age from 13–18. The ethnic descents of the young men included African-American, Guyanese, Eastern European, and Dominican. The young men differed not only in age and ethnicity, but also in defenses and capacity for insight. At first this group was fragmented and subtle disrespect and testing were common. During their first session each member wrote down his favorite song, so that a music mix could be created and played during art-making. The selections included rap, R&B, heavy metal, rock 'n' roll, and Latin music. This music mix helped them to tolerate each other's interests and backgrounds. The group initially laughed and made fun of each other's songs, but the students were encouraged to respect each other's songs, no matter how different they sounded. The music represented who they were, and as they came to accept each other's songs they began to accept each other as individuals. This intervention established a common ground and allowed them to see that one thing they had in common was a love of music. The group came to accept very different sounds and styles of music, and so were able to discuss racial and ethnic differences.

During the early, fragmented stages of the group, using clay seemed a logical way to ground them. The group was curious to work with clay and it literally gave them something to hold onto. As they began their own creative processes, they turned their focus inwards, rather than on each other. It seemed to unite them, and they became explorers in this uncharted territory of clay creation. To help facilitate collaboration, group members were encouraged to seek assistance from two young men in the group who had some previous experience with clay. These two young men were able to help guide the others, which led them to working together, mutually seeking and giving assistance and building group cohesion. Encouraging the students to help each other built group cohesion. Instead of depending on the therapist for help and competing against each other, they worked together. Clay establishes a common ground (Henley 2002) and this united the group, and helped them to bind together.

As the group came together, conflicts were redirected to the clay rather than to specific group members. Though clay is very grounding and exciting to work with, it can be frustrating to build something that will stay together. Clay is very malleable and can be easily transformed, but, paradoxically, this quality also makes it difficult to form. The young men had to work through conflict within the art process in order to make clay creations that were successful. When using clay there are certain rules and processes to follow in order to successfully create a ceramic object. For instance, the clay needs to be "wedged" so that there are no air bubbles which could break the piece during firing in the kiln. Additionally a technique called "scoring" is used to attach pieces together in such a way as to remain intact. The rules for using clay became metaphors for the rules of the group – as the students respected and followed the rules for working with clay, group rules were more fully adhered to.

During one group session the students joked about race and shared that if they didn't joke around about race, there would be "so many more fights in the school." They were able to talk openly about themselves and how they were "cool" with each other despite being different. They related to each other and accepted each other through joking. This was important, because in so doing they disclosed their own coping skills for racial conflict. Riley (1999) notes that group process and sharing can be a way to address ethnic, cultural and racial issues.

As the eight-week group drew to an end, an interesting event occurred. When the students glazed their clay pieces, they each chose their own color for their base under-glaze. One student chose a top glaze called "snapdragon" that produces pops of color all over the original base color. This glaze was a risky choice, compared with the clear glaze, which simply makes the original color shiny. After he chose this glaze, the others followed suit one by one. This could have been owing to a desire to conform and fit in, a negation of their own "colors", or a metaphor for the previous discussions about race. On the other hand, it could also be seen as a unifying process of them coming together as a group. The young men were all relating and connecting, and this glaze choice seemed to mirror their behavior.

The participants in the boys' group were able to deal with conflicts that arose and create a collaborative and creative space where, no matter how different they were, they could get along and support each other. Riley (1999) states, "Group cohesion demonstrated in a teen group is covert, it is verified by behaviors, not by words" (p.81). When a group gels together and works though conflict, there is a nonverbal expression of peace within that group.

Anger management

Anger is a feeling that can manifest in many ways. It can be projected onto group members or the leader, or can become obvious through voluntary absences from the group. It can be seen or unseen, latent or manifest, direct or indirect, passive or aggressive. The more students learn how to express their anger appropriately and safely, the better they can cope with and accept their feelings. Kaplan (1994b) has shown that art can be used to modify images of anger in a constructive manner and that there is a relationship between how angry a drawing appears and how angry its creator feels.

Art therapy groups facilitate anger management by providing a supportive atmosphere in which to explore the topic. The artwork itself provides a place to release anger, sublimate frustration, and express feelings in a non-threatening way. The art product and processes allow for projections to occur, and this reduces the projections that occur between group members. If students are enabled to turn their anger into something meaningful, the experience becomes transformative rather than simply cathartic. Kaplan (1994a) calls the "catharsis theory" into question and suggests that unlimited catharsis can result in increased hostility. It is suggested that anger needs to be not only expressed, but understood, owned, transformed or channeled into positive action.

Malekoff (2004) states, "Group work with kids is rarely neat. It is more abstract than still life, more jazz than classical (p.19)." The mistakes, surprises, and unexpected nuances that occur in the group process are often the ones that produce the best moments for growth and understanding to occur.

Anger management Case Study 1: Mandalas and mask-making

The art therapy group described here included male and female students ranging in age from 14–18. This group had a transformative experience using art to work through mistakes made by the therapist, group anger, and frustration. The creative art-making process transformed group anger and frustration into something positive.

Session A

Facilitating cohesiveness was initially challenging, as the group members varied widely in their interests and investment in the group. There was also a level of disrespect that needed addressing. In response to this, the group created a group mandala. Group members were given pre-cut pieces of a large circle that fit together like a puzzle. They were asked to color their piece in any way they wished and with any colors. As this happened, the students explored the idea of "respect," and they all indicated that being disrespected made them feel angry. We agreed that since this was an anger management group, the members would try to respect each other so as not to make each other angry. As they put the pieces together we explored how this large, circular image signified all the different group members coming together and working as a team, despite differences (in the images and in themselves). The circular image of a mandala represented the group coming together as a whole. After this session the students seemed to be more comfortable and respectful of each other.

When running groups it is important to provide a safe space for growth. Winnicott (1971) describes the importance of the environment that a mother provides for an infant as one which protects and contains while allowing growth to occur, similar to the safe space that a therapist provides for a group. When youth are given a safe place to play, experiment, and work through difficult emotions like anger, they are able to grow emotionally (Webber 2003). The growth in this group allowed for further exploration of anger.

Session B

In a subsequent session the art directive was ceramic mask-making. Rolling, wedging, pounding, and molding clay can provide a physical opportunity to discharge the energy of anger, and can aid in channeling group aggression (Henley 2002). Students began by wedging and pounding out the clay and discussed how this process helped to release anger and energy. Students rolled their pieces out into clay slabs. They helped each other with this process, producing a sense of accomplishment, pride and protection for their masks.

They were directed not to make their clay slabs too thick, because they would be too heavy. This proved to be bad advice, however, because the two thinner masks ended up breaking, while the thicker ones were all stable. Additionally, there was some delay in the kiln schedule, so the masks could not be glazed on the expected day.

These two mistakes on the part of the therapist proved to be opportunities for growth. The therapist took responsibility and let the group members know that it was her mistake for misguiding them. Adult responsibility was not something these students were used to. The students did not react negatively to the news. They had worked very hard, and though they did voice disappointment, they did not express any anger.

During the next group the glazing had to be postponed again, because the fired pieces were not yet cool enough to glaze. Finally one of the quieter and newer members of the group said to the therapist in a very joking and light-hearted manner, "Ashley, you suck!" There was laughter but, more important, the students were able to understand that you can express anger honestly, without being disrespectful. Opportunities to discuss anger and ways of coping when disappointed by adults were created, since the group was cohesive, and because the therapist had acknowledged that she was at fault.

One student, whose mask had broken, took his pieces and contemplated them. He said, "I actually don't want to glue mine together, after all. It's kind of like two sides of a personality." He decided he wanted to display two sides of the mask to illustrate this. He glazed the inside of his mask with brilliant mahogany, purple, terracotta, tan, and maroon shades, and he painted a black-and-white pattern on the outside.

We took this metaphor and related it to life experience. Students discussed frustrating situations they had encountered, which they were able to turn into something positive. A few students related this to their suspension, relaying that initially they were angry and upset to have been suspended, but that since coming to the suspension school, they were trying to make the most of it and learn from it. Some even felt they had grown to prefer this suspension school to their old school. After the broken mask came out of the kiln, the student discussed a creative side of himself that he had discovered. This process seemed to transform his view of himself, as well as his ability to work through issues with art. As described by Ross (1996), the use of artwork can lead to verbalization of feelings and development of better coping skills.

The group understood that they were able to make something positive out of their anger by empowering themselves to take control. Working through anger with artistic expression encouraged deep understanding and transformation. Because adolescents often have difficulty finding words to express rage, anger, conflict, frustration, and fears, the art-making process serves as a profound experience for them to express and experience these emotions.

Self-esteem

Self-esteem can be improved simply by making an art creation and being in a supportive group. Young people who enter a group with low self-esteem can leave it feeling positive and excited about what they have made, and therefore about themselves. McManus (1993) writes, "Perhaps the most vital aspect of the art therapy process is the way the symbolic image begins to generate a more creative and responsive self (p.21)."

It is important to note in this section that self-esteem is an integral factor in working with the two previously discussed topics of anger and conflict. As a young person's self-esteem improves through the art-making process, she becomes more able to support her peers. Expression is empowering and freeing. When students feel happy about themselves, they are less likely to put others down and more likely to be supportive. In her account of an art therapy program with students who had excessive truancy problems, McManus (1993) describes the goals of the art therapy program as centered around building self-esteem, self-image, and self-expression, rather than specifically focusing on truancy. Liebmann (1996a) also notes that self-affirmation is a necessary foundation to be laid before any conflict resolution work can begin.

Self-esteem Case Study 1: Animal collage and mixed media

In the co-ed art therapy group described here, there was a wide range of ages (13–18), personality, ego-strength, and ability to express things metaphorically and directly. Some group members had the capacity to express their emotions directly, while others were not able to do this, and put up a defensive front.

An art directive was introduced, using photos of animals. Group members were asked to choose one that they felt connected to, or that represented them. Riley (1999) has used animal metaphors in her work with adolescents and describes this intervention as a place for projections of the adolescent self to occur. Choosing a picture is a metaphoric means of exploring how group members feel about themselves.

The group members thoroughly enjoyed sorting through the images, and some actually asked to use two or three animals. They glued their photos onto blank paper, and used art materials to create an environment around the photo. This process flowed easily, and they used chalk, pastels, and watercolors to create their images. One student picked a wolf, and said that the two colors he used represented the calm and the anger that a wolf possesses. His description showed a capacity for insight that he had not yet shared with the group. By using metaphor he was able to say something about his personality. Another young man chose many animal images, and used paint to make many different shapes around them. He explained the various animal images as representing a fighter, being strong, being tough, enjoying eating, and "chilling" or relaxing. This student was able to incorporate many different ways of "being," and therefore explore the complexities of his personality.

Franklin compares art-making to the early stages of human development:

> The unformed materials, much like the [mind at birth], begin to take shape as the artist engages in a decision-making process that documents change. To work with art materials is to transform their physical and symbolic potential. Thus art-making may be considered a simultaneous process of reformulating the self through the active formation of an object. (Franklin 1992, p.79)

This group began with a blank sheet of paper and the animal pictures opened doors to their creative selves. After they had formed their images, they were able to have an authentic discussion about how these animals related to parts of their personalities. The use of colors and shapes around the animals seemed to metaphorically represent a safe place for the animals to be, similar to the way in which the art therapy group provided a place where the students could creatively express, and really "be" themselves.

Self-esteem Case Study 2: Printmaking

It is difficult for adolescents to support their peers, because they are in an egocentric stage of development. They are trying to figure out who they are and how others view them, and are often unable to empathize with or understand how others feel. Often when students are in crisis or conflict, they are literally caught in their own internal world, and it takes time for them to see the other person's point of view. Helping them to collaborate and support each other is a big part of the art therapy group process. This can only happen when they feel safe and secure with themselves.

Making a print resembles leaving your stamp or making your mark. In pre-school, children often finger-paint or make imprints of their hands in plaster. It is an awing process to see a reflection of yourself. Developmentally adolescents are repeating stages that they went through when they were younger. Therefore it is no surprise that this more mature form of imprinting one's own authentic expression is so satisfying for youth.

Printmaking is immediate, easy, and structured, yet freeing, sophisticated, and surprising. One form of printmaking involves carving into a styrofoam surface and then rolling ink onto the surface and printing the inked surface onto a sheet of paper. When students carve in the styrofoam, they are creating a spontaneous expression. The inking process is fun and allows them to connect with and use one color. The actual printing is like a surprise: you never know exactly what will come out, so this process enables students to take a healthy risk, which is a natural part of adolescence. Muller-White (1988) conveys the importance of the printmaking process, which allows for an authentic and individual creation as well as freedom and a healthy loss of control.

Because this process is usually so successful, group members often comment positively on each other's artwork. Muller-White (1988) also talks about a component in printmaking that aids in "leveling the playing field" (p.36). This process is usually new to everyone and is such an adventure that even group members who are usually timid, shy, or more passive with art-making can produce wonderful prints that peers will praise.

One student who usually destroyed and recreated much of his art found this process very satisfying and easier to master than other projects. He was usually quiet and was often picked on in the school. After many attempts at shapes and words he didn't like, he finally produced a print of the word "Africa" with his own mix of brown, gold and orange colors that he himself had created by combining inks. After this, he moved gracefully to the next art directive with much more ease and confidence, and the group acknowledged his success and gave him compliments about his print. Franklin (1992) discusses how the struggles and subsequent accomplishments in art-making improve an individual's self-esteem. By mastering an art process, one can begin to integrate a sense of self-worth, which can be extended to other areas of life.

In this particular group there had been much banter and teasing each other previous to the printmaking activity. After printmaking, group members began to compliment each other and were able to see each other in a different light. They seemed to take much pride in their creations and in the positive responses they received. Social roles were checked at the door, and instead, they took on the role of "artists".

Conclusions and considerations

As this chapter illustrates, art therapy groups are meaningful and effective ways to work on conflict resolution, anger management, and self-esteem through the collaborative group process and the creative art-making process. The combination of these two elements makes it possible to address the three issues as they relate to students who have been suspended from school.

There are many successes in the suspension school. Students grow in their capacity to express themselves, manage their emotions, and cope. The growth in therapy groups often translates into other areas, making school a more enjoyable and successful experience for them. As they learn to collaborate with each other and create art, they become able to resolve conflict and cope with their anger in healthy ways, while building their self-esteem. Students leaving the school are usually better equipped to function in the regular school system.

One challenge that often occurs is that by the time group cohesion is established and the group has reached the potential to work more deeply, it is often time to end, owing to the short-term nature of the program. Schaefer-Schiumo and Ginsburg (2003) discuss the importance of violence prevention programs, and how effective programs should include long-term alternatives for youth to communicate their views on violence. Though the art-making groups are short-term, one positive aspect of this structure is that students get to experience termination in a healthy way. This helps them to better cope with loss, and to rework previous experiences of saying goodbye that may have been unresolved. This is particularly fitting, since many students did not have a chance to resolve the conflict that got them suspended in the first place, or to say goodbye to their friends and teachers in their previous school.

One recommendation to therapists is to know yourself and know how you work best. I personally found that the more I got back to the basics of the art process and the group relationships, the better the groups flowed. As I empowered myself to deal with my own self-esteem, anger, and conflict within the workplace, the better equipped I was to empower these young people.

Malekoff (2004) says that group work with adolescents often includes elements of chaos, excitement, angst, fun, noise, and challenges, all wrapped up in one package. These elements are present in the suspension school groups, but are not tied up in pretty boxes with bows. They are more like bouncing balls, with bows and paper flying everywhere. Sometimes I feel like I am grabbing onto the ends of the bows as the balls pull me along. However, this is the nature of adolescence as well as the nature of group work.

I learn more and more about what these young people need and how best to work with them by really trying to see who they are and where they are coming from. The more honest I am with myself about what is best for them, the more I can slow the ball down and provide a container of safety, structure, limits, empowerment, authenticity, freedom, creation, and collaboration. This becomes a place where conflict, anger, and self-esteem are explored and relationships grow within the group collaboration and the art creation.

Acknowledgements

Special thanks go out to an amazing art therapist, mentor, and inspiration: Eileen McGann, who supervised and helped me immensely with this chapter. Thank you also to my amazing team and supervisor, who give their support and energy daily to this suspension program: Jeff Samanen, Dawn Wechsler, Joel Avin, Jonathan Rust, Martin Rios, and Sue Davis. And, of course, thank you to the young people of the program who show so much strength, resilience, and creativity.

References

Blos, P. (1962) *On Adolescence: A Psychoanalytic Interpretation.* London and New York: The Free Press.

Franklin, M. (1992) 'Art therapy and self-esteem.' *Art Therapy 9*, 78–84.

Henley, D. (2002) *Clay Works in Art Therapy: Plying the Sacred Circle.* London and Philadelphia: Jessica Kingsley Publishers.

Kaplan, F.F. (1994a) 'The art of anger: Imagery, anger management, and conflict resolution.' *The Canadian Art Therapy Association Journal 8*, 1, 18–29.

Kaplan, F.F. (1994b) 'The imagery and expression of anger: An initial study.' *Art Therapy 11*, 139–143.

Kaplan, F.F. (1996) 'Positive images of anger in an anger management workshop.' *The Arts in Psychotherapy 23*, 1, 69–75.

Liebmann, M. (1996a) 'Introduction.' In M. Liebmann (ed.) *Arts Approaches to Conflict.* London: Jessica Kingsley Publishers.

Liebmann, M. (1996b) 'Giving it form: Exploring conflict through art.' In M. Liebmann (ed.) *Arts Approaches to Conflict.* London: Jessica Kingsley Publishers.

Lorion, R. (1998) 'Exposure to urban violence.' In E.S. Delbert, B.A. Hamburg, and K. R. Williams (eds) *Violence in American Schools.* London and New York: Cambridge University Press.

Lovett, K. (2005) 'City schools keeping suspension rate low.' *The New York Post.* Accessed June 2005 at http://www.nypost.com/news/regionalnews/50079.htm

Malekoff, A. (2004) *Group Work with Adolescents.* New York: The Guilford Press.

McManus, A. (1993) 'The effectiveness of art therapy with Grade 7 and 8 students in a special attendance (s.p.a) curriculum, established by the Toronto Board of Education.' *The Canadian Art Therapy Association Journal 7*, 1, 15–29.

Muller-White, L. (1988) *Printmaking as Therapy: Frameworks for Freedom.* London: Jessica Kingsley Publishers.

Riley, S. (1999) *Contemporary Art Therapy with Adolescents.* London: Jessica Kingsley Publishers.

Rosenthal B.S. (2000) 'Exposure to community violence in adolescence: Trauma symptoms.' *Adolescence 35*, 138, 271–284.

Ross, C. (1996) 'Conflict at school: the use of an art therapy approach to support children who are bullied.' In M. Liebmann (ed.) *Arts Approaches to Conflict.* London: Jessica Kingsley Publishers.

Schaefer-Schiumo, K. and Ginsberg, A. (2003) 'The effectiveness of the warning signs program in educating youth about violence prevention: a study with urban high school students.' *Professional School Counseling 7*, 1, 1–8.

Waller, N. (2004) 'Loaded punches: more fights result in school suspension hearings.' Accessed June 2005 at http://www.jrn.columbia.edu/studentwork/youthmatters/2004/edu_1_waller.asp

Webber, J. (2003) *Failure to Hold: The Politics of School Violence.* Oxford: Rowman and Littlefield Publishers.

Winnicott, D.W. (1971) *Playing and Reality.* London: Tavistock Publications.

Yalom, I.D. (1995) *The Theory and Practice of Group Psychotherapy.* New York: Basic Books.

CHAPTER 14

Prevention Interventions

Art and Drama Therapy in Three Settings

Laura Soble and Janet K. Long

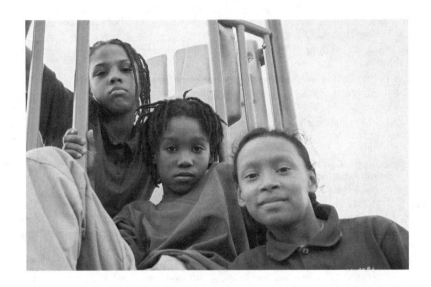

'Prevention' in this chapter refers to three major areas: 1) increasing emotional intelligence and critical thinking skills to increase self-esteem and school retention; 2) lowering the chance of participation in high-risk behaviors; 3) using mentorship to enhance a sense of self and community involvement. Prevention is presented through the lens of three settings in which therapeutic art, drama and poetry interventions are used with at-risk inner city children in California. The chapter covers 1) a six-week arts-based violence prevention project with a sixth grade class in a public school; 2) a case study of a 12-year-old boy living in two worlds – the inner city on weekends, and a middle-class neighborhood during the week; 3) a community arts program in Oakland, California, that uses photography as a mode to engage at-risk children, involve them with the arts, and expand their horizons beyond the challenges of their communities. The importance of prevention is discussed and prevention processes are outlined.

Introduction

The purpose of this chapter is to illustrate the importance of a prevention model in working with at-risk inner city children. Through the use of creative arts modalities, children are given alternative experiences of what life can be like. Helping at-risk children discover their own talents and creative energy, explore alternative options for their futures, and develop ways to channel their inner resources is an important aspect of prevention work.

LaCerva, who works in the field of violence prevention, believes that reinforcing characteristics of resiliency is critical for children to survive and cope in the world. He describes psychologist Suzanne Kobasa's three characteristics of psychological hardiness that contribute to positive outcomes for children: *commitment*, the capacity to be fully involved in whatever is happening; *control*, emerging from the belief that one has influence over the changing aspects of life; *challenge*, rooted in the belief that change is more prevalent than stability and that change can be a stimulating incentive for growth, rather than a threat to security. "The net effect of psychological hardiness is a reversal of the powerlessness and helplessness felt in response to unpredictable and unexpected events" (LaCerva 1996, p.145). He further describes how layers of protective factors at the individual, family, school and community levels can block negative outcomes. Examples he uses include the presence of at least one healthy adult and mentors who are readily available.

Prevention models using the creative art therapies with children and adolescents offer multi-modal approaches that have been shown to be more effective than lecture-discussion models (Larson 1994). In both urban and rural settings creative arts therapies have been used to help children manage cultural and environmental dilemmas caused by violence and chaos. Preventive use of the creative arts therapies in three diverse settings (a public school, private practice, and community-based) is described here.

1. Prevention in a public school environment: A six-week violence prevention program

A six-week violence prevention program was developed in California in 1996, and has been used throughout California, the United States and Europe. The aim was to assist sixth-grade students in managing the violence that they experienced in their communities. This interactive model utilized art and drama therapies to empower young people to make better choices about their actions and reactions. Long and Soble's (1999) account of the project forms the basis of this section.

In October 1996 the California Division of Kaiser Permanente supplemented a small Oakland Healthy Start grant to create an experimental violence prevention project in an inner city sixth-grade public-school classroom. The objective was to give students an enriched, hands-on and educational experience to help them identify and explore the effects of violence in their personal and communal lives.

The team of facilitators included four creative arts therapists and three educators. The team engaged in an open-ended creative planning process, in which the needs of the students in their school environment were taken into consideration. An integrated approach was formed that included art therapy, drama therapy, and health education interventions to address specific topics over a six-week period. Members of the professional team conferred with each other at the end of each week to discuss the themes initiated by the children and the feedback from the classroom teachers. Desired outcomes included creating safety and trust among all participants, exploring feelings, thoughts, and specific fears about the effects of violence (Landgarten 1981; Rubin 1978; Spolin 1986), and creating an educational action model that students could practice and use in their daily lives (Goleman 1995).

Each session began with an opening circle, followed by drama and/or art therapy exercises, and ended with a closure circle. An atmosphere of acceptance, respect and fun was communicated and modeled by the group leaders. Clear ground rules and agreements for behavior were introduced by the facilitators and added to by the students.

Each drama therapy group followed a similar format: a period of "warm-up" which involved group-building games and exercises relating to the theme of the day (Landy 1986); an "action" section in which students engaged in an activity, often culminating in sharing or performance; and a "closure/reflection" section in which to process, create safety, and ensure closure before returning to the larger group. Each session revolved around one of six project themes.

Session 1: Your world – how does violence impact on your world?

ART THERAPY EXPERIENCE

Students were asked to think of their world (school, home, neighborhood) and to draw something they would see there. Vivid images emerged that included streets, buildings or houses, family members, street violence, drive-by shootings, gun battles, car accidents, violent scenes from video games and TV, street fights, gang portraits, people engaged in violent arguments, and the end results of fatal violence – cemeteries.

DRAMA AND POETRY THERAPY EXPERIENCE

Groups brainstormed around specific words such as "angry" and "violence" and created poems, which were then read aloud by students. One group created a short group cinquain poem about the feeling "Angry":

Angry

UPSET UNHAPPY MAD

SMOKING SELLING KILLING

I FEEL REALLY UNCOMFORTABLE

WEED

Another group wrote about a related topic brought up by one of the students: "Saying 'no' to drugs". Each line represents words of an individual:

Violence

I love myself so much

Sad angry unhappy scared No to drugs No to drugs

Sad angry scared sad angry scared unhappy

Drive by shooting

I think drugs are bad and people shouldn't do them because they can damage the brain.

Good happy

Happy angry

Alcohol unhappy scared sad

Just say No to drugs and alcohol

Scared, lonely, dead, "R.I.P."

Bad hate

Hurt pain

Unhappy, you're scared, say No

I'm scared.

Session 2: What "builds you up?" and what "tears you down?"
ART THERAPY EXPERIENCE

Pre-cut or torn pictures from culturally diverse magazines (people, alone and in groupings, man-made objects, background scenes from urban and natural environments) were provided for the students. They were asked to fold a piece of white paper in half and create on one half a collage entitled "What builds you up" in your environment, and on the other a collage of "What tears you down" in your environment. They could use pastels and chalks to enhance the images in the collage.

On the "What builds you up" side of the collage, students chose images of peaceful nature settings, people engaged in positive interactions with each other, athletes and other heroic role models, elders, groups of children playing, and multi-ethnic groups of people being together. Words such as "peace", "happy", "love", "fun" and "help" were cut from magazines or written on the collages.

On the "What tears you down" side of the collage, images such as worn-down urban environments, people standing in groups looking angry or bored, people in prison or at war, dictators and other violent leaders, guns and other weapons, people fighting, wounded and dead people, people crying and in pain, illness and hospital scenes were included. Words included, "help", "war", "stop", "sad", "violence", "anger", "fear" and "hate".

DRAMA AND POETRY THERAPY EXPERIENCE

In small groups, the subject of self-esteem was discussed. Students were encouraged to write down words that "built them up" and "tore them down." Each student wrote a two-line passage (one statement indicating how they were "built up" and one showing how they were "torn down"), and these were combined to create one group poem:

> I felt happy that time I made a goal.
>
> I felt angry the time my cat bit me.
>
> I felt happy with family.
>
> When somebody hits me, I felt bad.
>
> Good, happy, justice, ice cream, reading
>
> Bad, frustrated, squirmy, Richard Allan Davis.
>
> I felt good when I am happy.
>
> I don't feel good when people smoke!
>
> I feel good when I get things.
>
> I feel sad when I get lonely!!!

Session 3: Creating shields of protection and introducing the Stoplight Model

ART THERAPY EXPERIENCE

Acrylic paints were set out so that each child could create his or her own palette of colors. Some 14" x 28" shields were made in advance out of white railroad board, with handles attached to the back. The Stoplight Model, based on Goleman's work (1995), was pasted on the back of each shield. This method allowed for containing of emotional vocabulary, as well as developing problem-solving abilities.

The Stoplight Model

STOP: Breathe. Be calm. What's happening?

FEEL: Name the problem. Say how you feel.

THINK: Think of alternatives.

CHOOSE: Decide what to do. "I want to _____."

ACT: "I am willing to _____." Try it!

Students were asked to decorate the shields with symbols that gave them strength and courage and that protected them when they were tempted by others to act in dangerous and violent ways. The painted symbols appearing on the shields included trees, mountains, flowers, waterfalls, streams, rain, rainbows, suns, moons, animals, birds, family crests, houses, and people.

DRAMA THERAPY EXPERIENCE

Students were asked to answer the question, "What is peer pressure?" Students gave examples of specific types of peer pressure, role-played the situations, and brainstormed alternative responses. They gave voice to strong feelings of helplessness, fear, and having the courage to choose. Facilitators encouraged them to use the Stoplight Model, having someone call out "Stop!" when the conflict was presented, and discussing the "think" and "feel" steps, leading to enactment of an alternative.

Session 4: Practicing the Stoplight Model and the Crisis Hotline

ART THERAPY EXPERIENCE

Students folded a piece of paper into four parts. Starting at the top left space, they began to draw a situation in which they might use the Stoplight Model. In the top left space they drew the "stop" part, indicating what was happening. In the top right space, they drew the "feel" part, indicating what they were feeling. In the lower right space they drew the "think" part, showing what ideas they came up with to deal with the situation. In the lower left space they drew the "choose and act" part, which showed what they decided to do to handle the situation.

DRAMA THERAPY EXPERIENCE

Students formed a circle, holding their shields. Using a drum to lead them, students posed in each of the Stoplight Model steps (stop, feel, think, choose, and act). Students were then introduced to the Crisis Hotline drama therapy exercise. One student would be a caller who had a problem. To help with choices, a prepared scenario was drawn from a hat. The caller would call the Hotline for help with the problem, and another student would play the role of the counselor at the Hotline. The rest of the group would be the audience experts, who would help the counselor brainstorm suggestions for the student with the problem. Throughout the role-plays certain themes were considered safe: smoking, pressure to steal, and hitting other people. Riskier situations to enact were gangs, drugs, and family violence.

Session 5: The clay bridge-building project and enactment of the crisis hotline

ART THERAPY EXPERIENCE

Students had decided during a previous session to build a bridge like the San Francisco Bay Bridge. The art therapist placed glossy blue paper on a table surface to represent water. At one end of the table was an 18" x 24" collage of a chaotic, violent world. On the other end of the table was a collage of an idealized world of peace. Wet clay was used for sculpting personal symbols. Students created sculptures representing their strengths, interests, symbols of safety, and spirituality, and placed these sculptures on, around, or under the bridge that the group built together (Ault 1986).

DRAMA THERAPY EXPERIENCE

Each group was given two pretend telephones. "Issues" were written in advance on small pieces of paper and put in a hat for each group. Students created a Crisis Hotline and played out different roles and scenarios. Scenarios included peer pressure (around drug, alcohol and tobacco use), loyalty issues with friends making risky choices, and issues within the family.

Session 6: Enacting a vision of peace

The objective during this last session was to give students another chance to acknowledge and express more fully their feelings about the impact of violence on their lives. Closure for the six-week program was provided through art and enactment of this theme.

ART THERAPY EXERCISE

The students made feeling-masks, using collage. They were told to notice how they were feeling and to portray it in their masks. Collage materials such as paper plates, drawing tools, pipe cleaners, feathers, and sequins were made available to decorate the masks. Masks portrayed feelings such as despair, rage, outrage, disappointment, frustration, joy, happiness, sadness, sarcasm, hiding, and secrets. When the masks were completed the students had a masked parade (peace march) to celebrate their six weeks together doing art and drama.

DRAMA THERAPY EXERCISE

To review the Stoplight Model, small groups enacted scenarios, creating new coach characters, who were responsible for stopping the scene in progress and highlighting a phase of the model.

During this closing session, the students were unusually tense and the therapists sensed their anticipation of saying goodbye. Feelings of loss were expressed. A pizza lunch was shared with the students while they looked over a photo album documenting the entire six-week project. The closing circle seemed to provide a healing space for everyone to review their participation and to say goodbye. Each student was validated for being a part of the process, and invited to take away a small mineral stone as a transitional object. Students also chose artwork from the past weeks to hang on a display board outside their classroom. This art display became a sounding board for the students to share their experiences and pride with the entire school population.

Conclusion

Prior to this project, therapists had received feedback that purely cognitive models of anger management and violence prevention had not been successful in this school system (Larson 1994; Leighninger and Niedergang 1994). Combining interactive art therapy, drama therapy, and health education models to engage children in exploring their attitudes, thoughts, and feelings about violence provided a living laboratory in which they could express themselves. Students learned problem-solving strategies by actively communicating with each other and by exploring the unspoken through art activities. By creating safety through ground rules, community-building activities, and a strong sense of inclusion (Gibbs 1995), even initially shy and uncooperative students participated, contributed their ideas, and created, each week.

Students volunteered real-life experiences of violence in their schools, homes and neighborhoods. They created vivid imagery and powerful enactments as a way of expressing and sublimating the feelings and thoughts arising from this sharing. The positive communication between facilitators and students about violence and its effects was a constructive experience that empowered students to share this project with their peers. Kaiser Permanente's video documentation of the project, *Speaking a Language of Peace* (1997), was duplicated, so that each student had a personal copy to share with family and friends. This video was also shared with other classrooms and other schools. This project evolved into one of mentoring and support for burgeoning creativity.

2. Prevention in a private practice art psychotherapy setting: The boy who lived in two worlds
by Janet K. Long

This case study describes how individual art therapy provided a safe and neutral space for an 11-year-old boy who lived in a dangerous inner city on weekends and in a safer middle-class neighborhood during the week. Art therapy provided a bridge between the two worlds, where artistic self-expression gave non-verbal form to inner experiences.

Allen, an eleven-year-old African-American boy, was referred to art therapy by his county social worker. He lived in the "ghetto" on weekends with a drug-addicted mother in a gang-infested neighborhood, and was temporarily staying with a professional middle-class couple referred to as "godparents" during the week so that he could attend a better school and have the structure that he needed to succeed. Anger and frustration developed in response to his experiences, and held the potential for self-sabotaging and violent behaviors. The art therapy process helped to transform these negative feelings into more positive self-esteem and better coping skills.

Allen had recently been diagnosed with ADHD and was medicated with 60 milligrams of Strattera. He was additionally being evaluated for agitated depression. He had failed the previous school year, had low self-esteem, and played the clown to cover his real feelings. He said he did not like people who were happy all the time, because he was uncomfortable showing his anger around them. He described himself as "tough" but was himself a victim of violence and was gentle with younger children and animals. The fights for which he had been punished were started by others. He defended himself with physical violence. If anyone insulted him, he became violent.

His family history included three generations of multiple-substance abusers, with domestic violence and other crimes leading to jail time for his biological father (whom he had never known and who was now dead), his mother, aunts, uncles, and grandparents. All he had known was welfare dependence, neglect, chaos, and violence. He had been emotionally and physically abused by his mother, his uncle, and his caretaking grandmother (a functioning alcoholic who took care of him when his mother was in prison). He was used by his mom to receive a welfare support check from the county, even though he spent weekdays away from her. He was put down by his mother as worthless because he had failed in school. His mother was now HIV-positive and was still using drugs. His only brother, a three-year-old, was the mother's preferred child and still lived with her in subsidized housing. An uncle he looked up to "socked" him in the face when he saw his poor report card. All of these people had dropped out of school before high school and seemed to live with constant rage. Allen was expected to babysit for his brother while his mother was on the street. He continued to do this when he returned home on weekends. The social worker was concerned that he would be recruited into a gang if he stayed in his mother's neighborhood all week and no prevention intervention was implemented.

When he moved in with the godparents at age eleven, adjustment to the middle-class neighborhood was difficult: Allen would get mad and slam his bedroom door, play loud music until the house shook, and refused to go along with the new routine, which included adequate hygiene, helping with chores, getting up in the morning and going to bed early, so that he could be up on time and have energy for school. This rebellion against the structure at his new home and school continued until he began to trust enough to say what he needed and learn some basic communication skills that were respectful and mutual. After several months he learned the rules, and began to experience weight gain, better sleep patterns, and a sense that the people in this new situation wanted him to do well. Testing the limits was now the game, but academic gains at school became an intrinsic reward. He still wasn't comfortable with these new feelings, and defended the good intentions of his mother, always wanting to see her on weekends.

During art therapy sessions he was a gentle and loving child and enjoyed playing with Sonia, a dog who acted as co-therapist. He was shy at first, and very respectful. He did not like talking about his past, but after a few sessions he shared information about his brother and mother. Mostly he talked as he made art or played cards and board games.

Allen was having a hard time adjusting to his new school and living with his godparents. He would become frustrated and did not know how to handle his feelings except by going into his room and blasting music. To address this, communication skills were worked on during initial stages of therapy. This stage of therapy with children from violent and neglectful homes is slow and needs the therapist's full attention and commitment (Malchiodi 1990).

During one session he was directed to draw a kinetic house–tree–person image (Figure 14.1). He drew a vertical representation of himself with his hands behind his back, wearing a red shirt and tight-fitting blue jeans. He drew the face as a younger child might, with dots for eyes, a one-line mouth, no ears or nose, black hair only on the top of his head, and no skin color. In this drawing he is standing next to his godparents' house. He is more than half as tall as the house, with the yellow and red sun between himself and the house. All of these symbols are in the lower half of the paper. From an analytic point of view, this boy experiences himself as latency-age, with his square shoulders having born much responsibility, yet with the ego strength of a young child. He is adjusting to his new weekday surroundings and feels warmth from his environment, but continues to feel socially lonely. The house is drawn with no color and he is standing alone next to it. No tree was drawn, even though he was asked to include one. This indicates lack of psychic support (Allan 1988; Malchiodi 1998).

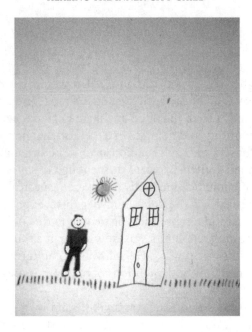

Figure 14.1 Allen's house–tree–person drawing

In a free art experience he painted himself on the ground, full-bodied, with a baseball mitt, ready to catch a ball. This painting includes a high skyline, which can be a sign of depression (Allan 1988), but it is a much more realistic representation of himself as an African-American boy, as he includes brown skin and depicts himself playing a sport he enjoys watching. No nose or ears are included, which are items that a younger child may omit. Allen's immature drawings may be the result of his emotional development having been interrupted by stress and neglect.

Next, he drew a bridge going away from Oakland, where his mother lived, towards San Francisco (Figure 14.2). The bridge had no supports on either side, and he drew an arrow going in the direction of San Francisco, symbolic of him leaving his home and escaping to some unknown place. The black and red colors denote his anger, and the empty line presentation may indicate depression (Rubin 1978).

After this drawing, he was asked to describe what would help with this situation. He drew a black and blue line drawing of himself being held up by balloons attached to his shoulders as he flies over the water (Figure 14.3). Analytically, he may be asking for help with his burdens, as he shows himself with no hands or feet to help himself.

By this point in therapy, he has become more trusting and able to disclose information about his mother's drug and alcohol abuse, about his brother being the "perfect" child, and how he feels criticized by his mother regarding his school problems.

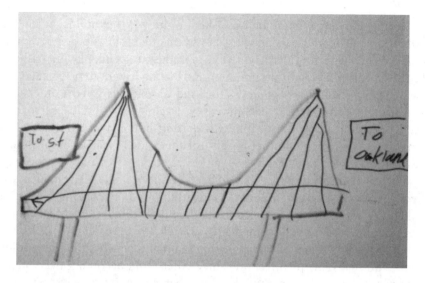

Figure 14.2 Allen's drawing of the bridge

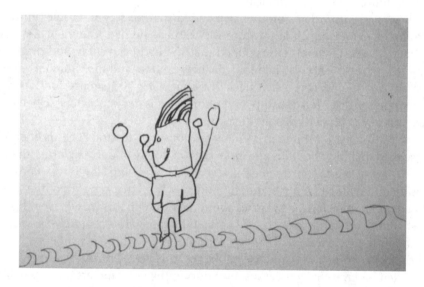

Figure 14.3 Allen flying over the water

How people express their feelings to each other became the next topic in therapy. Allen drew his idea of "love", creating a yellow sun on the upper left of the page, representing his mother, a black square to the right, representing himself, and his brother as an orange square sun to his right. He drew a green line under these figures and then drew L-O-V-E in block letters and doodled around these colorful letters with yellow, red and blue pencils, as he described feeling loved but also feeling very alone most of the time. In the drawing it appears that the word "love" is walking along by itself.

During the next session, he was asked to draw "What builds me up?" and "What tears me down?" His drawing shows that he is built up by good grades, getting approval from adults, having lots of money to spend, playing basketball like the stars, having family around him, and having friends to play games with. A bright yellow sun shows good weather and warm times. On the other side of the drawing he shows what tears him down: a cloud full of rain (tears), failing grades, people making fun of him and putting him down, being alone, and being poor. His struggle for better self-esteem, pride at real accomplishments, and a sense of belonging becomes very clear as he discusses his everyday life.

Easy-to-control art media seemed best for him at first, and he made a series of collages using magazine photos (Landgarten 1993), expressing his feelings, his identity conflicts, and his need for faith and nurturance. Eventually, he felt safe enough to use more fluid media (Lusebrink 1990; Malchiodi 1998; Long 2003). In the first stages of therapy, using familiar media (e.g. markers, colored pencils and magazine pictures) prevented Allen from becoming overwhelmed and frustrated with too many risk-taking behaviors. Introducing paints and clay was a natural progression, with him wanting more challenging media to express more feeling and intensity.

Unexpectedly Allen's mother demanded that he stay with her full-time. Overnight he was taken away from the stability he had known at the god-parents' house. The mother explained that she had been sober and drug-free for a few months since she had joined a new church, and the church members had advised her to take Allen back full-time. The godparents continued to worry about Allen's relationship with his mother as her unpredictable behavior was part of his life with his mother.

Without any warning, art therapy sessions had to stop. The mother was persuaded to allow the child one more session, to say goodbye. During the last session, a world was constructed out of colored modeling clay. It was a positive world that included family and friends and a school that supported him. Allen did not want to include his worries about the future in this world, even though he shared that he did not know what would happen now that he was with his mother full-time. He took this clay world home with him in a shoebox with a lid on it, "so no one at the house could get to it" (i.e. destroy it).

Allen had traveled a great distance during the year, and art therapy helped him to bridge the gap between his two homes. He was able to concentrate better on school work, his grades improved, he was talking more about how he really felt, he was problem-solving via art (Lowenstein 1999), he was partici-pating in swimming and other sports, and he had made friends who shared common interests with him at both of his residences.

Positive progress was made during one year of art therapy sessions, allowing for building of ego strength, shoring up of developmental gaps, and building up of a positive identity. Art therapy provided the ground and the building materials that were used to construct a more realistic inner world for

Allen. It provided an outlet for thoughts and feelings, as well as a symbolic and real foundation for future growth and hope.

3. Prevention in a community art program: FOCUS Youth Photography Project

Project Yield (Youth in Education and Leadership Development), a community-based arts program, gives urban children the opportunity to choose from a variety of arts modalities (digital video storytelling, theatre arts, spoken word, studio art, 3D sculpture, hip-hop, dance) in a school-based after-school arts education and youth development program. Professional artists teach classes in the visual, literary, performing, media, and public arts. Classes provide mentoring and are linked to school district curriculum standards, reinforcing the connection between in-school and out-of-school learning. The Project Yield program, staffed by teaching artists, is focused on youth development and building relationships with parents or guardians. All teaching artists in the Project Yield program meet for weekly staff meetings to avoid isolation, to talk about students, to share information, and to receive support. This team approach lets students know that there is an active network that holds them accountable for their actions, as well as maintaining regular contact with families.

An after-school arts mentoring photography program, Focus Youth Photography Project, funded by MOCHA (Museum of Children's Art in Oakland, CA), is one of the Project Yield interventions. Founded in 1999, Focus is committed to offering interdisciplinary, photo-based art education to young people in Grades 4–8 from economically challenged communities. Focus students are mentored while learning about and creating public artworks with photography.

Visual artist Carolyn S. Carr helped launch the Focus Project in West Oakland with founder Michelle Longosz:

> We are artists, educators and community activists. We do the work we do because we love art – the process of making it, thinking about it, and being in a community where it is valued. We do the work we do because we love mentoring young people as they discover their distinctive vision through both individual and collaborative work. (Focus Youth Photography Project 2005)

The Focus program's mission is to develop and enhance students' ability to see, observe, and pay attention to the world around them. As students learn basic photographic skills, they are encouraged to increase their visual, verbal, and written literacy skills. In addition, a broad range of art skills and, perhaps most important, life skills are taught.

A Focus photography class begins with a meditation. Students sit in a circle and focus on discovering their inner life through imagination. The facilitator guides them on a visual journey which encourages self-observation and helps to separate their school day from the after-school program. The meditation circle marks a time for slowing down. As growing artists these young people learn the importance and necessity of observing and then articulating what they see. They start by self-observation and move to looking at images in books by well-known photographers. As they look at images they increase their visual literacy.

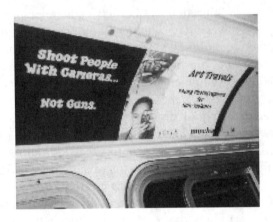

Figure 14.4 "Shoot people with cameras...not guns." (Photograph by Carolyn S. Carr, copyright 2005)

They learn to work in a darkroom, nicknamed by students "The Sanctuary". The process of printing their *own* photographs is a transformative one, involving many steps, each of which takes time and patience to create. Choices must be made along the way, such as how to focus, enlarge, and crop their image for best effect. Students using darkroom equipment learn transferable skills and also benefit from an increase in mastery, pride, self-esteem, and responsibility.

The program provides opportunities for students to see new places and people, and to expand their horizons within and outside their own communities through photography. The photography of Focus students has graced several community art projects in Oakland, CA. "Honoring Our Ancestors: Past, Present and Future", featured the creation of digital photomurals, which hang at two local schools. The Youth Voices Project featured the photography and writing of students on street banners hung along a major entry corridor into West Oakland. The Art Travels program featured student-created bus posters promoting non-violence. Three different posters were created: "Pack a Camera – not a gun", "load film...not bullets", and "Shoot people with cameras...not guns" (Figure 14.4)

Layers of mentoring underlie the work of the community artist working with students. Boundaries are important, as well as maintaining a sense of clarity and confidentiality. LaCerva (1996) would frame this ideal by stating

School protective factors consist of a caring and supportive environment with high expectations as well as numerous opportunities for participation. Among them is an extensive after-school program in keeping with the interests of a diverse group of students." (p.147)

The Focus Youth Photography Project creates opportunities for increased mastery, improved self-esteem, and increased responsibility. By examining the world within and outside of their communities, students are given access to alternative views and preventive outcomes. Teaching students new technical and life skills using the arts empowers them to make better choices. Students are encouraged to move away from teen pregnancy, gang involvement, and drug use, and toward a sense of hope and success.

Conclusions

The examples described above have shown how art and drama therapy interventions have been used to educate, empower and motivate youth. These vignettes show how creative pathways were opened up for youth to engage in dialogue about their feelings and thoughts in safe and creative environments. Art and drama therapies are, by their nature, transformative: children become aware, and are able to express, externalize, and transform difficult cognitive and emotional material, which allows them to formulate new approaches and attitudes to life. The skills acquired (e.g. learning the language of emotional intelligence, learning new critical thinking and problem-solving skills, becoming aware of self and others using new cross-cultural ideas, expressing conflicts about high-risk behaviors, and participating in mentorship relationships) serve as prevention interventions.

As creative arts therapists, we provide mentorship and a container within which awareness and self-expression can occur. The arts act as a mode of communication, giving students a possibility to express feelings of despair and fear and an opportunity to receive positive feedback about strengths. Expressive arts programs create opportunities for youth to explore and practice new problem-solving and self-esteem-building strategies. Young people connecting to themselves and the community through the arts, during school, after school and in creative arts therapy treatment, enjoy an artistic and multicultural experience that can inform them throughout their lives.

References

Allan, J. (1988) *Inscapes of the Child's World: Jungian Counseling in Schools and Clinics.* Dallas: Spring Publications.

Ault, R. (1986) *Art Therapy: The Healing Vision.* Topeka, KS: The Menninger Clinic, Menninger Video Productions.

Focus Youth Photography Project (2005) Accessed 2005 at www.focusyouthphoto.org/about.us.html

Gibbs, J. (1995) *Tribes, a New Way of Learning and Being Together.* Sausalito, CA: Center Source Systems.

Goleman, D. (1995) *Emotional Intelligence.* New York: Bantam Books.

LaCerva, V. (1996) *Pathways to Peace: Forty Steps to a Less Violent America.* Tesuque, New Mexico: Heartsongs Publications.

Landgarten, H.B. (1981) *Clinical Art Therapy: A Comprehensive Guide.* New York: Brunner/Mazel Inc.

Landgarten, H.B. (1993) *Magazine Photo Collage: A Multicultural Assessment and Treatment Technique.* New York: Brunner/Mazel Inc.

Landy, R. J. (1986) *Drama Therapy: Concepts and Practices.* Springfield, IL: Charles C. Thomas.

Larson, J. (1994) 'Violence prevention in the schools: A review of selected programs and procedures.' *School Psychology Review 23,* 151–154.

Leighninger, M. and Niedergang, M. (1994) *Confronting Violence in Our Communities.* Pomfret, CT: Topsfield Foundation, Inc.

Long, J. (2003) 'Medical art therapy: Using imagery and visual expression in healing.' In P. Camic, and S. Knight (eds) *Clinical Handbook of Health Psychology* (2nd edition) Cambridge, MA: Hogreffe and Huber.

Long, J. and Soble, L. (1999) 'Report: An arts-based violence prevention project for sixth-grade students.' *The Arts in Psychotherapy 26,* 5, 329–344.

Lowenstein, L. (1999) *Creative Interventions for Troubled Children and Youth.* Toronto, Ontario: Champion Press.

Lusebrink, V.B. (1990) *Imagery and Visual Expression in Therapy.* New York: Plenum Press.

Malchiodi, C. (1990) *Breaking the Silence: Art Therapy with Children from Violent Homes.* New York: Brunner/Mazel Inc.

Malchiodi, C. (1998) *Understanding Children's Drawings.* New York: The Guilford Press.

Rubin, J.A. (1978) *Child Art Therapy: Understanding and Helping Children Grow Through Art.* New York: Van Nostrand Reinhold Co.

Speaking a Language of Peace (video). (1997) Oakland, CA: Kaiser Permanente.

Spolin, V. (1986) *Theatre Games for the Classroom.* Evanston, IL: Northwestern University Press.

CHAPTER 15

Emotional Repair through Action Methods

The Use of Psychodrama, Sociometry, Psychodramatic Journaling and Experiential Group Therapy with Adolescents

Tian Dayton

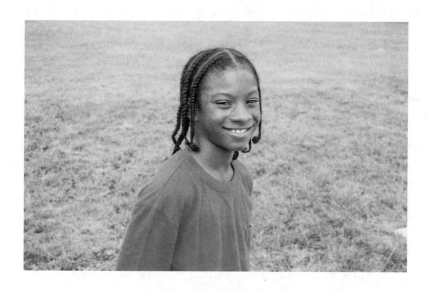

The urge to act out is inborn. The use of dramatic forms to communicate, teach, and heal, is as old as history. The Ancient Greeks used drama to illuminate issues close to the human heart. The stage became a safe arena in which to explore and explain psychological and emotional themes through role-play. Audience identification with the characters portrayed was one of our earliest forms of therapy. Psychodrama, sociometry and experiential group therapy provide for a controlled acting-out in the service of healing. They are modern adaptations of an ancient form. As illustrated by

concrete examples, the drama therapies described here offer methods that develop and repair issues related to the development of emotional intelligence, regulation, and literacy.

Overview

Being able to attach words to feeling states is a cornerstone of developing emotional literacy and consciously regulating behavior. Emotional learning is a mind–body phenomenon. The limbic system, which is the brain–body system associated with the regulation of our psychological and emotional states, can become deregulated in individuals who grow up in less than optimal environments. Children who have grown up without appropriate emotional decoding by caring adults may lack emotional literacy. Such emotional deregulation can lead to moodiness, depression, and acting-out behaviors such as bullying, violence and addiction.

An increasingly significant aspect of experiential therapies is their ability to allow the body to be a part of the therapeutic process. Young people who are asked to "describe" their inner world may not have any idea how to do so. Action methods enables them to enter the therapeutic milieu through action, allowing words to follow. Psychodrama, sociometry and group psychotherapy are parts of a three-tiered healing system developed by Moreno (1964). He believes that what was learned in action must be unlearned in action, and what was learned in relationship must be unlearned in relationship. The goal of undoing problematic patterns of thinking, feeling, and behaving through action, and learning more adequate ways of experiencing and expressing the self in a relational context, is the work of psychodrama, sociometry (the study and investigation of group dynamics), and experiential group therapy.

Drama therapies provide therapeutic approaches that allow children to mobilize strengths and qualities, experience and express themselves more coherently, connect with others in constructive rather than destructive ways, and gain a sense of hope and faith. A thoughtful integration of drama therapies can allow young people to express and process emotional and psychological pain symbolically and creatively. The physical, emotional and psychological benefits are numerous. The creative arts therapies:

- enhance qualities associated with resilience such as independence, creativity, ingenuity, humor (Wolin 1993)

- offer an arena in which the nuts and bolts of developing emotional intelligence and literacy can be revisited and reworked (Greenspan 2000)

- regulate the limbic system through experience of the self in relationships within a healing context (Lewis, Fari and Lannon 2000)

- expand and train the ability to attend and focus on specific goals and activities

- allow for a creative and symbolic expression of thinking, feeling, and behaving that can lead to enhanced creativity and spontaneity and increased ability to perceive and take action toward desirable life choices

- allow for a controlled "acting out" of pain and anger in the service of healing

- provide practice in connecting with others in meaningful, purposeful and healthy ways

- lift the spirit and instill a sense of hope and beauty

- offer a healthy way to attain "feel-good" states and a sense of oneness and intimacy with others

- offer alternative ways to boost the immune system through sharing and writing to resolve inner conflicts (Pennebaker 1997).

The exercises in this chapter are designed to enhance the client's ability to connect with others in positive ways, find safe ways to share thoughts and feelings, and break patterns of isolation. The psychodramatic empty chair exercises are intrapersonal approaches that explore the inner world of the client. The interpersonal sociometric exercises explore relationships and preferences within the group context. Psychodramatic journaling has been included as a method that allows theoretical concepts of role-play to be explored through writing, thus allowing for containment and safety. Some of the exercises are a combination of drama therapy and psychodrama. Drama therapy allows for a more distanced approach to healing. A story, for example, might be told or acted out by the client in the third person rather than the first. This can allow the client to work through issues symbolically or with an emotional distance that is particularly well suited to work with children and adolescents.

How behavior becomes infused with emotional intention and meaning

Gesture, our first language

Gesturing, or action, is our first language. It is the mind–body communication upon which all subsequent language is built. Before language formally enters the picture, we have learned a rich tapestry of gestures and actions to communicate our needs and desires. This gesturing comprises non-verbal communication that informs our ability to express ourselves and understand others. The expression of concern or alarm on a mother's face, for example, causes the child to feel "held" or alerted to danger. A child's screech accompanied by an arm motion may signal a wish to be picked up or cuddled. Body language is part of an action-oriented, gestural communication that contains important meaning. Each tiny gesture is double-coded with emotion and is stored by the brain and body with emotional purpose and meaning attached to it. Through this interactive process of communicating our needs and desires, we can build emotional intelligence and literacy as surely as we can learn math in a classroom.

Because gesturing is our first form of communication, much of this language becomes part of our unconscious and surfaces in the form of "automatic emotion". Alan Schore (in press) in his research on affect regulation writes, "this 'automatic emotion' operates in infancy and beyond at non-conscious levels and... shape[s] subsequent conscious emotional processing." Our emotional unconscious is formed through interactions with our family and caregivers (our first social atom) and this lays a foundation for later emotional growth and language development.

What occurs between people as subtle exchanges of emotionally laden signals occurs so quickly that we hardly know it is happening. Evolution has made the processing of emotions and their communication to others very rapid. Nature has favored this speed for obvious reasons. The mother who can "feel fast" and sense danger can communicate this to her child in order to get him out of harm's way.

These unconscious processes help us to walk, digest, self-regulate and remain grounded within the self, in relationships and our environment. They allow us to operate on automatic. Children who have grown up in environments where feelings were not talked about, or behaviors were inconsistent with expressions of emotion, have a hard time identifying their emotions and intentions when they try to self-reflect. They may be all action, with little awareness of what is driving their behaviors, and they may misread subtle non-verbal signals (Dayton 2005b). This emotional history travels with children into the educational system and affects their ability both to have successful relationships and to regulate themselves within the learning environment.

The obvious emphasis on intellectual learning in school masks the extent to which emotions inform and drive our relationships within the school environment and our ability to learn. Greenspan (2000) feels that emotional development is not simply a base or foundation for important capacities such as intimacy and trust. His research has demonstrated that it is also the foundation of intelligence and a wide variety of cognitive skills. At each stage of the child's development emotions lead the way, and the learning of facts and skills follows.

The nuts and bolts of developing emotional intelligence and literacy

The following is a progression of emotional development outlined by Greenspan (2000). It describes how a developing child translates the raw data she gathers from her senses and inner feelings into images and modes of communication. These are the foundations of sound emotional development.

THE SIX DEVELOPMENTAL LEVELS OF THE MIND

1. **Self-regulation:** Self-regulation is a primary developmental task that allows children to regulate themselves emotionally and physically. Regulating the self involves learning to organize sensations and body responses. From a jumble of sounds, sights, smells and tactile feelings, patterns begin to emerge. Sounds become rhythms and sights become recognizable images. Physical and emotional self-regulation are at the core of healthy functioning on all levels.

2. **Engagement:** Engagement represents the first stage of building the capacity for relationships. It begins with the child's emotional awareness of a fellow being's presence.

3. **Intentionality:** The ability to connect with at least one other person leads to intentionality – a willed exchange of signals and responses. Children who have successfully completed the passage into deep engagement gradually come to perceive that the actions passing between themselves and others are part of a two-way exchange.

4. **Purpose and interaction:** Once a child connects sensation and emotion to intentional action, more complex, pre-symbolic communication equips him to find his way in the world of social interaction. He can now distinguish facial expressions and body gestures, and discriminate among basic emotions, distinguishing those meaning safety and comfort from those meaning danger.

5. **Images, ideas and symbols:** The child begins to deal not only with behavior but with ideas. She begins to understand that one thing can stand for another. This realization enables her to create an inner picture of her world.

6. **Emotional thinking:** Experience now can be linked into sequences of inner images that allow a child to consider actions before carrying them out. Words and ideas can link up to emotions, for example, "I am sad because it is raining and I want to play outside." These skills make up basic personality or ego functions. They include reality testing, impulse control, and the ability to see connections among many different feelings and ideas.

Without this structure the mind cannot function coherently, but only in a fragmented, jumbled fashion. The drama therapies offer methods that synthesize this progression of developing emotional intelligence, regulation and literacy.

Significant emotional repair can occur when therapeutic methods permit a full and integrated mind/body engagement that accesses and incorporates these six levels of mind development.

The fear factor: how trauma affects us and deregulates the limbic system

Neurobiological research provides a much needed window into working with those whose neurological systems have become deregulated through less than optimal relational experiences, such as familial neglect, abuse or living with addiction.

The body can't tell the difference between an emotional emergency and physical danger. When the emergency response is triggered a child will either seek safety or stand and fight. In cases where the family itself is the source of stress, there may be no opportunity to flee or fight. Children in these situations may find escape impossible, and this causes them to shut down their inner responses by numbing or dissociating. Though this strategy may help them to get through a painful situation, it teaches them to reject their authentic emotions. In so doing, they lose access to valuable information that would help them to navigate their relational world and regulate their emotional reactions to it.

The ability to escape or take oneself out of harm's way is central to whether or not a child develops long-term trauma symptoms (post-traumatic stress disorder, or PTSD), (van der Kolk 2005). If escape is not possible, the intense energy that has been revved up in one's body to enable fight or flight, becomes thwarted or frozen (Levine 1997), creating a feeling that the stressor is ever-present.

Children do not have a fully developed capacity to understand what is happening around them and to regulate their intense emotional responses accordingly. They depend on the adults around them to hold, reassure and restore them to a state of equilibrium, to help them contain their excitement, and to calm and soothe intense fear. If this modulating occurs at the time when painful circumstances are occurring, the child is unlikely to become symptomatic because the parent is wooing him back toward balance and a sense of safety. However if the parent or family environment are the primary stressor, the child is left to live through repeated ruptures to his developing sense of self, with little ability to make sense of it, interpret the level of threat, or use reasoning to regulate and understand what is going on.

Adolescents may enter school without having developed the skills needed for sound emotional regulation. They may develop defensive walls designed to keep potentially overwhelming pain from emerging. To avoid feeling vulnerable on the inside, they may act "tough" on the outside. This prevents them from ever receiving the support they need and distances them from the kind of closeness that would lead to healing rather than continuous rupture.

Exercises to do with adolescents and teenagers

A. Choose a picture and share: picture sociometry

Goals

- to offer a non-invasive way to talk about what's going on
- to focus on what is going on inside of a person, bring it to conscious awareness, and talk about it.

Steps

1. Provide pictures that represent different mood states. The pictures can be cut from magazines or can be art postcards or reproductions. The idea is to provide emotional variety, e.g. a lion (aggression, power, strength), a sunrise (hope, renewal), a landscape (peace, serenity), a sad face (sadness), and so on.

2. Scatter the pictures on the floor.

3. Invite the students to stand next to a picture with which they identify.

4. Invite the students to share about why they chose that picture.

5. Invite participants to walk over to someone who said something they identified with and tell them what it was.

6. Return to seats for continued processing.

B. Locograms

Locograms involve designating locations on the floor (with words written on pieces of paper) to signify particular elements such as group preferences, feelings, or roles. Locograms get participants out of their seats and help them to connect with each other in small, controlled increments. "Other" is a constant category in locograms, as it allows participants to respond with their own words.

Goals

- to provide a safe way to share something personal, meaningful or authentic.

Steps

1. Determine the subject to be explored (eg: feelings, roles, etc.)

2. On large pieces of paper write feeling words or roles, always leaving a few pieces of paper blank for the group to write their own words.

3. Place the words a few feet apart on the floor.

4.   Invite participants to stand on or near the word that best describes them or their feeling.

5.   Invite participants to share, in a sentence or two, why they are standing where they are.

6.   The group can repeat the process, stand on another word and share as before.

7.   Invite participants to place their hand on the shoulder of someone who shared something that they identified with. Participants share directly with that person why they came over to them.

8.   The group shares about the process and what came up in the course of it.

Variations

Although the therapist can come prepared with words on pieces of paper, choosing words as a group allows the participants to get engaged, warm up and bond. Putting words into a locogram can be a useful way to explore thoughts and feelings and to deepen awareness about how these are affecting relationships. Identifying with more than one word allows participants to define themselves in different ways. Locograms can help the therapist to recognise who is ready to share with the group if a piece of paper is used to represent each of the following:

- I have something I'm burning to share.
- I have things to share.
- I can take it or leave it.
- I am not feeling like I want to share.
- Other.

The same activity can be done by laying out masks that represent a variety of emotions and asking participants to stand near the one that they identify with. This allows them to identify with something outside of themselves, and helps them to creatively connect with an emotion. Masks appeal to the imagination, encourage spontaneity, and allow for emotional distance.

C. Choose a song and share

Goals

- to provide a fun way to share about one's inner world and life experiences
- to begin bonding as a group.

Steps

1. Provide recordings of several songs that represent different musical eras. Put the CDs in the center of the circle.

2. Invite one participant to choose a song that represents a period from their lives or has a special meaning for them.

3. Invite that participant to play the song and share about why she chose it. Ask, "What was going on for you at that time in your life?" or, "Why does this song have special meaning for you?"

4. Repeat the process for each participant.

5. After all have finished, continue sharing and processing.

Variations

You may vary the criterion questions according to the needs of your population. This exercise can be used as a warm-up for further work.

D. Share a memory

Goals

*   to provide a bonding experience for participants
*   to allow participants to share something personal in a non-threatening manner
*   to strengthen resilience.

Steps

1. Invite participants to recall a memory that they would like to share. The criterion for choosing the memory may vary according to the thrust of the group.

2. Invite each participant to share their memory. The leader may suggest a time limit.

3. After each person has had the opportunity to share, the group may share about the process or may journal about what the memory brought up for them.

4. Return to the group for sharing and closure.

Variations

This can be used as a strength-based exercise by focusing the memory on "a time you felt proud of yourself" or "a time you felt good about things". Participants can also be asked to "try on the role" of a person who is happy and speak from that role.

E. Psychodramatic journaling

Psychodramatic journaling is a translation of psychodramatic role theory to the written page. It allows the benefits of techniques such as role reversal to be used creatively through journaling. It has the advantage of providing opportunities for self-expression, as well as for deepening our understanding of others by standing in their shoes. Psychodramatic journaling can be used to extend experiential exercises and create more opportunities for personal exploration. It can be inserted into the process at the discretion of the director (i.e. after group action, after the sharing, or as a warm-up to action). Sharing the material itself, and further sharing about the experience of writing and what it brought up, should accompany psychodramatic journaling. If used as a warm-up, the action can grow out of the journaling (e.g. writing a letter can be a warm-up, and reading the letter can be the action component of the group).

F. Journaling with photographs

Goals

- to allow work to focus itself naturally around the context and content of photographs that clients have chosen themselves
- to gain practice in expression of personal issues through the safe and creative vehicle of writing.

Steps

Participants are invited to select a photograph of themselves that speaks to them and to answer the following questions:

- What feelings come up as you look at this picture?
- What do you imagine the people (including yourself) are thinking?
- What do you imagine they would like to say?
- What would you like to say to yourself or to anyone in this photograph?
- What does this picture mean or symbolize to you?
- What part of yourself in this photo would you like to keep?
- What part of yourself would you like to let go of?
- If you could be the "inner voice" of yourself or anyone in the picture, what would it say?
- What strengths do you see in yourself in this photograph? Reverse roles with yourself in this photograph and write a monologue describing your inner experience. *Example:* "I am Laura and I am feeling…"

Variations

Participants may put the photograph of themselves on an empty chair and talk to it. Role reversal and doubling may be incorporated into this.

Other journaling ideas include:

- Write a journal entry as yourself at the time of this picture. *Example:* "I am Catherine. I am eight years old and I am feeling…"

- Write a journal entry as another person in the picture (reverse roles). *Example:* "I am Gerald (Catherine's father). I am feeling lost at this moment. I am 42 and have recently lost my job…"

- Write a letter to someone in the picture to whom you have something to say.

- Write a letter you would have liked to receive from someone in the picture. *Example:* "Dear Catherine,…"

- Write a journal entry as the spirit of the picture, or the inner voice of the picture that gives voice to the overall mood of the time. *Example:* "I am the voice within the photograph and it is a time of confusion, change…"

These journal entries can be read out loud in the group or in sub groups.

G. Writing a letter

Goals

- to enable group members to say what they need to say in a safe format that is used for emotional processing

- to provide a contained form of expression that can lead into a contained form of experiential work.

Steps

1. Ask group members to write a letter to anyone to whom they feel they have something to say, or to a part of themselves – for example, themselves at a time in their past or their future; an imagined or desired self; their depression, their addiction, their successful self, and so on. The letter is for emotional processing only. It is not to be sent.

2. Invite group members to share their letters in the group, or in dyads or small groupings. Other ways the group can share letters are:

    - use an empty chair to represent the person or aspect of self, and read the letter to the empty chair

    - choose a role-player to represent the substance or behavior and read the letter to the role-player.

3. Continue sharing in the large group about how it felt to write the letter.

Variations

Letter-writing can be used to extend experiential work, as a warm-up, or as an exercise in and of itself, and can include sharing the letter and how the whole experience felt.

H. The empty chair

Goals

- to release feelings toward a particular person in a safe way
- to create a situation in which deep feelings can be expressed in a spontaneous fashion, thus bypassing intellectual resistance and avoiding censorship.

Steps

1. Set up two chairs facing each other. Have a participant who is ready to share sit in one, and face the other empty one.

2. Ask the participant who they have put in the other chair, and then invite them to say anything they need or want to say to that person. Ask them to reverse roles if it is clear that more feelings would be expressed from the opposite role. It is important that they actually get up and take the other chair, then speak from that role. They can reverse roles as many times as is appropriate.

3. If this is done in a group, there may be other participants who have strong identifications with what is being said by the person working (the protagonist). Invite the people who feel this way to stand behind and slightly to the side of the protagonist as their "double" and to say a few things that they feel might further the feeling action of the protagonist. They can stand up and "double" when it seems appropriate, and sit down when it feels appropriate.

4. When you feel the protagonist has spoken fully, say, "Say the last thing you need to say," and when that has been done, end the action.

5. Allow participants to share what came up for them as witnesses or contributors to the action. Ask anyone who played a role to de-role. In this way everyone gets a chance to do personal work and share from their own experience. Keep the sharing on a personal basis, as this is not a time for giving advice or questioning. The people who played roles can share from the point of view of the role if they wish.

Variation
Participants can put parts of themselves in the empty chair – for example, their "anger", their "fear", their "scared self" their "strong self" – or they may put someone else in their chair who they wish to talk to. This can be used as an exercise to further explore what comes up from previously detailed exercises.

I. Facing the inner self: sculpting the self

Goals

- to allow the protagonist to concretize and explore their inner world

- to reduce the sense that someone else is to blame or has all the control.

Steps

1. Ask the protagonist to choose someone to represent himself, and auxiliaries to represent internal roles (for example, his angry self, his strong self, sad self, resilient self, resentful self, rebel, artist, student).

2. Ask the protagonist to place first himself and next his roles (close or far in relationship to himself). He can place them in any way, relate them to one another, or sculpt them in ways that physicalize their inner meaning and impact.

3. Ask the protagonist to double for any or all parts of himself, talk to them, reverse roles with them, or talk back to himself.

4. After all work has taken place, invite the protagonist to resculpt the scene as he would wish it to be with the roles in a new configuration.

5. Return to seats for sharing and processing.

J. Working with masks

Goals

- to give the protagonist the sense of being anonymous, allowing more candid and honest expression

- to concretize both mood and feeling.

Steps

1. Make masks or use prefabricated masks. Participants are asked to choose one that they are drawn to.

2. When all participants have masks, ask them to wander around the room until they find somewhere they wish to settle, and then sit down.

3.   Ask them to spend some time looking at the mask and paying attention to the feelings that arise.

4.   After they have had a few minutes to do so, ask them to take turns introducing themselves to the group, either from where they sit or using a designated stage area. They should say who they are and describe themselves, speaking as the character represented by the mask. Everything should be spoken in the first person present, regardless of when it may have occurred. The director may wish to double in order to further or deepen the action, or may introduce an empty chair to represent the real self if the protagonist wants to reverse roles.

5.   Allow each person to speak fully from the character role and to take the time to move through his feelings.

6.   When everyone has shared, ask the group to share what came up for each of them, or to make a sociometric choice and walk over to the person with whom they felt identification and share with that person. Afterwards they can come back to the larger group to continue sharing.

Variations

- *Mood masks:* make masks representing a mood you often find yourself in, a mood you avoid, or a mood you wish you felt more often.

- *Many selves:* more than one mask can be made to represent aspects of the self (e.g. inner self and outer self) in order to explore levels of dissonance or integration between the two.

- *Addiction masks:* for a case that involves addiction (either a recovering addict or the child or spouse of an addict) people can make a "clean" mask and a "high" mask, and then introduce them in role reversal.

- *Life stages:* masks can be made to represent different stages of life. People who are coping with life transitions might find it useful to revisit themselves at various stages throughout their lives in order to promote integration.

- *Idealized selves:* a client might make a mask of her idealized self or the idealized parent, spouse, child, and so on.

In all of these cases, journaling might be a useful way to follow up on feelings that continue to arise. Journaling can be done in the first person, the third person, or in role reversal (journaling as another person).

Excerpts from my book are used in this chapter with permission from Health Communication, Inc. *The Living Stage* (Dayton 2005a)

Drama therapy exercises in this chapter were provided by Alex Dayton, Masters candidate at New York University.

References

Dayton, T. (2005a) *The Living Stage: A Step-by-Step Guide to Psychodrama, Sociometry and Experiential Group Therapy.* Deerfield Beach, FL: Health Communications.

Dayton, T. (2005b) *Modern Mothering: How to Teach Your Kids to Say What They Feel and Feel What They Say.* New York, NY: Crossroads Publishing.

Greenspan, S. (2000) *Building Healthy Minds.* New York, NY: Perseus Publishing.

Levine, P.A. (1997) *Waking the Tiger: Healing Trauma.* Berkley, CA: North Atlantic Books.

Lewis, T., Fari, F., and Lannon, R. (2000) *A General Theory of Love.* NewYork: Vintage Books, a division of Random House, Inc.

Moreno, J.L. (1964) *Psychodrama Volume 1.* Ambler PA: Beacon House.

Pennebaker, J. W. (1997) *Opening Up: The Healing Power of Expressing Emotions.* New York: Guilford Press.

Schore, A.N. (in press) *The Right Brain, the Right Mind and Psychoanalysis.* New York, NY: Guilford Press.

van der Kolk, B. (2005) 'The body keeps score.' Lecture presented by The Meadows, New York City, 23 October 2005.

Wolin, S.L. (1993) *The Resilient Self.* New York, NY: Villiard Books, a division of Random House, Inc.

Further reading

Amen, D.G. (1998) *Change Your Brain, Change Your Life.* New York, NY: Three Rivers Press.

Brazelton, T.B. and Greenspan, S. (2000) *The Irreducible Needs of Children: What Every Child Must Have to Grow, Learn and Flourish.* New York, NY: Perseus Books.

Damasio, A. (1999) *The Feeling of What Happens.* New York: Harcourt, Inc.

Dayton, T. (2000) *Trauma and Addiction.* Deerfield Beach, FL: Health Communications.

Howard, P.J. (2000) *The Owner's Manual for the Brain.* Atlanta: Bard Press, 2000.

LeDoux, J. (2002) *The Synaptic Self.* New York: Viking Penguin Group.

Lewis, T., Fari, F., and Lannon, R. (2002) *A General Theory of Love.* New York: Vintage Books, a division of Random House, Inc.

Pert, C.B (1999) *Molecules of Emotion: Why You Feel the Way You Feel.* New York: Simon & Schuster.

Rosenthal, N.E. (2002) *The Emotional Revolution.* Secaucus, NJ: Citadel Press/Kensington Publishing.

Russell, P. (1979) *The Brain Book.* New York: Plume.

van der Kolk, B. (1987) *Psychological Trauma.* Washington DC: American Psychiatric Press, Inc.

CHAPTER 16

"Make Me Wanna Holler"

Dramatic Encounters with Boys from the Inner City

Craig Haen

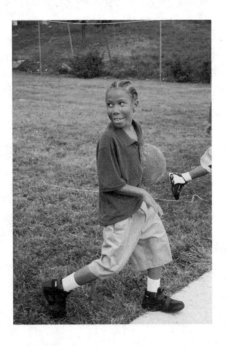

Informed by gender theory, role theory, and postmodernist thinking, the author examines some of his experiences as a White, male therapist working with predominantly minority inner city boys in New York City. The author outlines key features specific to this population, discusses transference and countertransference dynamics, and suggests drama therapy treatment goals and interventions.

Introduction

On a sunny evening in May, just as the days were getting longer and the city was getting warmer, I left the after-school program in the Bronx where I was conducting anger management groups. As I stepped out of the building, one of the bright spots on an otherwise industrial block, the sensory signs of summer in New York City drifted from the nearby neighborhood. I walked to my car, which was parked nearby. Along the way, I heard the booming of hip-hop from an upstairs window, smelled the Cuban food from the *bodega* on the next block, and was taken with the rhythm of life that was palpable on the street.

As I rounded the corner, a young Latino boy brought his bike to a screeching halt at the end of the street. He stared at me from a distance with curious fascination (equal parts amazement and fear). As I met his gaze, he said to me, somewhat incredulously, "You're here???"

I responded with a simple, smiling "Yes." He countered with a quiet "Wow!" and then hurtled his bike back into motion, presumably riding off to tell his friends about the alien he had seen. As I continued to my car, I found myself wondering about this boy. Was he incredibly sheltered or incredibly wise? I began checking in with my perceptions of being a visiting White man in this largely minority-inhabited, inner city neighborhood, and I started to think about the steps and turns I had taken in my life that had led me to this moment.

The short scene the boy and I had played out on the street corner seemed to speak volumes about my role as "other" in this neighborhood. I began to wonder: What during our brief interaction were we projecting onto each other? How much of our own cultural lessons had informed the interaction? And what could it teach me about the challenges and potentialities of being a White, middle-class man working in an impoverished neighborhood with minority boys? What do I represent? What do I carry with me? And where does the potential for change lie?

Personal history

I spent my own boyhood in a largely White, middle-class community in the midwestern portion of the United States. My first experiences of the inner city were driving through urban areas in Milwaukee and Chicago during family vacations. My young eyes would be glued to the car window, enthralled by the diversity of people and places. I imagine that my fascination matched that of the boy on his bike. My memory also includes my parents anxiously checking that the car doors were locked and commanding me not to stare, in a tone that suggested that we were in an environment of danger.

When I moved to New York City, I was introduced to the many neighborhoods while employed with an educational theatre company that performed workshops in classrooms throughout the five boroughs. I was one of the few White men who belonged to the company, and the implicit message from my supervisors seemed to be that I would not be able to understand where the young people were coming from. My first few weeks were filled with a self-imposed attempt to be "down" with the students and to pick up their terminology, cultural references and mannerisms. I envied my colleagues of color who had grown up in New York, wishing that I could find a way to access their unique ability to connect and understand.

As I became increasingly secure with who I was and embraced my position as outsider, an important lesson took shape. I found that playfully exaggerating my "Whiteness" served an important educational purpose. The students began to laugh at me, which made them feel at ease. Because I was so pathetically "uncool", they would allow me to question the phrases and beliefs that they took for granted. I would ask them to explain their ideas and terminology to me. In response, they would go deeper into their processing, diving into the important issues that we were there to discuss – sexuality, race relations, violence, and literacy.

They often projected their fears and anger onto me and I was able to embody these feelings within the context of scenework by playing characters once-removed from their fears: bullies, dominant authority figures, and helpless victims. Staying present during these difficult moments, as when an 11-year-old boy yelled, "Go back to Manhattan, White boy!", allowed us to move into important discussions. In addition, through equal co-leadership with my colleagues of color, we were able to model cross-cultural collaboration in which there was no power differential.

As I became a therapist, I carried these lessons with me: the importance of my role as "other" and of embodying and being with discomfort. I found myself working with minority clients from the inner city so often that when I finally ran a group with suburban, White, middle-class boys, it felt like I was doing cross-cultural treatment! I had become so accustomed to the inner city client population that when I worked with clients more similar to myself, I found that I had to adapt my treatment approach.

Choosing to work with clients from the inner city has at times felt like a political act. I have found myself modeling advocacy and assisting clients in navigating the system in order to meet concrete needs. If the political aims become too present, though, they have the danger of dominating the clinical space, and relegating minority and impoverished clients to the status of objects whose lives can become fetishized by the White therapist's voyeuristic fascination or need to triumph over the system.

In contributing to this volume, I wrestled with how to present children from the inner city in a way that honors their challenges, without walking the reductionist line that many writers have trodden. Too much emphasis on the client's race, ethnicity and socio-economic status can lead to over-generalization. It is important to bear in mind that while there are themes that run through the lives and treatment processes of children from the inner city, each child remains a unique individual who internalizes and integrates his or her surroundings differently.

In this chapter, I will present some of the knowledge gained from my clinical experiences with boys from the inner city. I will view these experiences through a cultural lens informed by gender theory, role theory and postmodernist thinking. Finally, I will present some applications of drama therapy that may prove beneficial in work with boys from the inner city.

The White male therapist

At the beginning of this chapter, I asked several questions about being a White, male drama therapist in the inner city, such as what I represent for clients, what internalized messages inform my own biases and behavior, and what the intersection of the two means for the therapy process. Therapists who utilize a relational framework continually analyze the dynamics between therapist and client, honoring what both bring to the table and recognizing the importance of the resulting patterns of interaction.

Javier and Herron (2002) define "Whiteness" as a social construction built from the components of economic and educational status. These authors assert that even therapists of color can fall under the Whiteness category when they have the means to live in a world to which the poor do not have access. 'Being White' means that one can avoid the inner city because one has more choices.

Clinicians who choose to work in urban areas open themselves up to an intensity of affect and experience that may be unfamiliar (Altman 1995). In addition they become an outsider, a role that is well-known to their clients. This choice requires therapists to accept being an object of projection and to realize that their gender and skin color may evoke a range of reactions. These reactions are frequently informed by clients' past experiences and are often part of an emerging transference. Or the projections may represent pieces of the clients that they are unable to hold and therefore need the therapist to contain. Transference reactions and projection are particularly heightened in the beginning stages of treatment, when the person of the therapist has not yet developed in the client's mind and trust has not yet been established. Instead, the therapist represents "just another White guy" or "another therapist-type."

Countertransference feelings might also manifest strongly during this beginning stage. For example, often with new groups of clients from the inner city, I find myself feeling flashes of fear, evoked less by the reality of the clients than by memories of a being a young boy who was taught that people who looked different than myself might cause me harm. These early life lessons can become deeply imbedded and require careful self-monitoring and effective supervision in order to make them a useful part of the treatment relationship, rather than a detrimental one.

Psychoanalysts have often described transference–countertransference phenomena by using terms drawn from drama and the theatre. I frequently refer to the transference process as one of being cast in the client's life drama. In my work with boys from the inner city, I have tended to represent some of the following:

1. A symbol of power, authority and oppression: Western society is structured such that the vast majority of those in power are both White and male. Institutions that control clients' lives, and that are responsible for traumatic events such as the removal of children from their biological families, are largely seen as White (Altman 1995). In addition, violence is largely, though not exclusively, perpetrated by men (Lisak 2001). I have been cast as a variety of perpetrators and have often been the focus of authority struggles within the therapy space that are informed by transferential feelings.

2. An embodiment of homophobic fears: Creative arts therapists advocate emotional expression through the arts, two areas that are seen to reside in the "feminine" realm and may be threatening to male clients, particularly those who subscribe to traditional gender roles. Similarly, boys may fear the intimacy of connection that can come with engaging in therapy with a male clinician. In a memorable session with a boys' group on a day when my female co-leader was absent, the group members, who had previously flirted with intimacy by playing gay lovers, this time played out a scene in which they killed a homosexual bank robber. The dramatization of the murder was particularly detailed, violent and affectively charged. When my co-leader (who often contained the affect for the group) returned, the members were able to process how the scene was a projection of their own heightened sensitivity to, and fear of, vulnerability in a suddenly all-male group.

3. A father figure: Given the importance of fathers in the lives of boys, it is not surprising that they transfer their feelings toward fathers, both negative and positive, to the male therapist. Negative feelings can play out in the form of authority struggles, fear of abandonment, and withdrawal. Altman (1995) wrote about how the women he treated in the inner city frequently cast him in the role of "the male knight in shining armor who had come to rescue them from their evil male villains" (p.5). Many of my male clients have similarly put me on a pedestal, casting me as an idealized father figure, more heroic and less human than the adult males with whom they have had contact.

4. A symbol of wealth and prosperity: Many boys from the inner city see the attainment of wealth as the key to separating themselves from the shameful aspects of their neighborhood. Designer clothing, cell phones and money are important symbols of this distancing. Clients often assume that I have wealth, or that I am able to grant them access to it. They have cast me in varied roles that reflect this theme, including a talent agent, a banker, an affluent man who they rob, and an aristocratic king.

It can be difficult to bear the transference, particularly when informed by the therapist's race, but it provides important ground on which to work. These projections can stem from a client's internal working model of how the world operates, or can represent a resistance to connecting with the therapist or the drama therapy process. Rosenthal (1987) discussed the importance of joining with and supporting the client's resistance, assisting him in building the ego strength necessary to move past it. Once trust is established, the therapist can partner with the client in exploring other possibilities about who the therapist is, to separate him out from the projections and to see him as a more complete person. As the client begins to see the therapist not just as "other", he is able to recognize a role model with whom he can connect and identify.

During a particularly challenging moment in the beginning stages of a group's development, one 16-year-old member marked his entrance into the second session by pointing at me and shouting, "You're a child molester!" Though taken aback, I was fortunately able to react with humor, remarking that no one had ever quite described me in that way before. In scenework, I was able to embody this projection by playing a character who misused his authority to denigrate someone else. My co-leader guided the action and maintained safety in her role as director. It was in the later stages of group development, once trust had been established, that the group member who had shouted the remark was able to talk openly about his history as a victim of molestation. He was able to begin to see the differences between his abuser and me, and eventually suggested a scene in which we played brothers.

Culture

The term "cross-cultural therapy" is often used to describe a treatment process in which the differences between client and therapist are significant. However, if one takes into account the fluid and individualized nature of culture, then most therapy could be considered cross-cultural. Therapists always grapple with differences, whether their clients are older, younger, of another ethnicity, race or gender, or from another geographic region. The greater the differences that exist between therapist and client, the greater the opportunities for misunderstanding and projection, but also for learning and growth.

Definitions of culture vary, but it is frequently defined as the sum of views, beliefs, attitudes and behavior patterns that serve to distinguish a group of people and to inform their sense of identity (Tseng and Stretzler 2004). Tseng (2001) noted that culture is learned and communicated through symbols, influencing both verbal and non-verbal expression. Its influence in people's lives can serve both adaptive and maladaptive purposes.

Culture is not a static entity; rather, it is both dynamic and improvisational. Laird emphasized the performative nature of culture and noted its fluid and emergent properties. That is, culture is expressed through interpersonal engagement, and its expression can depend on the context in which the people are operating. She wrote, "Who we are changes from moment to moment in shifting settings. We are all multiple cultural selves" (Laird 1998, p.24).

This multi-dimensional view of culture is compatible with the role theory perspective, one of the foundational drama therapy theories. Role theory, originating in the work of social psychologists Goffman (1959) and Mead (1934), and articulated by Landy (1993), views the self as composed of a collection of roles, each representing different facets of a person. While Landy initially questioned the existence of a core self, more recently he has added "the guide" to his conception (Landy 2001). "The guide" functions as an internal regulator who is able to negotiate between role and counter-role, providing direction and integration.

As with cultural expression, the roles one plays shift depending on the setting and the other people with whom one is interacting. In a system, roles become mutually dependent; for example, one cannot be a victimizer without a victim (Zur 2005), nor can one act in a victimizing way without denying the victim in himself. The role theory perspective leads one to consider the presence of the therapist as both a container and an influencer of the roles expressed by the client. In a relational context, the therapy space provides a laboratory for role expression and exploration, with the client and therapist functioning as co-creators of an emergent improvisational drama (Cattanach 1999; Way 2004).

In considering the challenges of difference in the therapist–client interaction, Emunah (1994) wrote:

> My background in acting taught me to find parts of myself in every character. Likewise, being a therapist involves reaching inside myself in search of what is in me, in my experience, that will enable me to understand and connect with the client more deeply. The boundaries between self and client in therapy, as between self and character in acting remain clear. But they are boundaries, not barriers. (p.49).

Boys from the inner city

In recent years, mental health literature has focused on male development and the male experience. Certain themes have run through these texts: the societal pressure on boys to be independent rather than affiliative; normative separation from the mother as premature and potentially traumatizing; anger as the only socially acceptable emotion for boys to express; male attunement to hierarchy, competition, and success; and the difficulty in attaining solid male role models (Garbarino 1999; Kindlon and Thompson 1999; Newberger 1999; Pollack 1998).

While these texts provoked an important cultural focus on the needs of male children, the authors largely based their studies on White, middle-class boys, generalizing their findings to all boys. In doing so, they often failed to articulate the unique experiences of minority youth from the inner city (Kimmel 2004). Males from the inner city face many of the same challenges as other boys and men, but the development of their cultural and gendered self is impacted by the inner city experience. Of particular significance are the topics of self-protection, disempowerment, male role models, and rage.

Self-protection

One dominant focus in the lives of boys from the inner city is that of protecting vulnerability (Chu 2005). Boys in Western cultures often internalize the message that they must be tough and avoid expressions of weakness. Inner city neighborhoods fraught with violence reinforce this need for protection as a means of survival. The "inner city warrior" or "angry male minority" have become popular mass media images which can captivate inner city boys who lack other role models.

For the boys described here, protective roles are well-honed and are an active part of self-expression. While developed out of necessity, these roles can often be rigid and can limit possibilities for meaningful connection with others. One sixteen-year-old client stated that he didn't have friends, "only associates: people who have money, who will buy me stuff, and who have wheels." Frequently my clients speak of their inability to trust anyone, a dictum often taught by their families (Way 2004) and reinforced through real-world experiences of betrayal.

While the original conception of development described movement from dependence to independence, recent writing and research have advocated a more balanced view, framing development as a move toward dynamic auton-omy. In this state, men and women are able to access both differentiation and relatedness and are able to balance roles of protector and protected (Sheinberg and Penn 1991). In the inner city, as in the rest of the world, one must be able to function autonomously, but also be able to find connection and community. A balanced role repertoire allows people to respond to an increasingly complex world with spontaneity, accessing different parts of the self to meet differing demands. This is consistent with one neurobiological model of health that views mental health as the ability of a self-organizing system to respond to maximal complexity (Siegel 2003). Seventeen-year-old Gage hints at the con-flicts engendered by self-protection in his poem:

In this cold world, I stand alone,

People say they know me as if I had a clone,

Every girl I been around thinks that I want to bone,

So I stand alone because my life is so cold,

I can't get home because I always been alone,

I stand alone like a New York shadow,

I made it all alone just by standing alone,

Females hate me but then they want to date me because I stand alone,

I am the man that gets along, because I am here then I am gone.

{You will find someone}

Disempowerment

Another concrete reality for the boys described here is the limited array of life choices available to them. Poverty limits choice (Javier and Herron 2002), as does being a minority in the inner city without a clear view of a way out. While conducting anti-violence workshops in inner city schools, I was approached by a 14-year-old in the hallway after one session. He said, "Craig, I like what you guys are sayin' about walkin' away and all, but for me, if I'm not in a gang then I get hurt." Similarly, I was confronted with the difficulties of teaching self-care during safe-sex workshops with students who firmly believed they would die by the age of 20. During a moment of honesty in a group therapy session at a crisis shelter, a 16-year-old said, "I can sit here and talk about change, but I know in my heart that in the end I'm gonna go back to the hood and make the same old choices." This young man could not envision a way out, could not imagine a different community in which he would fit in, and could not imagine employing any roles other than his finely developed role of "thug" while on the streets.

Those boys who do aspire to something more can experience role strain: wrestling with the conflicting values of mainstream society and those of their own culture (Tolan *et al.* 2004). The lack of choices and discrimination based on class and race can lead to a general lack of empowerment. Stevenson (2004) wrote, "They are not 'leading a charge' or 'making a mark' so much as they are following a script that is not as developed and broad as the scripts that the rest of the adolescent world have to follow" (p.64).

Recent critiques of writing on male development emphasize the way in which writers such as Pollack (1998), in focusing on the difficulties of boys, have presented a model in which boys are passive in the gendering process: victims of socialization or objects, rather than players. Chu (2004) presents an alternative model in which boys take an active role in determining which societal, familial and cultural messages they choose to incorporate into their gender schema (Bem 1987). By placing boys at the center of their development, Chu seeks to empower them, making them participants in their own lives. This reframed model is a therapeutic ideal to strive for, as clients learn to question both the conscious and unconscious messages they receive about who they should become.

Male role models

I have written elsewhere of the absent father and the effect his absence can have on the lives of male children (Haen 2002; Haen and Brannon 2002). In inner city neighborhoods, boys are often raised by mothers and grandmothers, with their fathers either physically or emotionally absent (Altman 1995; Way 2004). Frequently, absent fathers are not discussed in families, particularly when the absence is owing to death, imprisonment, or desertion. As a result, many boys utilize fantasy to provide a more complete story for the loss (Sklarew et al. 2002). For example, one five-year-old boy told fellow group members a detailed and compelling story about how he witnessed his father being gunned down on the street by a drug dealer as a result of the father's heroic attempts to rid the neighborhood of crime. In actuality, the father had abandoned the family when the boy was an infant. The fantasy was likely culled from the two neighborhood shootings the boy had witnessed, as well as his own need to hold an idealized vision of his father.

Affiliation with male role models is tremendously important for a boy's development, as these figures serve as cultural initiators. Research has demonstrated that boys from the inner city whose fathers are involved have less frequent suicidal ideation than those whose fathers are absent (Tarver et al. 2004). Similarly, in other studies, paternal support is correlated with decreased aggression, increased social competence, and improved academic performance (Parke and Brott 1999). When fathers are absent, other males can provide buffering. Florsheim, Tolan, and Gorman-Smith (1998) found that the involvement of male family members in the lives of boys from the inner city served as a mitigating factor in whether or not the boys developed externalizing behavior disorders.

Another interesting finding indicates that there may be a greater degree of intimacy in the friendships of minority boys from the inner city than in the friendships of other boys (Way 2004). In an environment of distrust, these boys frequently find friends who "have their back" and whom they can trust wholly. They often use family terms such as "blood" and "brother" to refer to their friends, and frequently prioritize them above all else, including romantic relationships. Way (2004) noted that friendships are also the area in which boys from the inner city struggle the most. Boys who are unable to negotiate the challenges of friendship and unable to establish trusting, interpersonal connections, are more likely to adhere to bravado, traditional gendered behavior and delinquency (Cunningham and Meunier 2004). Chu (2004) found that relationships can be a strong determinant of how a boy from the inner city internalizes peer and societal pressure, as well as assumptions about who he is and what he has the potential to be.

Rage

A final challenge for boys from the inner city is the staggering amount of rage they can harbor. Rage is frequently a response to having been repeatedly devalued, traumatized, neglected or abandoned (Haen and Brannon 2002), and is a strong correlate to violence (Hardy and Laszloffy 2005). Often this emotion serves a defensive function, masking the more vulnerable feelings of grief, shame, and fear that boys try to avoid. Expression of rage can also successfully distance boys from others, protecting them from the risks that come with connection while distinguishing them as someone who has power.

Treatment goals

Creative arts therapists working in the inner city must remain mindful of issues of power and authority, recognizing that in many circumstances, clients have been mandated to attend treatment (Gersie 1995). Even boys who have not been mandated to attend may fear that therapy will derail their sense of self and take away their right to choose (Cohen 2003), or make them vulnerable to the imposition of White, middle-class values. These dynamics can be heightened in residential and in-patient settings, where a client often gets the message that in order to move on he needs to change essential aspects of himself or play the role of "healthy person" as defined by the treatment team. In these controlled settings, the focus on pathology can lead to an incomplete understanding of the client's needs and strengths, and the survival skills that the boys have developed can be pathologized and mis-labeled as "maladaptive" (Haen 2005a).

Walsh (1998) notes the difference between "treatment", which is something the therapist does to the client, and "healing", a word that refers to an internal process that literally means "becoming whole". A creative arts therapist who views his job as that of supporting healing is able to witness and bolster the strengths of the client, helping to place him in the position of power (Nash and Haen 2005; Tyson and Baffour 2004). The therapist creates a partnership with the client and is able to see his humanity, honoring the co-existence of vulnerability and strength, victim and perpetrator, role and counter-role (Lisak 2001).

Drawing on the thoughts of other practitioners (Emunah 1994; Hamburg and Hamburg 2004; Hardy and Laszloffy 2000, 2005; Tolan *et al.* 2004; Tyson and Baffour 2004; Walsh 1998) and integrating them with my own clinical experiences, I would suggest the following treatment goals when working with boys from the inner city:

1.   increasing the client's role repertoire and expanding a sense of hope and possibility for the future

2.   supporting strengths and identifying talents

3. strengthening support networks and community (particularly male role models), as well as the client's ability to connect with and internalize them

4. assisting the client in finding and owning his voice

5. developing appropriate pathways of expression for rage

6. supporting the client in critically examining cultural assumptions and messages

7. helping the client to make meaning of adversity and to integrate his experiences.

Drama therapy

This volume is filled with chapters outlining creative arts therapy approaches to working with clients from the inner city. Creative arts therapy modalities can be effective with boys from the inner city to the extent that they provide an active means of self-expression that is compatible with boys' natural propensity toward action rather than words. Drama therapy's use of metaphor allows for themes that may be intolerable in discussion to be explored in an active, embodied way that aids in creating novel associations in the brain and in forming new synaptic connections that can lead to altered perceptions, increased feelings of connection, and an expanded sense of self (Haen 2005b; Siegel 2003). At its core, drama therapy is about connectedness: to other people, other perspectives, and one's own internal landscape and role repertoire.

Clients will bring themes and needs to sessions and gradually unpack them when they begin to feel safe. An attuned therapist is able to recognize these themes as they emerge and honor them by co-creating scenes that help to fulfill the aforementioned clinical goals. Role-play can be built from issues endemic to the inner city male experience, such as fatherhood, protection, abandonment, closeness, fear, identity, community, poverty, and adversity.

The dramatic space, when properly established as one of pretend and safety, can provide a container for expressions of rage. When utilizing role or narrative, the client has an embodied experience of exposing rage and having it witnessed, validated and respected. Through repeated channeling of rage through the arts, clients learn to control and master this strong affect, rather than having it silenced. This experience disconnects the rage from shame and lessens the need for it to be expressed through dysregulated violence.

Drama therapists can assist clients in examining cultural pressures and biases safely through the distance of metaphor. Hare-Mustin and Marecek (1990) note that many culturally dominant meanings are embodied in language and metaphor. They describe the therapist's job as one of negotiating and reframing these meanings, expanding the more subtle, ignored aspects of the metaphor. Hardy and Laszloffy (2005) define this role as one of cultural translator. The therapist might choose to reframe a scene by casting a client in an alternative role, introducing ambivalence, projecting the scene into the future, exploring the inner thoughts and feelings of a less dominant character, or changing the setting so as to affect the role expression of the characters. Cultural messages such as "Walk like a man," "Boys will be boys," and others generated by the client can be explored through body and object sculptures, scenes and pictures.

Finally, drama therapy can serve as a coping strategy (Tyson and Baffour 2004). Casson (2004) wrote, "Creative therapy is not just about problems but about discovering strengths and the pleasure of creativity" (p.135). The boys I have worked with have never ceased to impress me with their capacity for creativity and discovery. A client who feels successful and accepted during sessions can carry those feelings of empowerment and connection with him as he walks out of the therapy space and onto the streets.

Case example

Robbie was an imposing figure. At 16 years of age he already weighed 250 pounds and often greeted the members of the drama therapy group in his residential treatment center with a sneer and a sarcastic comment. He had a streetwise swagger that spoke of his years living in a violent neighborhood in the Bronx where he had been involved in a variety of street crimes. He frequently would attempt to derail the group process with devaluing comments about my suggestions or through attention-seeking behaviors, and attempts to engage him by discussing his preferences were also aggressively shot down.

During one session, Robbie joined the warm-up activity, an improvisational acting exercise known as Hitchhiker. In this game three group members role-play driving in a car. They then pull over to pick up a hitchhiker, played by another group member. This member enters the car playing a strongly defined character. The other group members must join with the character (matching his affect, style of presentation and storyline) and play out a short scene, until a new hitchhiker presents himself. The group members then shift places in the car, with the "driver" rotating out of the scene so that the new character may enter and a new scene can begin.

When Robbie entered the car, he initiated a scene in which he was a bank robber running from the police. His peers joined him with enthusiasm to play out a brief scene. However, when it came time to switch chairs, Robbie refused to give up his chair. He sat in protest, and all attempts to assist him in moving were met with firm rejection. It became clear that he was vying with me for control of the session. I noted my internal reactions of anger, trepidation and frustration. The authority struggle became explicit when Robbie proclaimed with satisfaction, "I'm the king of this group!" I recognized this as the way in and began to build a scene around it, asking the king to tell us about his kingdom and to describe his style of ruling the land. Robbie beautifully played out the role of a sadistic tyrant, describing all of the things he would do to others, just because he could. (What Robbie was not yet ready to connect with was how much this role was an embodiment of his own father, who had physically and emotionally abused Robbie and his siblings for a period of three years in between two prison sentences).

After we expanded and gave voice to Robbie's brand of power, I wondered aloud if anyone else in the group might enjoy being king. The other boys, who typically stayed out of Robbie's way, admitted that they might like that. "Clearly," I said, "this king will not readily give up his throne. So, here is how you can become king…" We then developed a game in which the other group members could raise their hands and, one by one, the king would summon them up. They could then use any tactic (except for touching him or the chair) to attempt to convince the king to give up his throne. Gradually, a very interesting drama played out. Members attempted to cajole, bribe, and trick Robbie into giving up the throne. They were all dismissed in turn, while I supported the king's absolute authority and right to choose for himself.

I noted that Leron, a quieter group member, seemed to be wrestling with his desire to participate. I said that it looked as though he might have an idea of how to win the throne and encouraged him to overcome his reluctance. Leron walked up to Robbie and whispered in his ear. Robbie paused and appeared to be thinking over what he heard. He then stood up and allowed Leron to take the throne. The group demanded to know what Leron had said. Leron responded, "I told him that his grandma was in trouble and needed his help." The session proceeded with other members vying for the throne.

The group closed with a discussion about what was so important to the members that they might give up their own power for it. Though Robbie continued to have difficulties in successive sessions, something shifted slightly. He joined the group more frequently, utilizing the dramatic space to play characters who were often consumed by rage. However, in time, he also gradually was able to take on other, more vulnerable roles, most memorably volunteering to play a loving and gentle mother in a family scene. This role allowed the group to connect to Robbie in a new way, and they accepted and supported the risk he was taking in playing the part.

Drama therapy provided Robbie the space in which to safely enact his distrust, anger, resentment, and fear. It provided a space in which his whole self, not just the self-protective aspects, could be expressed and honored. Finally, the group allowed him to begin to connect with peers and an adult role model in ways that he had not been able to before, providing him with a community.

Concluding thoughts

One distinctly magical piece of the therapy process is the gradual transition of the therapist from the position of outsider to becoming accepted and internalized by the client. In order to reconcile the dilemma of both wanting and fearing connection, clients often creatively alter the emerging drama. As I write this chapter, the adolescent boys in the crisis shelter where I work have developed a myth that allows them to incorporate me into their realities despite their distrust of White people. The story they have developed is that I grew up as the only White boy in an inner city neighborhood (or, as one boy metaphorically described it, "the only vanilla in a sea of chocolate"). They have speculated on what my life must have been like, what adversity I faced, and how I must truly understand what it is like for them, even though I am not their color. This retelling has allowed me to experience being cast in a new role of "the exception". As with other roles I have taken on as a therapist, I welcome this new one and the possibilities it holds.

References

Altman, N. (1995) *The Analyst in the Inner City: Race, Class, and Culture through a Psychoanalytic Lens.* Hillsdale, NJ: The Analytic Press.

Bem, S.L. (1987) 'Gender schema theory and its implications for child development: Raising gender-aschematic children in a gender-schematic society.' In M.R. Walsh (ed.) *The Psychology of Women: Ongoing Debates.* New Haven, CT: Yale University Press.

Casson, J. (2004) *Drama, Psychotherapy and Psychosis: Dramatherapy and Psychodrama with People who Hear Voices.* New York: Brunner-Routledge.

Cattanach, A. (1999) 'Co-construction in play therapy.' In A. Cattanach (ed.) *Process in the Arts Therapies.* London: Jessica Kingsley Publishers.

Chu, J.Y. (2004) 'A relational perspective on adolescent boys' identity development.' In N. Way and J.Y. Chu (eds) *Adolescent Boys: Exploring Diverse Cultures of Boyhood.* New York: New York University Press.

Chu, J.Y. (2005) 'Adolescent boys' friendships and peer group culture.' *New Directions for Youth Development 107,* 7–22.

Cohen, E. (2003) *Playing Hard at Life: A Relational Approach to Treating Multiply Traumatized Adolescents.* Hillsdale, NJ: The Analytic Press.

Cunningham, M., and Meunier, L.N. (2004) 'The influence of peer experiences on bravado attitudes among African-American males.' In N. Way and J.Y. Chu (eds) *Adolescent Boys: Exploring Diverse Cultures of Boyhood.* New York: New York University Press.

Emunah, R. (1994) *Acting for Real: Drama Therapy Process, Technique, and Performance.* New York: Brunner/Mazel Inc.

Florsheim, P., Tolan, P., and Gorman-Smith, D. (1998) 'Family relationships, parenting practices, the availability of male family members, and the behavior of inner city boys in single-mother and two-parent families.' *Child Development 69,* 5, 1437–1447.

Garbarino, J. (1999) *Lost Boys: Why Our Sons Turn Violent and How We Can Save Them.* New York: Free Press.

Gersie, A. (1995) 'Arts therapies practice in inner city slums: Beyond the installation of hope.' *The Arts in Psychotherapy 22,* 3, 207–215.

Goffman, E. (1959) *The Presentation of Self in Everyday Life.* Garden City, NY: Doubleday.

Haen, C. (2002) 'The dramatherapeutic use of the superhero role with male clients.' *Dramatherapy 24,* 16–22.

Haen, C., and Brannon, K.H. (2002) 'Superheroes, monsters and babies: Roles of strength, destruction and vulnerability for emotionally disturbed boys.' *The Arts in Psychotherapy 29,* 31–40.

Haen, C. (2005a) 'Group drama therapy in a children's inpatient psychiatric setting.' In A.M. Weber and C. Haen (eds) *Clinical Applications of Drama Therapy in Child and Adolescent Treatment.* New York: Brunner-Routledge.

Haen, C. (2005b) 'Rebuilding security: Group therapy with children affected by September 11' *International Journal of Group Psychotherapy 55,* 3, 391–414.

Hamburg, D.A., and Hamburg, B.A. (2004) *Learning to Live Together: Preventing Hatred and Violence in Child and Adolescent Development.* New York: Oxford University Press.

Hardy, K.V., and Laszloffy, T.A. (2000) 'The development of children and families of color: A supplemental framework.' In W.C. Nichols, M.A. Pace-Nichols, D.S. Becvar, and A.Y. Napier (eds) *Handbook of Family Development and Intervention.* New York: Wiley.

Hardy, K.V., and Laszloffy, T.A. (2005) *Teens Who Hurt: Clinical Interventions to Break the Cycle of Violence.* New York: Guilford.

Hare-Mustin, R.T. and Marecek, J. (1990) 'On making a difference.' In R.T. Hare-Mustin and J. Marecek (eds) *Making a Difference: Psychology and the Construction of Gender.* New Haven, CT: Yale University Press.

Javier, R.A. and Herron, W.G. (2002) 'Psychoanalysis and the disenfranchised: Countertransference issues.' *Psychoanalytic Psychology 19,* 1, 149–166.

Kimmel, M. (2004) Foreword to N. Way and J.Y. Chu (eds) *Adolescent Boys: Exploring Diverse Cultures of Boyhood.* New York: New York University Press.

Kindlon, D. and Thompson, M. (1999) *Raising Cain: Protecting the Emotional Life of Boys.* New York: Ballantine.

Laird, J. (1998) 'Theorizing culture: Narrative ideas and practice principles.' In M. McGoldrick (ed.) *Re-visioning Family Therapy: Race, Culture, and Gender in Clinical Practice.* New York: Guilford.

Landy, R.J. (1993) *Persona and Performance: The Meaning of Role in Drama, Therapy, and Everyday Life.* New York: Guilford.

Landy, R.J. (2001) 'Role theory and the role method of drama therapy.' In R.J. Landy (ed.) *New Essays in Drama Therapy: Unfinished Business.* Springfield, IL: Charles Thomas.

Lisak, D. (2001) 'Homicide, violence, and male aggression.' In G.R. Brooks and G.E. Good (eds) *The New Handbook of Psychotherapy and Counseling with Men: A Comprehensive Guide to Settings, Problems, and Treatment Approaches, Vol. 1.* San Francisco: Jossey Bass.

Mead, G.H. (1934) *Mind, Self and Society.* Chicago: University of Chicago Press.

Nash, E., and Haen, C. (2005) 'Healing through strength: A group approach to therapeutic enactment.' In A.M. Weber and C. Haen (eds) *Clinical Applications of Drama Therapy in Child and Adolescent Treatment.* New York: Brunner-Routledge.

Newberger, E.H. (1999) *The Men They will Become: The Nature and Nurture of Male Character.* Cambridge, MA: Da Capo Press.

Parke, R.D., and Brott, A.A. (1999) *Throwaway Dads: The Myths and Barriers that Keep Men from Being the Fathers They Want to Be.* Boston: Houghton Mifflin.

Pollack, W. (1998) *Real Boys: Rescuing our Sons from the Myths of Boyhood.* New York: Random House.

Rosenthal, L. (1987) *Resolving Resistance in Group Psychotherapy.* Northvale, NJ: Jason Aronson.

Sheinberg, M. and Penn, P. (1991) 'Gender dilemmas, gender questions, and the gender mantra.' *Journal of Marital and Family Therapy 17,* 1, 33–44.

Siegel, D.J. (2003) 'An interpersonal neurobiology of psychotherapy: The developing mind and the resolution of trauma.' In M.F. Solomon and D.J. Siegel (eds) *Healing Trauma: Attachment, Mind, Body and Brain.* New York: Norton.

Sklarew, B., Krupnick, J., Ward-Wimmer, D., and Napoli, C. (2002) 'The school-based mourning project: A preventive intervention in the cycle of inner city violence.' *Journal of Applied Psychoanalytic Studies 4,* 3, 317–330.

Stevenson, H.C. (2004) 'Boys in men's clothing: Racial socialization and neighborhood safety as buffers to hypervulnerability in African-American adolescent males.' In N. Way and J.Y. Chu (eds) *Adolescent Boys: Exploring Diverse Cultures of Boyhood.* New York: New York University Press.

Tarver, D.B., Wong, N.T., Neighbors, H.W., and Zimmerman, M.A. (2004) 'The role of father support in the predication of suicidal ideation among black adolescent males.' In N. Way and J.Y. Chu (eds) *Adolescent Boys: Exploring Diverse Cultures of Boyhood.* New York: New York University Press.

Tolan, P.H., Sherrod, L.R., Gorman-Smith, D., and Henry, D.B. (2004) 'Building protection, support, and opportunity for inner city children and youth and their families.' In K.I. Maton and C.J. Schellenbach (eds) *Investing in Children, Youth, Families, and Communities: Strengths-based Research and Policy.* Washington, DC: American Psychological Association.

Tseng, W. (2001) 'Culture and psychotherapy: An overview.' In W. Tseng and J. Streltzer (eds) *Culture and Psychotherapy: A Guide to Clinical Practice.* Washington, DC: American Psychiatric Press.

Tseng, W. and Streltzer, J. (2004) 'Introduction: Culture and psychiatry.' In W. Tseng and J. Streltzer (eds) *Cultural Competence in Clinical Psychiatry.* Washington, DC: American Psychiatric Press.

Tyson, E.H., and Baffour, T.D. (2004) 'Arts-based strengths: A solution-focused intervention with adolescents in an acute-care psychiatric setting.' *The Arts in Psychotherapy 31*, 213–227.

Walsh, F. (1998) 'Beliefs, spirituality, and transcendence: Keys to family resilience.' In M. McGoldrick (ed.) *Re-visioning Family Therapy: Race, Culture, and Gender in Clinical Practice.* New York: Guilford.

Way, N. (2004) 'Intimacy, desire, and distrust in the friendships of adolescent boys.' In N. Way and J.Y. Chu (eds) *Adolescent Boys: Exploring Diverse Cultures of Boyhood.* New York: New York University Press.

Zur, O. (2005) 'The psychology of victimhood.' In R.H. Wright and N.A. Cummings (eds) *Destructive Trends in Mental Health: The Well-intentioned Path to Harm.* New York: Routledge.

CHAPTER 17

"Sit Down and Be Quiet!"

Dance and Movement Therapy in an Inner City Elementary School After-care Program

Susan Kierr

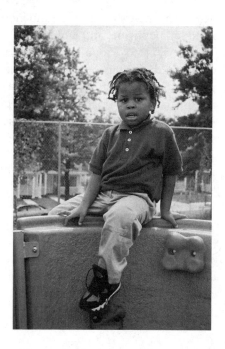

This chapter describes the use of Dance and Movement Therapy (DMT) as a means of "healing the classroom" by establishing the classroom as a safe holding place and a place to safely express strong feelings. The children described here attend a public elementary school in inner city New Orleans. To various degrees, they are exposed to threats and punishment in the mild to intense chaos that exists at home, at school, and in the community at large. This chapter looks at the impact of DMT interventions offered in an after-school care setting. Using a humanistic framework, a model of health rather than pathology is presented that focuses on increasing a sense of safety, support, belonging and intimacy.

Background

Mark Twain's *Huckleberry Finn* popularized a romantic vision of how education could be acquired in unconventional settings, beyond the regular classroom day and away from academic judgments and requirements. Twain wrote about real life adventures on the Mississippi River. His narratives demonstrate that the untamed impulses of young people can connect with real experiences and result in adventurous learning (Cohen 1988). Dance and Movement Therapy (DMT) can be used for this same purpose, allowing children to embark on adventures through creative movement, fostering learning of body, mind and spirit.

The public school system reflects the understanding that physical activity is appropriate in an educational setting. The academic day is usually designed to include physical education and playground time. Physical exercise has proven to be an important means for relieving physical and mental tension, enhancing psychological well-being and encouraging social behavior (Aahperd 2003). This is owing to the increase in energy production and monoamine synthesis in the brain: more serotonin, epinephrine, and endorphins.

After-school programs want to capitalize on this in order to support academic goals and reinforce the values of public education. However, after-school programs often consist of more school, run by tired teachers often doing little more than baby sitting, with the goal of keeping children safely off the streets (Schwarz 2004). For after-school care to be effective, children need the program to be fun, as well as different from school; parents need it to provide safe care; schools need it to help with homework and skill building; the broader community needs it to instill values, build leadership skills, and help prepare children for success (Schwarz 2004). DMT therapy in an after-school program potentially meets all these needs.

In this chapter we will discuss how DMT can meet presenting needs, and address specific goals of establishing safety, developing attuned attachment and channeling aggressive behavior. We describe experiences in which children have fun, feel safe, build skills that are helpful in the educational process, and clarify values that are connected to higher achievement.

My experience

For the past six years I have worked as a DMT therapist in after-school class-rooms, in a small elementary public school in Marrero, Louisiana, located five miles from downtown New Orleans. This excellent program was sponsored by the Jefferson Youth Foundation, a grassroots organization supported by grants. Unfortunately the grants that sustained the program and many of the children that it served ceased due to Hurricane Katrina in 2005. The children lived near the school in what can be described as a low-income urban neighborhood. The children's lives were characterized by loss owing to divorce, separation and death, witnessing and experiencing violence in the home and in the neighbor-hood, lack of consistent caretakers in the home, and financial hardship.

I entered the classroom one afternoon a week and received enthusiastic greetings from the children. My arrival indicated that homework time was over, and that the day had shifted to another kind of learning experience. The after-noons were arranged so that the first hour was spent doing homework and the second hour was for playground time, gym, video entertainment, computer time, or a visit from an "artist". This last alternative was a visit from a qualified person under contract to bring dance, music, writing, photography or drama activities to the program. I worked with children ranging from first to sixth grade over the years. All grades rotated among the artists each year, and all the classes received music, art, creative writing, or drama sessions during the second hour of the afternoon.

When I arrived in the after-school classroom, the children were usually instructed by the teacher to put away all pencils, papers, and books and were usually given a warning about their behavior: "Sit still, be quiet, and do what Ms Susan tells you to do, or she will leave." These instructions were typically given during the first few sessions of the semester, and when not modified by countermeasures, continued as the teacher's mantra.

Ironically, I was trying to build a sense of trust and acceptance. My goal was to encourage creative expression of feelings in a safe holding environment. I wanted the children to know that the only unacceptable behaviors were those that would hurt themselves or others. However, I was faced with classroom policies in which the teacher would judge student behavior and discipline them accordingly. If the teacher felt that the student was being too loud or impulsive, the child's name was often listed on the board, or the child was moved to the back of the room or the hallway. The child was often barred from further partici-pation for an undetermined length of time. Occasionally, and apparently when the teacher was especially worn out from his or her regular teaching day, children were sent to the office of an administrator to receive instructions on how to behave.

During my first year as the DMT therapist in the program I worked with first-graders and was dismayed by the number of interruptions from the teacher. The students were constantly being reprimanded for being "wild". The class was threatened with disciplinary action and told that they did not deserve to work with Ms Susan. The teacher banged on the desk, raised her voice to deafening levels, and even grabbed children by the arm, dragging them to remote parts of the room or hallway.

Six years later, once I had rotated through the other five grades, I returned to the first grade again and did not have this problem. Over the course of the intervening years, I had experienced similar classroom conditions and had learned ways of using DMT to increase the tolerance of exasperated teachers who wielded inconsistent punishments. I had come to understand that the

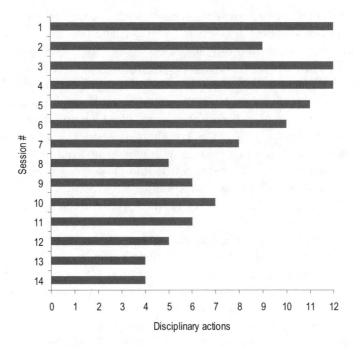

Figure 17.1 Decrease in number of disciplinary actions during 14 sessions of DMT – Year One

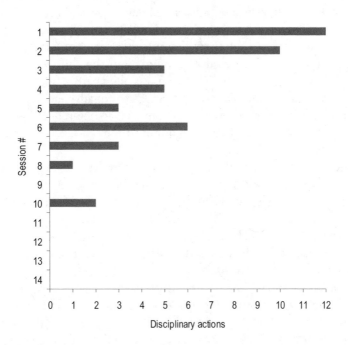

Figure 17.2 Decrease in number of disciplinary actions during 14 sessions of DMT – Year Six

classroom needed healing. Over time I acquired ways to strengthen the positive connection between the teachers and the students, while building an environment that nurtured and permitted expression of feelings.

This experience highlighted the healing effect that DMT can have in an after-school program, in that teachers came to trust and tolerate impulsive expression of feelings through the use of movement. This became evident in documenting a significant decrease in the number of disciplinary actions taken by the classroom teacher from the start of the semester until the end (Figure 17.1). The first year of DMT with the first grade was characterized by numerous disciplinary actions in the classroom, not changing significantly through the semester. Each week was marked with lectures and punishments by the classroom teacher.

By the sixth year of the program the disciplinary actions, though present at the start of the semester, were reduced to zero (Figure 17.2).

DMT goals

Establishing a sense of safety

The goals identified for DMT in this after-school care program begin with the creation of a safe holding environment. By the time the child enters the classroom, he or she has had up to six or seven years of informal learning. The child's brain and body know far more than is actually available consciously, and much more than the child can verbalize. There is a subliminal knowing, a felt sense, which Gendlin (1981) has described as sensing with the body, or a bodily knowing. The DMT program described here addresses the issue of safety, which school-age inner city children are already familiar with, since they have learned to recognize safe and unsafe situations.

The concept of making the classroom a safe place for the spontaneous expression of feelings in movement is not consistent with the academic setting described here, in which teachers judge what is right or wrong in a child's performance and harshly discipline "bad behavior". For this reason, the therapist's first goal was to increase the sense of safety in her relationship with the children. A DMT session should be used as a laboratory in which children can try new ways of moving and behaving, free of judgments or expectations (Levy 1995).

Clear and reliable rules that were agreed upon by the children, the therapist, and the teacher generally helped maintain feelings of safety and trust. One important rule was that all dance and movement would be acceptable as long as no one got hurt, even if it was noisy. This rule was stated during each session and became a therapeutic contract. A movement ritual was added to help establish the therapeutic contract, and a handshake with the therapist was used to affirm that each individual acknowledged the rule. With the handshake, the therapist used verbal cues to encourage eye contact. She made use of first names, and verbally acknowledged the presence of a firm grip.

Attuned attachment

A second and equally important goal was the development of a sensitive rapport intended to help build positive regard between the therapist and the children. This rapport fosters a connection called attuned attachment. Attunement begins with attachment opportunities before birth, as well as through the quality of the gaze between the newborn/infant and caregiver (Loman 1992). Securely attached children are found to have had early experiences with parents or caretakers who demonstrated a predominance of accessible, cooperative, accepting, sensitive and easy-to-read behaviors. When sensitive mothers interact with securely attached babies, the mothers instinctively do everything they can to maximize joyful and interesting experiences (Chodorow 2005).

In the DMT sessions, eye contact, tone of voice, and interactive rhythms are elements intended to reinforce attuned, secure attachment. In addition, use of mirroring fosters the kind of attunement identified as part of healthy early childhood experiences. This mirroring may happen in pairs (dyads) reminiscent of the original pairing of mother and child, as well as in groups. The DMT therapist identifies characteristic steps, gestures, and postures of participants and invites others to try them out, so that each individual has an opportunity to see his or her movement reflected back by a partner, or by the whole circle. This use of the circle originated with Marion Chase, founder of DMT, and is often referred to as the Chase circle (Bernstein 1972). The therapist may mirror movements of both teachers and children and the children are given opportunities to mirror the movements of their teacher, the therapist and their classmates.

Channeling aggressive behavior

A third and final goal, congruent with the aims of both therapy and education, is that of channeling aggressive behavior into creative outlets. The ability to modulate affect may have its roots in early cycles of rupture and repair between parent and child, but higher ego functions continue to evolve and may be influenced by classroom activities that involve mixing and modulating affect.

The dance therapist used stories expressing emotional turmoil, progressing from symbolically representing unconscious distress to verbalizing and making it conscious, and so increasing the ability to deal with it (Simon 2005).

Storytelling through movement became a useful tool for channeling aggressive behavior. By asking the children to create a story, and encouraging their choice of movements to enact it, the therapist elicited material that was congruent with thoughts, feelings and images authentic to them. Embodied storytelling is a technique that creates opportunities for an upward spiral of excitement through playful interactions, followed by a return to a more calm posture. In this way, the children acquire and practice skills that help them to be centered after excitement (Tortora, 2006).

A humanistic framework

DMT offers an alternative method of working within the context of a system-atized theory of human behavior. Differences in theoretical conceptualization may alter the style or technique of DMT therapists, but the underlying movement theories are inclusive (Chaiklin 1975). In this section I will consider the theoretical framework of humanistic psychology and apply it to the use of DMT in the after-school care program.

Humanistic psychology emerged in the late 1950s as an alternative to psy-choanalysis and behaviorism, the two dominant schools of thought in the field of psychology at the time. Its aim was to address the fullness of human poten-tial, the capacity of humans for creativity, art, spirituality, self-realization, and transformation. It does not exclude the central aspects of object relations theory or behaviorism, but encompasses them. Maslow, a founder of humanis-tic psychology, also identified himself as a Freudian, a behaviorist, and an exis-tentialist (Maslow 1971). Maslow, and other humanistic psychologists, base their work on models of health rather than pathology, and view human nature as intrinsically good and healthy (Maslow 1968).

When a DMT therapist leads a group in an after-school care classroom, this is exactly the stance that is most appropriate. The group setting provides an opportunity to address needs that have not been satisfied in early life. Partici-pants can experience safety, acceptance, respect, support, a sense of belonging, and intimacy (Emunah 1994).

Humanistic psychology recognizes two innate forces: fear of the unknown and the desire to grow. As fear of the unknown yields to a sense of safety, a desire for growth emerges, such as when healthy infants take risks when they sense the reassuring presence of their parents. They move forward when there is a secure base from which to venture, knowing that a retreat back to that base is always possible. DMT sessions are useful in the therapeutic pursuit of provid-ing this sense of a safe place. The concepts of humanistic psychology elucidate the relevance of DMT as it is used to promote safety in the classroom situation. It is also substantiated by object relations theorists, including Winnicott (1960) in his descriptions of good-enough mothering and adequate holding environ-ments, and Mahler (1975) in her analysis of separation and individuation.

The dance and movement therapy contract

In the DMT experience described here, an agreement was formed among the children, the teachers, and the therapist. The DMT session was to be a time to move freely, have fun, and express feelings, in such a way that no one got hurt.

These terms were emphasized so as to help establish a holding environment that was accepting, supportive, and caring.

Because the DMT sessions took place in a school setting, it was expected that roll be called at the start of each session. This was used as the basis for an opening ritual that included shaking hands, making eye contact, and using voices. The ritual of the roll-call handshake encouraged characteristics of a socially acceptable greeting. Children learned to identify their right hand as the one to offer, reciprocating the extending of the therapist's right hand to them. There was no wrong hand, simply a differentiation of right from left. Eye contact was reinforced as children began to mirror the therapist's steady gaze, smile, and voice, as she pronounced their name with clarity and purposefulness. Frequently the teacher engaged in this greeting as well.

The group agreed to move together with safety and control. The process of promoting this principle was designed to include teachers as well as students, and the following three steps were identified:

1.   At the start of each session, in what is sometimes called a "check-in" in group therapy and "attendance" in an educational setting, each child heard his or her name and was expected to respond. In this case, the child was asked to walk over to the therapist and to shake hands. The goal was to make eye contact as well as physical contact. The therapist said, "Hello, Desmond," and the child responded, "Hello, Ms Susan." Developmentally appropriate social skills were being developed by engaging in a gaze that affirmed mutual awareness and acceptance.

2.   The contract was verbalized at the start of each session with words like "Let's dance together in a safe way, so that none of us hurt ourselves or hurt someone else. Agreed?" Including the teacher in the contract was crucial. The therapist might ask, "Mr Donald, is it alright with you if the students move and dance and make noise, as long as no one hurts themselves or someone else?" The teacher's agreement allowed the therapist to encourage escalation of energy and excitement during sessions so long as the children remained safe from injury. It was made clear that hurting feelings or bodies was included in this agreement.

3.   Safety and control were further encouraged with "movement and freeze" dances. The ability to release energy in movement and to pause the movement and regain control when the music stopped was a skill used throughout sessions. When a child was expressing or acting out strong feelings that resulted in either physical or emotional pain, the group "froze" the movement. By pausing, the group was able to review the safety contract, individuals were able to build impulse control and everyone in the room was able to

increase their understanding of how the contract made the classroom a secure holding environment.

In summary, the DMT contract is an instrument applied to group activities designed to be congruent with the goals of humanistic psychology. Goals include creating safety and showing individual participants acceptance and respect – with handshakes, eye contact, smiles, and a personalized greeting using names, high fives (which is when the raised hands of two people meet and clap mid-air) or a knock fist to fist.

DMT activities

Positive regard

Activities which help heal the classroom include those that encourage positive regard for individual expression. To futher that experience, the group can be asked to stop its movement to watch a classmate's movement combination, and then applaud. Applauding is a sign of approval in the broader culture in which we live, and appropriate to use in this circumstance.

Positive words can be used to describe the movement. For example, getting shaky and losing balance during a "move and freeze" activity is described as taking a risk and learning more about balance. The shaky moment is reframed to emphasize the learning opportunity and to generate positive attention for the mover.

Spatial boundaries

Spatial boundaries are explored as the children discover ways to move and freeze without getting in the way of another person's balance. The teacher and therapist can demonstrate this (which does not require that the teacher be an experienced dancer or even a confident mover, merely that she understand the goal of freezing in a shape that does not bump into the therapist).

Leadership

The humanistic goal of experiencing a sense of belonging is also increased by sharing leadership. Each participant is encouraged to take a turn leading. The child sees his circle of classmates mirror his movement. This is a structured version of a Chase circle in that the leadership role passes around the circle, to each group member in turn, starting with the therapist and including the teacher. The participants know that they will each have a turn to lead. If an individual feels shy, there is always a peer eager to suggest a movement, a gesture, or another response that the hesitant person could use to lead the group. No one is left out. Every movement is named after its originator, such as "Kesha's wavy arms", "Roland's bouncy legs", "Anthony's clapping hands", "ShaQuielle's big whole self". Using music can add flow to this activity.

Safety and control

Moving with safety and control can be structured in many ways. One of these is to clear enough floor space for a run and slide. The children can slide in socks or on the seat of their pants. A drum roll is used to accompany the run, and a louder final beat is used to mark the landing. Mark Twain's Huckleberry Finn might have had the same grin as the first-graders when they accomplish a safe and condoned way of tearing across the room, with a big, loud, percussive drumroll to celebrate the landing.

Expression through storytelling

Storytelling is an excellent way to generate expression. The leader, in this case the DMT therapist, begins with "Once upon a time a group of children went for a walk…" and turns to the child next to her to continue the story. Leadership is passed around the circle, each child adding to the story. Every child belongs in the story, so even the shy or inarticulate child is credited with an element of the story. In some cases, the therapist may have to interpret a shrug or gesture as a viable piece of the plot. When the telling travels around the entire circle, the last child's contribution becomes the ending.

The story is then retold in a smooth but faithful version by the therapist. At this point it can be written down, which often impresses the children. First-graders who are just beginning to read find having their story put into print especially significant. The stories can be carried around in a book, which communicates the message that their thoughts and feelings are valued and safe.

The story can then be read from the written page. This emphasizes the role of reading and writing, thus personalizing the value of academic achievement. An expressive tone of voice is used, along with postures and gestures to highlight the storyline. Children's movements are used in the retelling, and, as in a Chase circle (Chaiklin 1975), movements that help illustrate the story's theme are clarified and exaggerated. Everyone in the circle can then stand up and embody, by enacting, the story that they created.

These stories inevitably include great adventures, monsters, heroes, weapons, blood and gore. It is required that all the enactments keep to the agreement that no one gets hurt. Whenever this seems precarious, a freeze stops all action. The story can include, for example, monsters being decapitated, but the children are reminded that all the battles are imaginary. In one situation one part of the story was intolerable for the classroom teacher: a boy in the class declared that the hero cut off the "balls" of the scary villain. The teacher panicked and squelched that part of the story. He insisted that the imaginary castration be deleted. An interaction like that can be processed as an example of a way in which imaginary things can scare a grownup too.

The escalation of emotion in a story is essential to good drama. The ability to devise a story that is close to home, that captures the hopes, wishes, and fears of the storytellers and their audience, is essential for good catharsis. The disclosure of frightening fantasies builds intimacy and trust. The story belongs to everyone in the circle. The management of the ensuing emotions, the endurance of disruption and the return to calm, are the goals of the classroom experience.

The enactments, and even the move and freeze activities, frequently result in children spinning, falling, and collapsing. The children often find ways to land on top of one another, grabbing and pulling each other off balance. This is not always a safety issue because the children seem to be creating ways to touch one another by landing one on top of the other. They may be seeking more contact or closeness. It is important to help them find safe ways to experience age-appropriate intimacy which feels controlled, is not overstimulating, and is less likely to lead to physical injury.

Cooling down through belly breathing

Belly breathing is a cool-down activity that permits safe physical intimacy. First, the children practice lying on the floor, each in their own space, breathing from the bottom of their lungs. As the lungs expand, the belly moves outward. Children can feel and see their bellies rise up on the inhale and go down on the exhale. Over the course of two weeks, other elements of this breath awareness exercise are added. Each child is given a small stuffed animal to perch on his belly, to watch rise and fall. Then each person finds another child's belly on which to rest the back of his or her head, creating safe physical contact. All heads can be seen gently moving up and down.

The children are calm and comfortable during belly breathing. This can be used for energy modulation and to close each session. Children can take their stuffed animal home with them as a reminder of the power of breath, as an instrument to practice body awareness, and as a transitional object to maintain connectedness to the group.

Cool-down activities are important in the academic classroom. The young brain's emotional centers can overwhelm the pre-frontal voice of reason. Strong emotion and arousal can hijack decision-making (Dahl 2005). The teacher may explain and threaten consequences to disruptive behavior, but the child who is emotionally charged and excited does not remember these rational consequences. Belly breathing helps children, just as it helps adults, to gain control when feeling overwhelmed. Slowing down breath and breathing from the bottom of the lungs reverses the cascade of excitement, and lowers heart rate and blood pressure. The gentle rise of the belly with each inhalation can capture the attention of young children, promoting focus and body awareness.

James S. Gordon, MD, founder and director of the Washington DC-based Center for Mind–Body Medicine, has a successful six-week training program using breathing exercises with children to alter the fight-or-flight response (Gordon 2004). His, "Art of living", program is used to reduce post traumatic stress in troublespots around the world, which have included Bosnia, Kosovo, and Israel (Evans 2005).

Conclusions

Teachers often want students to "Sit down and be quiet", whereas dance therapists understand the importance of emotional expression and movement. To address this conflict, the DMT therapist works towards making classrooms safer for expression. The therapist establishes that DMT works best if children move the way they feel like moving, remembering that there are no right or wrong ways to move. This clarification is an essential part of the therapeutic process, as it helps to build a safe container and is intrinsic to developing a secure and safe attachment between the child and therapist. A DMT contract further helps to heal classroom stress and conflict.

Data from the after-school care program described here showed that disciplinary actions taken by teachers in efforts to control student behaviors decreased when the therapist, teachers, and students agreed that it was permissible to express feelings with movement and make noise, so long as no one got hurt. What was measured in this study was how the classroom environment changed when it was no longer organized by disciplinary attempts to keep children quiet and orderly, but instead became a container for expression. The healing effect on the classroom was seen in increased teacher efforts to tolerate emotional excitement and the development of tools for stress management for children. The children felt supported and protected, the teachers saw new skills emerge, parents understood that the children were safe, and the children acquired tools for positive social interactions and constructive community values.

This study shows that DMT is an effective addition to after-school programs. It further demonstrates how DMT in the regular school classroom can be a learning experience congruent with the educational process.

Note

Portions of this chapter appeared in *Moving On* (the quarterly journal of the Australian Dance Therapy Association) Vol. 4, No. 1, 2005. The material here is used by permission of the Association.

References

Aahperd (2003) 'Women, physical activity, and leisure: jeopardy of wheel of fortune.' *Journal of Women in Sport and Physical Activity 12*, 1, 113.

Bernstein, P. (1972) *Theory and Methods in Dance-Movement Therapy.* USA: Kendall/Hunt Publishing.

Chaiklin, S. (1975) 'Dance therapy.' In S. Arieti (ed.) *American Handbook of Psychiatry*, Vol. 5. NY: Basic Books, 701–720.

Chodorow, J. (2005) 'Early development and symbolic physical action.' *Dance Therapy Association of Australia Quarterly 14*, 1, 8.

Cohen, David K. (1988) 'Teaching practice: *plus ça change*.' In Phillip W. Jackson (ed.) *Contributing to Educational Change.* Berkeley: McCutchan.

Dahl, R. (2005) 'Looney teens.' Interviewed for *Sky Magazine* by Sophia Dembling, September 2005, Atlanta: Delta Airline Publication.

Evans, Karin, (2005) 'The art of breathing.' *Health Magazine 10*, 4, 111–113. Birmingham, AL: Southern Process Corp/Time Inc.

Emunah, R. (1994) *Acting for Real: Drama Therapy Process, Technique, and Performance.* New York: Brunner/Mazel Inc.

Gendlin, E. (1981) *The Focusing Book.* New York: Bantam Books.

Gordon, James S. (2004) 'Treatment of posttraumatic stress disorder in postwar Kosovo high-school students using mind–body skills groups: a pilot study." *Journal of Traumatic Stress 17*, 2, 143–147.

Levy, F. (1995) *Dance and Other Expressive Therapies.* New York: Routledge, 127.

Loman, S. (1992) 'Fetal movement notation: a method of attuning to the fetus.' *The Body/Mind Connection in Human Movement Analysis.* New Hampshire: Antioch New England Graduate School.

Mahler, M. (1975) *The Psychological Birth of the Human Infant: Symbiosis and Individuation.* New York: Basic Books.

Maslow, A, (1968) *Toward a Psychology of Being.* Princeton, NJ: Van Nostrand Reinhold.

Maslow, A. (1971) *The Farther Reaches of Human Nature.* New York: Viking Press.

Schwarz, E. (2004) 'After-school time.' *Lesley Magazine*, Spring issue, Cambridge: Lesley University Press, 15-17.

Simon, R. M. (2005) *Self-Healing Through Visual and Verbal Art Therapy.* London: Jessica Kingsley Publishers.

Tortora, S. (2006) *The Dancing Dialogue: Using the Communicative Power of Movement with Young Children.* Baltimore, MD: Paul H. Brookes Publishing Co.

Winnicott, D. W. (1960) 'The theory of the parent–infant relationship.' *Maturational Processes.* New York: Basic Books.

CHAPTER 18

Operatic Play: A Drama and Music Therapy Collaboration

Maria Hodermarska and Suzannah Scott-Moncrieff

For the children who make us sing.

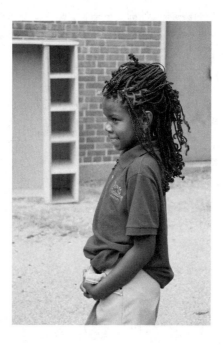

This chapter describes a drama and music therapy collaboration in a therapeutic childcare program located in Brooklyn, New York, within a comprehensive family support program for mothers in substance abuse treatment. This collaborative therapy embraces the chaos of the playroom and ranges broadly in its energy, focus, and narrative aspects. The result is operatic play, which incorporates improvised arias alternated with recitative (a style used in opera, in which the text is declaimed in the rhythm of natural speech with slight melodic variation) and dialogue.

Lisa

"She dies. They all die. The girl dies because the house is a mess," sings Lisa, a five-year-old girl, during the final moments of her improvised opera. Her drawing of the dead family lies completely obscured beneath four sets of hands criss-crossed over sheer scarves, resting on top of a pile of toys.

The therapists gently introduce the closure ritual, indicating that it is time to transition back from play to rest time. The therapists want to support safety and provide containment. The drama therapist, the music therapist, and Lisa's two-and-a-half-year-old brother Michael await Lisa's instructions for what to do next.

The therapist asks, "Can we bury the story here in this magic garden we have made? Bury it for next time?" Several alternative choices are proposed, to offer her, and all of us, some possibility for containment, rebirth, renewal, or change. Lisa replies, "No it can't."

Lisa removes the scarves and sifts through the pile of plastic junk to expose the image of the dead family. She gets up and grabs her chips and drink from her cubby. Imperturbably, chin and chest thrust forward, she struts away and readies herself in another part of the room for a video and rest time.

There is no containment or safety that can be provided with words or deeds. She won't help clean up. Michael and the therapists put everything away – "back to being toys" (Weber 2005, p.33) – in the symbolic transition back to real life. Lisa's tragic opera ends in a literal mess: life imitates art, which imitates life.

Introduction

Our collaborative operatic play method emerged from our need to create a safe space out of the divergent chaotic elements in the playroom. Neither drama therapy nor music therapy alone was big enough to take over the scale or the chaos of the space, and the chaos of the lives that inhabit it. When the combined therapies met the worlds of the playroom and the people they served, there was a combustion that resulted in operatic play.

The drama and music co-therapy creates within the physical space of the disruptive playroom a musical play-space that helps to contain and support the children's expressions and emotional and developmental growth. The children's home environments are mirrored in the children's program environment: chaos, disruption, lack of privacy, and lack of containment. Privacy and confidentiality rarely exist for the therapists and children, making a therapeutic play-space difficult to establish. In this work, the music becomes the "holding environment" for the play, and visa versa (Winnicott 1965).

Although our treatment strategy developed organically from circumstance, elements of this intervention have been previously described. Drama therapist Johnson (1986, 1991) references a technique called "psycho-opera", an exaggerated drama therapeutic intervention used by the therapist, as part of unstructured play. Klein (1974) writes about a music therapy and psychodrama collaboration also called "psycho-opera", which emphasizes the use of song over spoken word in psychodramatic enactments.

Life inside the fish bowl

To understand operatic play, one first has to understand the setting in which it occurs. The physical and emotional space of the playroom reflects the complexity and chaos of the lives swirling through and around it.

The room itself is a well organized, bright, colorful, and child-friendly space. Like any well thought out playroom, it is arranged into sections: gross motor and sensory play, a library, a manipulatives area, shelves of toys, a house-play area, and plenty of open space. It is a wonderful distraction from the sandy-colored, dimly lit institutional corridors beyond the doors. The windowed double doors of the playroom open onto the main corridor of the outpatient program. Adults receiving treatment constantly walk by, and the din during break-time can be overwhelming.

The soundscape of the room is a condensed hubbub of urban life. The constant noise is mirrored by visual interference, as faces of passers-by in the corridor constantly peer in. Counselors from other departments come and go as they check in on their clients and their clients' children's progress.

An aquarium sits on the opposite side of the playroom, on the "grown-ups' side". A large table functions as the great divide. The tank is in the part of the room that children are only allowed to enter with staff permission. The serenity and rhythmic pulsing of the aquarium beckons to the children, but this real fishbowl is inaccessible. As in the great banquet scene in Antwone Fisher's recurring dream in the movie by the same name (Washington 2002), the children can see before them but cannot "eat from" this aquatic feast. An apt metaphor for the inner city child, the fishbowl is a thing of beauty, calm, and life that calls to them, like sirens, to cross the invisible line to see it. It's irresistible. Rule-breaking, born of desire and longing, is engendered in this playroom from the very beginning.

All families receiving daycare services through the program have an active Administration for Children's Services (ACS) case. This means that the children have already been identified by child protective services as being at risk for, or victims of, abuse or neglect. The therapeutic childcare program at the hospital is part of an effort to keep families in crisis together. The children served range in age from three months to 13 years and they receive nursery, preschool or after-school services.

Mothers and their families enter the program in crisis. Disentangling the knot of issues facing the family (child abuse, criminal justice, addiction, domestic violence, lack of entitlements, poor nutrition, poverty, or homelessness) is challenging. The process of recovery for the family is fraught with backsliding and ongoing crises typical of addiction and its social, emotional, physical, and spiritual fallout.

With monitoring by numerous bureaucracies, including child protective services, the criminal justice system, and chemical dependency organizations, mothers and their children, like fish in a tank, are under steady scrutiny. Child protective services, addiction counselors, child counselors, and parole officers are all watching. This is humiliating for a mother: the unintended message is that she is incompetent, and that "the system" will do better than she will in caring for her children.

A culture of entitlement and institutionalization is bred of the absolute necessity for child abuse prevention. Like Bentham's prison structure (Foucault 1995), in which the prisoners are under constant observation and therefore must self-regulate in a system within which they have no power, life in the fishbowl for these women and children is an experience of constant invasion, disempowerment, and hypervigilance.

Like the mothers whose children we play with, we, the therapists, are also under intense scrutiny. We too feel invaded. We too are hypervigilant, as every small encounter with a child is staged or performed before the eyes of any passer-by peering in through the glass doors or entering the space.

Children in the program are pathologized from birth and by birth. They have complicated prenatal and perinatal developmental histories, including exposure to alcohol or other drugs in utero, and premature birth. Some are born HIV- or HBV/HCV (Hepatitis B Virus and Hepatitis C Virus)-positive. Most children are born with positive toxicology screens for illicit drugs. If the results of postnatal blood work don't already draw the child to the attention of the protective services system, their early months at home do. Neglect, abuse, poor nutrition, and developmental delays, common by-products of ongoing maternal substance abuse, may lead the child to the program.

The children exhibit difficulties with initiation, concentration, and verbalization. They present with conduct disorders, mood disorders, and developmental disabilities, with the playroom as their performance space. The "actors" perform in their roles in front of "audiences" of ghosts, internal demons, strangers, professionals, and various oversight authorities. It's a congregation befitting an opera.

Music therapist Pavlicevic writes about group music-making while working in a Soweto clinic and describes how there, not so different from an inner city playroom in New York, "the notion of privacy is spurious." (p.15). She writes, "Bit by bit, folk trickle in – and trickle out – and somehow the group music goes on regardless" (Pavlicevic 2003, p.16).

It helps to think of the playroom as a public space. The musical play "goes on regardless", allowing the children to play in spite of the myriad of sights and sounds. The secure child plays without regard for things around her. In this playroom, one that perhaps mirrors the child's own living space or social environment, the dramatic musical play creates the security that the insecure child so desperately needs.

Hope for these children lies in their ability to play. Just as the singer in a staged opera continues despite the audience's coughing, a torn costume, or a forgotten line, so does the child in her play. Once a child begins her song, the music allows her to continue. The operatic play becomes a means to carry on in the face of chaos or interruption. It is important for these children to see, recognize, and affirm the presence of others, but not stop the flow of feeling and expression in midstream. The music creates the stage, the bubble, the alternative reality. Kenny, writing about this kind of space created by music, describes how "Initial entry into this space is gained when participants are motivated to make the first sound, a creative gesture…[and] the space is 'sealed off' or contained, when both participants have joined each other in these first sounds" (Kenny 1991, p.344–345).

Definition of operatic play

> …whereas in poetry the words themselves lift the poem, in part at least, out of pure play into the sphere of ideation and judgment, music never leaves the play-sphere. (Huizinga 1955, p.158)

The term "opera" comprises many works. The music, drama (as it is reflected in action, conflict, character or role), human voice, sets, and costumes combine into one larger work. While experts disagree about what makes an opera an opera, most would agree that in opera the many works are held or contained by the music. Even Wagner, who early in his career claimed that poetry and drama "were of equal importance with the music", had abandoned this principle by the time of his first great opera, *Tristan and Isolde*, in 1859 (Pletsch 1991, p.128).

The music creates the world. In Wagner's *Rheingold*, for example, the holding environment of the music ranges from the sustained opening chords of the opera, which so compellingly and wordlessly open out into the primordial and eternal world of the Rhine, to the cacophonous clanging of hammers on anvils to greet Woltan's descent into the underworld of the Niebelungen.

Our goal is to create a safe space for exploration to occur. With chaos on every level we intuited from the beginning that our work had to harness the energy of the turmoil rather than fight it. Without thinking about it, we began our collaboration by singing, banging on tables (our own hammers on anvils), vocalizing, and harmonizing.

Hence, drawing from the drama, conflict, and forces of fate that abound, we create in operatic play our very own "wall of sound" with the children. The elements of operatic play include full-voiced singing, rhythm and melody making instruments, the potential for constant movement through the room, and use of materials (props, puppets, drawing tools) that we need in the moment.

We shape a new space with each other, within the room, and with our audience, which establishes a force-field that feels strong and safe. The force-field itself incorporates the turbulent energy around us in the free-flowing dynamic interplay, akin to what play therapist Axline (1969) referred to as a "kaleidoscope" (p.11) in her play therapy with children. It is our hope that the mutual whole is greater than the sum of its parts. When we are engaged in operatic play we are stronger than ourselves individually – unrepentant, unashamed, and emboldened.

The sessions begin where the child is, both emotionally and literally. They flow in a stream of consciousness, based upon what Axline (1969) called "permissiveness [to the child] ...to chart his own course openly and above board. " (p.15). The freedom of her developmental approach is echoed by drama therapist, Johnson (2000) in his emanation theory of drama therapy. In this theoretical model, using a process he calls "developmental transformations", Johnson incorporates the "dynamics of free play [in an] embodied encounter in the playspace" (p.87). Additionally, Johnson's process seeks to "establish non-linear norms" (p.93) in order to focus the patient on the feeling thread of the therapeutic encounter rather than as the linear, narrative thread of the plot unfolding. The omnipresence of music in operatic play may provide a "non-linear" emotional accompaniment within the encounter. This allows for the possibility of an experience of the emergent and existing emotions and themes to which Johnson refers.

As the operatic play unfolds, the communication is sung, played on instruments, or spoken. If a child offers a direction in spoken words, it is often echoed back or mirrored through song in a musical version of active listening. This mirroring is similar to Austin's (2003) technique of vocal holding. Vocal holding is a form of vocal improvisation which comprises "the intentional use of two chords in combination with the therapist's voice in order to create a stable and consistent musical container" (p.212). Austin emphasizes the value of this technique in working through "traumatic ruptures in the mother–child relationship and/or empathic failures at crucial developmental junctures" (p.237).

Peter

Peter rolls his Lego train across the table. The plastic horse falls off the moving train. "The horse is crying," Peter says, with a sad face. "He's so sad, he is crying." "Why is he crying?" I sing. Peter responds, "Because he has been left behind... bad horse," and he hits the horse to the ground. "Oh that hurts," I wail in song. "It's OK horse, I won't hurt you," he responds, and the next moment, "Bad horse! Get out of my face!" "Get out of my face," we sing. He looks at us, as if surprised by our words. "Get out of my face. Get out of my face. Get out of my face."

"No music!" Peter orders, as he puts one hand over Maria's, and presses the off button on the keyboard with his other hand. I continue to make music on my guitar, and yet he does not command me to stop. It's as if my playing is not the music, but a part of the environment. The guitar's quiet familiarity allows him to transition seamlessly between and behind the scenes of his own operatic play. He moves back and forth; sometimes with us, and sometimes apart from us, sometimes singing with us as we accompany and mirror his play; sometimes

with his back to us, in his own rhythm. All the while, the same four chords on the guitar let him know that he can come and go, that he is witnessed, and that the stage is his.

Operatic play, then, is more than pure *drama* therapy, in that music is an essential organizing and omnipresent ingredient. The storyline or narrative, in this case Peter's experiment with aggression and control, is permitted and supported by the repetition of the same four chords and vocal reflections. It is more than pure *music* therapy, in that the children are not always given an instrument to play, or encouraged to sing. We do not separate the therapy into music or drama or play. Like Peter's play, in an all-encompassing way, the children's non-musical narratives, gestures and toy-play are supported and used. The therapy encompasses props, musical interventions, dramatic tools, the spoken word and all that is in the playroom space.

The holding environment

Ultimately, the major theme of our collaboration has less to do with sound or narrative than it does with space. We find ourselves using spatial terms to describe our goals of holding and expression and our objectives of expanding a vocal and storymaking capacity. This capacity does not occur in spite of, or separate from, the children's life experience, but in concert with it. We are shaped by the space and energies around us as we use them to fashion an intra-psychic and inter-personal play-space or holding environment with the children.

Aigen (2005) writes, "The constituents of musical experience are the common elements of our fundamental experiences as human beings" (p.226). He discusses specific musical qualities as providing people with an experience of being contained, being uplifted, being brought down, taking a journey, or being part of a whole. In the case of the playroom and the children within, there is a special need for containment and being held. He states, "The musical container, in its protective entailment, can provide a safe haven for people for whom life itself is felt as dangerous"(p.190).

While the music we use is mostly the container or vessel, it can, on occasion, become the thing requiring containment. In the operatic play this is exemplified when a shift in point of view occurs, when the narrator suddenly becomes the protagonist, or the reverse. This shift or movement between the worlds of the actor and the storyteller occurs when the child requires a change in her intra-psychic relationship to the text. She achieves this by seeking less or more distance from the action. According to Landy's (1994, 1996, 2000) concept of distancing in drama therapy, mental health is dependent upon the person's ability to establish a healthy range of psychic movement into and out of role, between roles, and within the role and its shadow or counter-role. This dynamic balance also offers the possibility for insight and catharsis. People can be under- or over-distanced in the role relationships, and the movement or plastic quality of transforming this distance is regulated and monitored by the therapist.

At times children will sing in the first person and suddenly move into a third person point of view, gaining distance from something or moving into an overdistanced relationship to the narrative.

Charity

Two-year-old Charity is playing in the dollhouse with the drama therapist, singing and playing three notes on the electric piano in the familiar children's playground chant, "NA-NA-NA-NA-NA" (based around the interval of the minor third). It is simple and rhythmic.

Therapist:	*I make dinner for baby.*
Charity:	*Dinner mommy.*
Therapist:	*I make dinner for baby.*
Charity:	*Dinner mommy.*
Therapist:	*Dinner for baby.*
Charity:	*She don't want no bottle from lafrigerator! She don't want no bottle. She bad baby. [Throws her baby doll to the floor with a mock angry face, which masks a slightly naughty smile, as the therapist continues to hold the moment by playing the three-note melody.]*

The child singing in the "I" suddenly transforms her sentient experience and sings in the "she." The more distanced role of narrator or storyteller may offer some safety. It is in these moments, we conjecture, that the function of the music may shift from container or holding environment, to that which requires containment (emotion). The music moves center stage as the beating or bleeding heart. The story becomes the container, and the music becomes the emotion requiring expression.

Lisa's sad story (self-titled)

Some parts of the aria below are sung, some are spoken, and all are accompanied by the guitar using C, D minor, F, and G7 arpeggiated chords, in common time. Throughout the aria Lisa is moving from drawing an image of the family on paper, to moving through the house play area banging dishes together, to sitting at the Lego building table. She uses the entire playroom.

Lisa:	*There once was a little girl who was a rat. She was sad. Look at her eyes. They are crying.*
Therapist:	*Why is she crying? Why so sad?*

Lisa:	*She's crying because her mother is a bogeyman and leaves her alone. The house is a mess. Her father is a spider. The rat girl dies and he saves her. He's a bogeyman, too. He hits her Mommy and he makes Mommy die.*
Therapist:	*And what happens to the little girl?*
Lisa:	*I don't know. [Smiles, long pause as the music continues]*
Therapist:	*We don't know. [Therapists look at each other.] We don't know.*
Lisa:	*She dies, too. They all die. No one is alive. She is burned in the fire.*
Therapist:	*And then what happens?*
Lisa:	*She comes back to life.*
Therapist:	*Does she have scars?*
Lisa:	*No, she dies.*
Therapist:	*How do we make the little rat girl safe?*
Lisa:	*You can't. She dies. They all die. The girl dies because the house is a mess.*

An example of need for less distance is found when Lisa sings, "I don't know." This shift in point of view is a moment of under-distancing. Lisa abandons the role of narrator and comes to center stage in the role of protagonist. She is the storyteller in an existential crisis, at a loss for meaning in the events in her story. She is simultaneously the actor or the "rat girl" speaking her truth, her existential *crie de coeur*. We mirror her operatic play. We don't know the answers either. In all operas comes the moment of high drama or transcendence, when everything seems to stop. The hero or heroine takes center stage and delivers his or her aria.

In an operatic aria the music emphasizes the emotions of the character, and the text is more reflective and less action-oriented. The aria actually pulls the listener away from the action of the story (like the therapist pulling the child away from the action of the playroom, and vice versa). The aria is the character's acknowledgement of the audience's presence, and the world beyond the stage.

For a moment, there is an intimate connection between the child and the witnessing therapists. Lisa pulls away from the action, and stays with the sadness that is the messy house, and the angry parent. For a moment, the child can stand still and give voice to her feeling.

The guitar itself is a kind of boundary, or an object that embraces a space and creates a space of its own. It is also an object that the therapist can cradle in her arms, and hold close. It has many potential projections for the child. For example, when the guitar is being held firmly against the therapist's breast, it is in itself symbolic of the therapist's ability to hold.

The very act of creating music together is a process of "fine interpersonal attunement" (Dixon 1992, p.128) and intimate creative interaction. Violence, disorder, and disengagement can be expressed in words, while connection and warmth are maintained in the musical relationship. While Lisa sings about acts of violence and separation, she is intimately connecting with the therapists in rhythm and pitch. Simultaneously, Lisa is grounded in her body; as she sings, her breath expands her lungs and lowers her diaphragm. Her body is thus more relaxed and open, rather than closed, to sensation (Austin 2002; Pinkola Estés 1992). Whatever the words, singing is for Lisa an act of embodiment, an act of connection to self and other, and a life affirmation.

Lisa doesn't need to make her emotional narrative "safe" for the purposes of closure, because resolution is inherent in the musical structure. The music is predictable, repetitive, and allows her narrative to remain intact: with everyone dead. The music itself is enough completion. She can live with the unknown in the words, because the music provides the known element.

In Lisa's operatic play, the music is simple and repetitive. Within the chord sequence there is movement toward tension and resolution or release. Its simple and flowing nature through the minor second chord to the dominant seventh, allows for tonal openness and exploration of a variety of feelings, none determined by the specificity of major or minor chords. Simultaneously the music holds her in space and time. The circling, harmonic movement and the steady rhythmic pulse act as a frame or container for her experience, and her consequent freedom of expression. There is familiarity and predictability, which Lisa can trust will be there, no matter what. Aigen describes this experience in music as "I know what I am doing, I am in a familiar place, I am in this song now, I know what will happen next" (Aigen 2005, p.296).

Within the boundaries and safety of musical structure there is the possibility for expansive and intense expression (Kenny 1991). A musical note means nothing and everything simultaneously. The single tone is stillness, yet it is alive with the potential for movement. The music can express felt emotions and be expressive of unfelt emotions. Music does not offer the child a clear direction; it does not lead, but has infinite possibilities for meaning.

Conclusions

Contemporary theater scholar, Stefan Rudnicki, references the Brechtian hierarchy of form in the theater, which has its apotheosis in song. We speak when we can no longer move. When physical gesture and words fail, we must sing (Rudnicki 1982). Operatic play actively engages the disorder and turmoil of the therapy space and the clients' lives. The result is a heightened creative therapeutic intervention which is full-voiced, able to engage with a breadth and depth of personal material, fully expressed physically, fully engaged in the space, and fully played musically. This magnified experience fashions a safe space out of the chaos by mirroring the chaos in a creative and containable form.

We enact our dramas in song, because there is nothing else we can do in response to pain and disorder. Mere words and gestures fail. But in this distillation of experience through operatic play, art transforms life, even if only for the moment of the encounter. Life experience and emotion are represented or presented in crystallized form. Word choice is streamlined, narratives succinct, gestures and movements strong and concise. Time is not measured but taken up or filled.

Paradoxically, in all this expansiveness, a simplification occurs. Or, as Brecht stated, "Let them here produce their own lives in the simplest way; for the simplest way of living is in art" (Brecht in Willett 1992, p. 205). These grand dramas in song, therefore, may offer children the simplest way of being seen.

Lisa

Lisa lies on the floor. Her brother Michael follows suit and throws himself down on the mat, giggling and squirming. Lisa lies still and sings, "Bury me," with intent in her voice. The music therapist sits above her in a chair, mirroring her words and accompanying her softly on the guitar. Lisa sings each line in a descending three-note scale (the "Three Blind Mice" melody) and we sing it back to her. "Bury me," she sings. "Bury me," we mirror. "Because I love you," she sings. "Because I love you," we sing. "I will miss you," she sings. "I will miss you," we reply. "I'm going to heaven," she sings. "I'm going to heaven," we respond. "Bury me," she sings. "Bury me," we sing.

As therapists, we are in the moment overcome with sadness, but in retrospect her song is one of rebirth and renewal. All at once she is mourning a dead part of herself, the 'rat girl' perhaps, and looking with hope to her life to come. We are reminded not to shy away from the child's sad, scary, deep, and challenging feelings expressed in the operatic play. We are reminded to carry on, despite the public nature of the space, and the shame onlookers seem to feel when they witness the sadness that the therapy can bring into the open. It reminds us to go through all Lisa's expressions with her, because rather than change her experience of the world, our only role is to witness it, help her give voice to it, and trust her unique journey.

We do not presume to change her life, but we can sit and sing with her, learn her stories, enact her dramas, show her that we hear her, and show her that all her feelings are right and good. There is much meaning in Lisa's words, in the melody she sings, in the way that she positions her body on the floor, and in her submission to the earth. By appreciating this opera that is her life experience, we feel love for all that Lisa is and will be.

Note

In order to protect their confidentiality we have changed all identifying information, including the names and, in some cases, the gender of the children.

References

Aigen, K. (2005) *Music-Centered Music Therapy*. Gilsum NH: Barcelona Publishers.

Antwone Fisher, film, directed by D. Washington. USA: Fox Searchlight Pictures, 2002.

Austin, D. (2002) 'The voice of trauma: The wounded healer's perspective.' In J.P. Sutton (ed.) *Music, Music Therapy and Trauma*. London: Jessica Kingsley Publishers.

Austin, D. (2003) *When Words Sing and Music Speaks: A Qualitative Study of In Depth Music Psychotherapy with Adults*. Unpublished doctoral thesis, New York University, New York, USA.

Axline, V.M. (1969) *Play Therapy* (2nd edition). New York: Ballantine Books, Inc.

Dixon, M. (2002) 'Music and human rights.' In J.P. Sutton (ed.) *Music, Music Therapy and Trauma*. London: Jessica Kingsley Publishers.

Foucault, M. (1995) *Discipline and Punishment: The Birth of the Prison* (2nd edition). New York: Vintage Books Inc.

Huizinga, J. (1955) *Homo Ludens*. Boston, MA: The Beacon Press.

Johnson, D.R. (1986) 'The developmental method in drama therapy: group treatment with the elderly.' *The Arts in Psychotherapy 13*, 17–33.

Johnson, D.R. (1991) 'The Theory and Technique of Transformations in Drama Therapy.' *The Arts in Psychotherapy 18*, 285–300.

Johnson, D.R. (2000) 'Developmental transformations: Towards the body as presence.' In P. Lewis and D.R. Johnson (eds) *Current Approaches in Drama Therapy*. Springfield, IL: Charles C. Thomas Publisher Ltd.

Kenny, C. (1991) 'The use of musical space with an adult in psychotherapy.' In K.E. Bruscia (ed.) *Case Studies in Music Therapy*. Gilsum NH: Barcelona Publishers.

Klein, T. (1974) 'Psycho-opera: A new concept combining opera and psychodrama.' *Group Psychotherapy and Psychodrama 27*, 1–4, 204–211.

Landy, R.J. (1994) *Drama Therapy: Concepts, Theories, and Practices* (second edition). Springfield, IL: Charles C. Thomas Publisher Ltd.

Landy, R.J. (1996) *Essays in Drama Therapy: The Double Life*. London: Jessica Kingsley Publishers.

Landy, R.J. (2000) 'Role theory and role method in drama therapy.' In P. Lewis and D.R. Johnson (eds) *Current Approaches in Drama Therapy*. Springfield, IL: Charles C. Thomas Publisher.

Pavlicevic, M. (2003) *Groups in Music: Strategies from Music Therapy*. New York: Jessica Kingsley Publishers.

Pinkola Estés, C. (1992) *Women who Run with the Wolves*. New York: Ballantine Books.

Pletsch, C. (1991) *Young Nietzsche: Becoming a Genius*. New York: The Free Press.

Rudnicki, S. (1982) Lecture to undergraduate students. New York University, Department of Undergraduate Drama, New York, NY.

Weber, A.M. (2005) ' "Don't hurt my mommy": Drama therapy for children who have witnessed severe domestic violence.' In A. Weber and C. Haen (eds) *Clinical Applications of Drama Therapy in Child and Adolescent Treatment*. New York: Brunner-Routledge.

Willett, J. (1992) *Brecht on Theater*. New York: Hill and Wang.

Winnicott, D.W. (1965) *The Maturational Processes and the Facilitating Environment*. New York: International Universities Press.

CHAPTER 19

Safe Expressions

A Community-based Creative Arts Therapy Program for At-risk Youth

Flossie Ierardi, Mark Bottos and Mary K. O'Brien

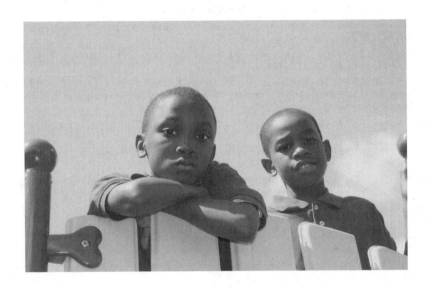

Safe Expressions was developed to determine the effectiveness of a multi-modality creative arts therapy program in addressing psychosocial needs of at-risk youth, in the Greater Philadelphia Metropolitan area. Over 200 twelve- to seventeen-year-olds from a variety of school settings participated in music therapy, dance/movement therapy (DMT), and art therapy sessions from 2002 to 2004. Participants were seen for a full or half an academic year. Based on a comprehensive evaluation protocol, results indicate that most participants demonstrated improvements in skill areas such as self-esteem, interpersonal skills, anger management, impulse control, and development of new coping strategies.

Background

Safe Expressions is a community-based creative arts therapy program that was initiated in September 2002 through a grant from the Pew Charitable Trusts. The program is currently in its second grant cycle. A previous Kardon Institute pilot project implementing dance/movement therapy (DMT) in a violent public school in Philadelphia revealed that students made observable improvements in self-esteem, social skills and academic achievement, as reported by their classroom teachers. The success of this project, combined with publicized information regarding increased violence and academic failure among youth in Philadelphia, prompted Kardon Institute to generate a participant-centered program grounded in creative arts therapy theory and community arts programs for at-risk youth.

Attendance rates in the Philadelphia public schools for the 2001–2002 academic year indicate a disturbing trend: elementary school – 91.1 per cent; middle school – 86.6 per cent; high school – 78.2 per cent (Philadelphia Safe and Sound 2003). The trend is obvious: as students get older, attendance rates decrease. Furthermore, "Students with attendance problems are more likely to become involved in delinquent behavior" (Philadelphia Safe and Sound 2003, p.58). In an urban school district with 185,000 children, continual financial challenges, and increased violence, there is a dire need for meaningful therapeutic experiences that encourage increased self-esteem, respect for self and others, and adaptive social skills.

The Pew Charitable Trusts, an independent non-profit organization, focuses on three major areas: advancing policy solutions, informing the public, and supporting civic life. They responded to the lack of successful programs for low-income children by developing the Children and Youth Fund, offering two-year grants to community agencies. The goal of the Children and Youth Fund is "to promote the healthy development of children and youth, especially those from low-income and vulnerable families, to help them realize long-term economic and social well-being" (Pew Charitable Trusts 2001, p.4).

The Fund has several stated objectives to meet the health, educational and vocational needs of at-risk youth. Objectives that could be addressed by creative arts therapy interventions included the following:

- to increase the supply, quality of, and access to, youth development programs
- to address the needs of adolescents for:
  - safe and nurturing environment
  - cognitive and social development
  - acquisition of life skills
  - prevention of violence, delinquency and pregnancy.

In response to the stated objectives, Kardon Institute for Arts Therapy submitted a grant proposal for Safe Expressions, identifying the following goals:

- to expand access to programming that addresses the needs of at-risk adolescents and prevents delinquency by providing creative arts therapy that will facilitate cognitive and social development and acquisition of life skills, thus enabling adolescents to develop academic skills

- to create a program that will develop and test programmatic approaches and evaluation tools, forge collaborations with community providers and schools, and demonstrate the effectiveness of creative arts therapy in delinquency prevention.

These goals directly addressed the objectives of the Fund, but there remained the challenge of presenting a creative arts therapy philosophy in language that meshed with the community and civic focus of the Fund. To address this, the program was presented as a curricular model for adolescents, with pre-stated therapeutic goals and a functional title (Safe Expressions). Based on the earlier pilot program at Kardon Institute, the following five domains of focus emerged:

- impulse control
- anger management
- self-esteem
- relationship skills
- coping skills.

While these domains are general, creative arts therapists could work within them to address specific psychosocial needs of participating youth. While creative arts therapists typically identify individual therapeutic goals for their clients, Safe Expressions combines individualized goals with pre-identified ones. In this context, therapists complete an assessment, identify goal areas, and create arts-based objectives for each participant.

Service delivery contexts

By the second year of the grant cycle, Safe Expressions therapists were providing services in eleven school and community programs. Delivery of services as well as method of referral differed depending on the setting. Some groups were mandatory for all students, some were comprised of students who were referred specifically for issues such as anger management, and some groups were court-mandated to address behaviors such as truancy, marijuana use and fighting in school.

Of these programs, one (delinquency prevention) had music therapy and DMT, two had DMT only, two had art therapy only and six had music therapy only. The choice of modality depended on agency requests and the availability of creative arts therapists. When the program was presented to facilities, there was a need for education about the work of creative arts therapists, as well as logistical clarification regarding group size, session length, and physical space. A typical commitment included two consecutive, one-hour sessions for six to eight participants, followed by an hour of documentation and meeting time for the therapist.

Safe Expressions implementation took place in a variety of settings, which differed in amounts of structure. Less structured settings included voluntary after-school programs.The most highly structured setting was a school program within a residential facility for girls with behavioral issues and histories of abuse and neglect. Figure 19.1 gives an overall view of settings that include specialized learning environments for youth at risk and mandated programs for those with identified behavioral issues, and flow of the diagram from left to right illustrates increasing levels of structure and support within the educational or therapeutic environments. The shaded areas indicate settings where Safe Expressions took place during this grant cycle.

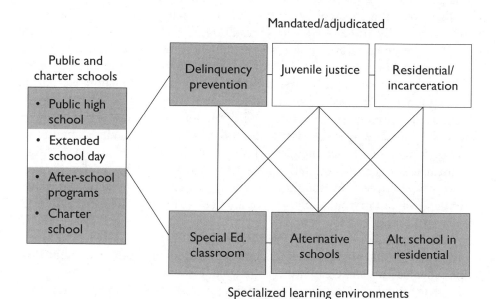

Figure 19.1 Service delivery contexts for Safe Expressions interventions (The shaded areas indicate settings where Safe Expressions took place during this grant cycle.)

As indicated in the diagram, students can move from one setting to another as their need for structure increases or decreases. The goal for all of these programs is to move students towards the left side of the diagram, i.e. the least restrictive settings. When creative arts therapy interventions took place in less structured environments, such as voluntary after-school programs, the goal was to prevent the emergence of serious issues related to the five domains identified by Safe Expressions (see page 257 above). As the setting became more structured, creative arts therapy interventions were more aimed at increasing awareness of maladaptive behaviors and encouraging new and healthier thought processes and interpersonal responses.

Theoretical context

The Safe Expressions program was influenced by community arts programs as well as creative arts therapy models, both of which utilize arts experiences to achieve goals that are personal and transcend the sphere of the arts. While community arts programs emphasize creation of an art product or performance, community-based creative arts therapy programs use the art-making process – and the group dynamics that evolve in the course of it – in such a way as to effect change. Community arts programs promote a sense of belonging as a goal area (Farber 2001). Community-based creative arts therapy programs tend to focus on intra-personal issues such as emotional expression and relief of anxiety (Schelly Hill and Howard Jones 2004).

One community arts program that influenced Safe Expressions was the YouthARTS Development Project for adjudicated and non-adjudicated inner city youth (Farnum and Shaffer 1998). The project, a collaborative effort among federal agencies, national and local arts organizations and arts-based delinquency prevention programs, used evaluation tools to document changes in social skills, feelings of mastery and competence, and risk-taking. Significant evidence was found that after-school programs that included arts instruction contributed to a reduction in delinquent behaviors (Clawson and Coolbaugh 2001). Safe Expressions sought to test a creative arts therapy approach using similar evaluation tools to measure outcomes in a participant-centered, process-oriented environment.

Students Against Violence Everywhere (SAVE) (Boxill 1997) is an inner city, creative arts therapy delinquency prevention program that mobilizes individual talents and creativity in a therapeutic environment in order to facilitate changes in behaviors and attitudes among youth. SAVE provides a creative arts therapy model that the authors integrated with the outcome measurement strategies of the YouthARTS Project in order to develop applicable implementation and documentation protocols for Safe Expressions. This combined approach responded to the assertion of O'Brien (2001), the public health consultant for Safe Expressions, that "one of the most fundamental problems with violence-prevention programs is the lack of theoretically driven program development and the paucity of carefully planned evaluation studies that measure programmatic impact on violence outcomes." (O'Brien 2001, p.389).

Amir (2004) describes community music therapy as an approach that "explores the universal human need for self-expression and creativity, addresses cultural and musical identity in order to enhance the quality of life" (p.251). She later states that community music therapy "looks at clients as cultural as well as musical beings, and as persons whose place within the community needs to be taken into consideration in music therapy" (p.251). While acknowledging that the physical environment of a community may be affected by violence, drugs and other risk factors, Safe Expressions seeks to use creative arts therapies to strengthen the participant's positive sense of self in relation to others in order to navigate the many challenges presented on a daily basis.

The contextual parameters of this program did not always allow for insight-oriented treatment. In some settings such as after-school programs, attendance was not consistent enough for interventions that would encourage safe uncovering of deeper issues. Some in-class settings, however, where confidentiality and containment were part of the daily routine, allowed the creative arts therapist to work more in-depth with students who felt safe sharing personal information. When in-depth work was contra-indicated owing to participants' lack of readiness, or inconsistency in the environment, therapists used here-and-now problem-solving interventions within the immediate arts experiences to test and reinforce coping skills and to increase awareness of positive and negative behaviors. This task was typically approached using verbal feedback. In all settings, therapists addressed immediate stressors as they arose. Examples of these included abandonment by a mother who returned to drug use, referral to a more restrictive program ("boot camp"), school suspension, and threats of self-harm.

Documentation of goals and outcomes

One innovative feature of Safe Expressions is the comprehensive evaluation protocol designed to document measurable outcomes. The evaluation component of this project was consistent with the requirements of the grant. Assessment included pre- and post-participant self-surveys and skills assessments, and treatment goals which were introduced to agency administrators and staff. Therapists also kept weekly progress notes. All documentation was specifically developed to measure skill development within the five psychological and behavioral domains identified for the program.

The self-survey was developed by the authors and a public health consultant. Some questions were adapted from existing instruments, while others were original items. The survey required participants to provide demographic information such as gender, age, race, and grade level, as well as pre- and post-responses to 92 questions categorized into five domains. Overall, the pre- and post-self-survey did not prove to be a statistically reliable measurement of self-recorded progress. In reviewing the self-survey responses to understand the low reliability co-efficients, response patterns appeared to suggest strongly that some participants did not provide genuine responses to questions. Their responses appeared to be random and lacking in consistency within the same domain. After further investigation of the participants' responses, evaluators concluded that the self-survey was too lengthy for the participants to complete with ease. In addition, the participants' reading comprehension levels may have contributed to the lack of genuine responses.

The pre- and post-skills assessments were conducted by the therapists for each participant. The skills assessment consisted of ten specific skill areas (see Table 19.1), which were rated on a Likert scale from 1 to 4 (where 1 = low and 4 = high). The assessment was adapted, using a therapeutic perspective, from a similar instrument used by the YouthARTS Development Project (1998).

Analysis of the pre- and post-skills assessments demonstrated encouraging outcomes. Across all groups, the assessment indicated improvement in all ten areas addressed. The most sizeable increases in skills were in the domains of relationship skills and coping skills – more specifically, communicating effectively with peers and adults and developing creative solutions for problem-solving.

Table 19.1 Ten skills assessed in the Safe Expressions program

1.	Engages in arts experiences from beginning to end.
2.	Responds without physical and verbal aggression.
3.	Communicates effectively with adults and peers.
4.	Cooperates with others in the group.
5.	Demonstrates ability to accept redirection from therapist.
6.	Demonstrates ability to share and take turns.
7.	Demonstrates appropriate use of objects in activities.
8.	Respects personal boundaries of peers and adults.
9.	Demonstrates creative solutions for problem-solving.
10.	Demonstrates initiative and leadership skills.

Therapists were asked to link their clinical observations to the five domains when creating goals for participants. While the long-term goals within each domain were frequently similar, arts-based objectives were generally modality-specific, as shown in Table 19.2. Goal areas most frequently identified by the creative arts therapists were the domains of self-esteem and relationship skills.

Table 19.2 Goals and objectives in the five domains of the Safe Expressions program

	Impulse Control	Anger-management	Self-esteem	Relationship skills	Coping skills
Art therapy	**Long-term goal** To increase strategies for controlling acting out and attention-seeking behaviors. **Arts-based objective** Participant will engage in structured art tasks that emphasize cause/effect relationships.	**Long-term goal** To develop appropriate strategies for safely expressing angry feelings. **Arts-based objective** Participant will wait for appropriate time to play or verbalize during turn-taking experiences and discussions.	**Long-term goal** To increase positive self-image. **Arts-based objective** Participant's art work and relevant verbal responses will indicate improvements in awareness of positive self-traits.	**Long-term goal** To increase positive interactions with peers. **Arts-based objective** Participant will offer support to peers during verbal processing of artwork.	**Long-term goal** To increase ability to deal with negative events. **Arts-based objective** Participant will use art media as directed to explore coping strategies in response to life events.
Dance/ movement therapy	**Long-term goal** To increase ability to think and plan before acting and speaking during group experiences. **Arts-based objective** Participant will demonstrate ability to "stop, think and act" during structured group movement tasks.	**Long-term goal** To increase ability to interact with peers without aggression. **Arts-based objective** Participant will demonstrate awareness of physical boundaries and respect for personal space during movement experiences.	**Long-term goal** To increase awareness of positive verbal and social skills. **Arts-based objective** Participant will take a leadership role within the group movement experience.	**Long-term goal** To increase positive/supportive interactions with peers. **Arts-based objective** Participant will verbally express positive comments to peers during turn-taking movement experience, utilizing props.	**Long-term goal** To increase problem-solving skills. **Arts-based objective** Participant will make contributions during group tasks requiring creative solutions.
Music therapy	**Long-term goal** To increase ability to listen to others' musical or verbal expression without interruption. **Arts-based objective** Paticipant will wait for appropriate time to play/verbalize during turn-taking experiences and discussions.	**Long-term goal** To increase ability to express angry feelings without physical or verbal aggression. **Arts-based objective** Participant will use verbal song material (original or pre-composed lyrics) to safely explore reactions of anger.	**Long-term goal** To increase confidence in personal opinions and abilities. **Arts-based objective** Participant will spontaneously offer opinions/ideas during group songwriting and musical problem-solving tasks.	**Long-term goal** To increase ability to listen to others. **Arts-based objective** Participant will take leadership role during group musical improvisation.	**Long-term goal** To increase frustration tolerance. **Arts-based objective** Participant will engage in musical experience that requires specific responses (e.g. assigned rhythms) throughout.

Clinical examples by modality

Art therapy

As in music therapy and DMT sessions, art therapy tasks were designed to address the intrapersonal and interpersonal aspects of the five identified therapeutic domains. In one school setting, students with anger management issues were referred to an art therapy group. The art therapist identified additional areas of concern such as relationship difficulties, impulsive behaviors, and limited coping skills.

Early in the sessions, participants were offered a large (11" x 18") piece of blank paper and a box of words that had been cut out of magazines to glue onto their paper. The materials and the task were chosen by the art therapist to provide structure and a non-threatening creative environment for those participants who generally presented with resistance in response to the involuntary nature of the group (as well as the scheduling of sessions during lunch). The participants' choice of words, size of words, and their placement on the paper were very telling of their histories and immediate issues, as described in the case example below. This task facilitated participant expression without concern for artistic technique, while giving the art therapist an initial "picture" of what the individual chose to reveal.

Another task involved life maps, or "a roadmap of your life". Participants were shown examples of drawn maps and were asked to create their own life roadmaps, including events from childhood, the present, and where they would like to see themselves in the future. The finished product provided opportunities for a safe and externalized review of perceived significant life experiences, balanced with the expression of positive ambitions. Artistic responses such as size of words, color, and intensity of the lines on the maps, as well as the events illustrated, were expressions of therapeutic interest. In addition to group tasks, the therapist assigned individually designed tasks as specific themes or issues emerged.

In this school setting, the art therapist had frequent communication with the on-site family therapist. This communication and added support provided opportunities for more in-depth therapeutic work. Participants were referred to an anger management art therapy group at varying times during the school term. The therapist noted an initial degree of resentment and resistance from most participants because the group shortened their lunchtime.

CASE EXAMPLE

Participants were initially given the opportunity to work within a provided structure, placing pre-cut words on a large blank sheet of paper. One female participant chose a large cutting of the word AUDACIOUS for the center of the page, with other prominent choices including PLANS, SAFE, SUCCESS and other positive words. Another participant chose a large cut-out of NO END IN

SIGHT for the center of her paper, surrounding it with other large choices of PAIN, NIGHTMARES, DAD, and SECRET. These were intermingled with smaller words: HOW TO WIN, FAMILY, LOVE, TANTRUMS and TRUE BELIEVERS. Verbal discussion which followed provided additional information for the therapist, including information that the participant chose to reveal "out loud". The therapist asked carefully chosen questions based on clinical judgment concerning how much "probing" the participant could tolerate at a given time.

Participants' artistic responses to the life map task included past events, such as losses, family births, and vacations. Participants then followed through with hopes for the future. One participant's life map revealed that her mother had recently returned to using drugs and living on the streets, leaving the daughter to live in the home with an adult male friend of the mother. While expressing feelings about her mother, this student was asked by the art therapist to draw a picture of "a significant memory with your mother." Her drawing included mother and daughter at a very large mall, and she spoke about how her mother took her to this mall once when she was younger.

The process just described allowed the participant to: 1) disclose information about her current living situation, which could then be reported to the family therapist; 2) safely express feelings about her situation to a trained therapist; and 3) externalize possible feelings of loss and abandonment in a non-verbal sub-task that provided an artistic "segue" to the original task (i.e. the illustration of the significant memory could be seen as a "detail" of the larger life map).

DMT

Dance/movement sessions usually began with a warm-up period during which the therapist assessed the participants' activity level, use of space in relation to each other, personal boundaries, and the emergence of themes to develop during the session. Warm-ups served to create an environment for movement expression and might include props to provide structure when needed – the tactile experience of a weighted prop, such as passing a ball, aided the grounding of energy, as well as the development of interpersonal relatedness.

The immediate physical experience of using the body for expression provided opportunities for the therapist to observe and address issues such as awareness of self, respect for personal boundaries and frequent aggressive tendencies. Also noted in early stages of intervention were regressive responses, such as dropping to the floor. The therapist worked with developing themes through movement experiences, sometimes in the form of role-playing or group "games". Sessions generally ended with a group discussion or a grounding movement task to provide closure and support the transition to non-movement-oriented activities.

CASE EXAMPLE

The pilot project for Safe Expressions included DMT sessions for middle-school students in a public school creative writing class. The teacher had requested creative arts therapy as a weekly intervention to stimulate verbal and written expression. He had observed that students often did not express themselves in complete sentences and had difficulty expanding on a topic as a result of a lack of opportunities for healthy self-expression. This school had been identified as one of the most dangerous middle schools in the city of Philadelphia. The dance/movement therapist observed difficulties with impulse control, poor personal boundaries, including frequent hitting, low self-esteem, and negative verbal interactions.

Movement experiences included structured tasks and games, often utilizing props, to encourage more positive verbal responses and awareness of boundaries. One experience involved passing or throwing a ball to a peer, followed by a positive comment to and about that peer. The dance/movement therapist implemented experiences that allowed for safe and contained expression of feelings in an accepting environment. Growth in self-esteem was encouraged through opportunities to initiate individual movement expression and to explore leadership skills within the dance/movement tasks.

As sessions progressed, the class of 22 was divided into subgroups, each of which developed a dance/movement project to videotape and to share with peers. The dance/movement therapist facilitated this project by ensuring that each subgroup member had the opportunity to contribute to the creative process. Sessions ended with verbal discussion of the experience, including roles, feelings of accomplishment, and reactions to the artistic component of the project. The students worked on their projects during sessions and as assignments. The therapist and teacher observed increased participant investment in the projects and the group experience, even among those who had been apathetic or unassertive in early sessions. The final "performances" included dance, singing, and movement games, and involved contributions by all members. Anecdotally, the teacher observed increased levels of expressivity, especially among students who had initially presented as withdrawn and unmotivated.

Music Therapy

Music therapy sessions most often consisted of active/expressive music-making with occasional receptive/listening experiences such as lyric analysis. All musical experiences were based on participants' preferences or culturally informed approaches by the therapist. In environments where explicit rap lyrics were not acceptable, participants were encouraged to write and perform their own rap songs. Improvization (spontaneous vocal and instrumental music-making), songwriting, and participant-initiated sharing of recorded music, accompanied by lyric analysis, were the most frequent musical interventions.

Based on group interest and the type of setting, there were occasional examples of musical instruction, as well as informal and non-threatening rehearsal and performance. In one high school setting, the classroom teacher and music therapist decided to separate the class by gender for music therapy sessions. The therapist noted that while the girls preferred lyric analysis and songwriting interventions with a high level of self-disclosure and peer support, the boys initially preferred the active discharge afforded by group drumming and other rhythm-based experiences, from which they developed a sense of group cohesion.

CASE EXAMPLE

T and G were 12-year-old boys who attended an after-school Safe Expressions program. Both had innate musical abilities and spontaneity. T's spontaneity often led to poor impulse control and he frequently confronted peers, demonstrating poor physical boundaries. G exhibited significant anger and had much difficulty diffusing it, often sabotaging his own participation as well as that of peers. Throughout the course of music therapy sessions, it was noted that G had difficulty participating in and completing positive group experiences.

T had independently written a poem about staying in school. The wording of the poem made it conducive to rap music, and both of the boys experimented with it in a rap format with rhythmic accompaniment. It was decided that they would perform the rap for a presentation to participants in several other delinquency prevention programs.

While preparing for the performance, G's tendency to avoid positive experiences made it difficult for him to remain committed to the project and he threatened to withdraw several times. T was upset and responded with a combination of anger and pouting. The group persisted with rehearsals, as each boy seemed to have different needs in order to complete the project. T, who reportedly received little recognition from his family for his talent and achievements, was given reassurance that he would have the opportunity to present his musical creation, whether or not G was able to do so. G seemed to require a more behavioral approach, with consistent redirection and encouragement from the music therapist and program staff. As a dyad, these boys were able to work through issues more effectively within the musical experience than through a verbal intervention.

At the presentation, the boys were supportive of each other in the music, and each felt the freedom to improvise within established musical and stylistic parameters – T with vocal/rap idioms and G with hip-hop dancing. They received thunderous applause and were visibly proud of their performance. G proved that he was able to participate in a healthy experience with positive results. T was able to work cooperatively with a peer, and demonstrated improved frustration tolerance regarding G's ambivalence. The musical experience for these two boys created an initial step towards the ability to resolve conflict using new and healthy behaviors.

Conclusions

Findings indicate that Safe Expressions had promising results in the identified therapeutic domains. At the end of the first grant cycle, participants demonstrated increased investment in the program, as shown in the post-program self-surveys. Their efforts and responses seemed more genuine, indicated by (for example) asking questions when they did not understand an item, and in the patterns of their answers, which appeared to be less random than they were in some pre-tests.

Administrators' feedback was generally positive. One teacher reported that a girl who had been a street fighter was relating better to others and expressing her feelings more appropriately after taking part in the program. There was one negative response from a setting that had provided little administrative support for the program and resulted in a chaotic environment. The lack of a coordinated effort presented a barrier to the development of the group cohesion that would have been required in order to address further psychosocial goals.

In its second grant cycle the program continues to thrive, with revisions that were made based upon lessons learned from the previous two years. Some changes were administrative and organizational, while others involved elements of implementation such as documentation. Obstacles that were encountered in the first two years included scheduling, participant surveys, therapists' introduction to the project and its community focus, and a cumbersome mechanism for reporting progress. In the first grant cycle, programming that was delivered during school hours tended to have more consistent results, thanks to a clear indication of support from teachers and principals who were willing to "sacrifice" valuable academic time. All programs now occur during school hours. The participant survey was shortened to nine questions, making it a more user-friendly instrument. Therapist documentation has remained the same, except for implementation of a more streamlined reporting system for individual participant progress.

Owing to the non-traditional nature of the program, in that it integrates clinical and community perspectives, it was found that a more formal training was necessary for creative arts therapists. Training materials now include documentation protocols, rationale for the five domain areas being addressed, and access to program description literature that parents and school staff receive. Since much of the program planning occurred at the administrative level, it was discovered that the Safe Expressions therapists needed to be informed about expectations in order to ensure a consistent, supportive and therapeutic environment.

As a community intervention, Safe Expressions has bridged the gap between community arts programs and community-based creative arts therapies programs in the Greater Philadelphia Region. With clinical knowledge and sensitivity to the psychosocial needs of at-risk youth, the program continues to promote therapeutic learning while embracing talent and creativity.

Acknowledgements

We wish to express our special appreciation to the Pew Charitable Trusts, the creative arts therapists, participants and the collaborating schools for making the Safe Expressions Program possible, and for their part in making the program a success.

References

Amir, D. (2004) 'Community music therapy and the challenge of multiculturalism.' In M. Pavlicevic and G. Ansdell (eds) *Community Music Therapy.* London: Jessica Kingsley Publishers.

Boxill, E.H. (1997) *Students Against Violence Everywhere – SAVE – through Music Therapy: A Manual of Guidelines, Music Therapy Interventions, Music Activities, Music Materials.* New York, NY: Music Therapists for Peace, Inc.

Clawson, H.J. and Coolbaugh, K. (2001) 'The YouthARTS Development Project.' *Juvenile Justice Bulletin,* May 2001. Office of Juvenile Justice and Delinquency Prevention. Accessed July 2005 at http://www.ncjrs.org/ html/ojjdp/2001_5_2/contents.html

Farber, K. (2001) 'Teaching adolescents about community, critical consciousness, and identity through movement.' P. O'Reilley, E. Penn, and K. Demarrais (eds) *Educating Young Adolescent Girls.* Mahwah, NJ: Lawrence Erlbaum Associates, Publishers.

Farnum, M., and Shaffer, R. (1998) *YouthARTS Handbook: Arts Programs for Youth at Risk.* Washington, DC: Americans for the Arts.

O'Brien, M.K. (2001) 'School-based prevention and education programs.' In C. Renzetti, J. Edleson, and R. K. Bergen (eds) *A Source Book on Violence Against Women.* Thousand Oaks, CA: Sage Publications.

Pew Charitable Trusts (2001) 'Request for proposals, programs to serve children, youth, and their families, October 2001.' The Pew Fund for Health and Human Services in Philadelphia.

Philadelphia Safe and Sound (2003) 'Report Card 2003: The well-being of children and youth in Philadelphia.' Accessed July 2005 at http://www.philasafeandsound.org.

Schelly Hill, E. and Howard Jones, C. (2004) 'Pilot year in a creative arts in therapy after-school program in an urban community health center setting.' Poster session presented at the annual conference of the American Dance Therapy Association, New Orleans, LA.

YouthARTS Development Project (1998) YouthARTS Toolkit, Appendix 24. Accessed July 2005 at http://www.americansforthearts.org/YouthARTS/appendices/appendix24/pre-.program_skills_assess.dot

CHAPTER 20

Rediscover, Reclaim and Rejoice

The Sesame Approach of Drama and Movement Therapy with Exploited Girls in India

Sonali Senroy and Priyadarshini Senroy

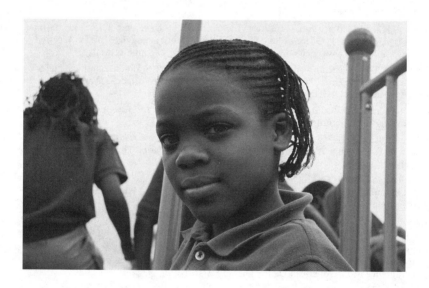

This chapter illustrates the use of the Sesame approach of drama and movement therapy with at-risk girls in the metropolitan city of Kolkata (Calcutta), India. The children described here belong to an increasing number of victims of the sex trade and child labor, often living on the streets. These children have been rescued from various forms of abuse and are currently living in a children's welfare home. An overview of the Sesame approach to drama and movement therapy and detailed case studies describe how the authors provide a therapeutic environment to reclaim and rediscover the inner child of these lost girls and enable the development of healthy and trusting relationships with adults.

India's population reached one billion in 2001 and the country has the most rapidly growing child population in the world. It is estimated that children up to 18 years of age number approximately 400 million, constituting about 40 per cent of the population (Ministry of Indian Human Resources 2002). Approximately 35 million children living in metropolition cities are said to belong to specific categories of at-risk children. Estimates suggest that there are about 4 million child prostitutes, 11 million street children, and about 15,000 children reported missing every year (Child Relief and You 2005a). The increasing number of at-risk children in inner cities in India is directly proportional to current socio-economic factors such as lack of adult employment, lack of access to education, and poverty, which result in migration from rural to urban areas by one or more family members (US Library of Congress 1995). This migration pattern often shifts the family structure from groupings of patri-archal families to single-parent nuclear families, where either the woman becomes the head of the household, or the women and children left behind by male relatives become absorbed into the extended family.

These changes impact on children in different ways, depending on their individual family circumstances. In many of these households, children are treated as the property of the very adults who are supposed to take care of them. Children in these situations are often ordered around, threatened, coerced, silenced, and denied basic rights and freedoms (Child Relief and You 2005b). Many run away from their homes and villages and end up living on the streets in big metropolitan cities.

These children live in environments devoid of the affection, love, caring and comfort of a family life. They have no permanent place to stay, no educational facilities, no facilities for hygiene, and no support system or resources. They are psychologically exploited and abused, and their basic needs for security and happiness are not met. These children lack opportunities for healthy recreation and social acceptance, work and live in unhealthy environments (often suffering from severe malnutrition and health problems such as venereal diseases and AIDS), are abused and exploited, are employed as cheap domestic or commercial laborers, or become involved in the sex trade, where they get lost in the vicious cyle of abuse and often death.

As described by UNICEF (2005), several non-governmental organisations provide services such as safe homes, educational programs, walk-in counselling centers, and vocational training programs to encourage rehabilitation of these children. The children are referred by shelter homes, police, social services, family members, or themselves, depending on the individual circumstances.

All Bengal Women's Federation (ABWF) is one such non-govermental organization in Kolkata which tries to ensure the survival, protection and development of exploited children, specifically girls. The organization runs three residential homes which house 130 girls between the ages of 6 and 14. Most of them are either lost, have run away from their homes, or have been referred through the Juvenile Justice Act. Some are orphans, have been abondoned, or have a single parent. Most have a history of domestic or commercial sexual abuse, along with exploitation and neglect of various kinds.

Their journey begins when they are arrested by the police for petty crimes or during brothel raids. They are kept in custody until they are ordered by the courts to temporary shelter homes. These homes then send them to ABWF for rehabilitation, which includes education, vocational training and therapeutic healing. The children are divided by age group in the residential homes and are primarily taken care of by house mothers. Once in the residential homes, the children are given complete physical, medical, social and psychological assessment. Psychometric tests are conducted to identify problem areas. They undergo medical tests, such as blood, urine, HIV, and skin test, and chest X-rays. After an initial assessment, they are seen by a physician and a psychiatrist who prescribe medication if required. The psychiatrist refers children with mental health issues such as post-traumatic stress disorder, depression, and suicidal tendencies to a team of psychologists and counselors who determine avenues for counseling and therapy.

During their stay the children are sent to integrated schools, which are neighborhood primary schools that accommodate children who have often missed out on their pre-school and kindergarten years. As young adults they are trained in various vocational skills such as sewing, machine knitting, block printing, bakery production, as well as nurses' training, which gives them skills that will make them self-reliant and able to lead their lives with dignity in the future.

The most challenging aspect of this research was the absence of authentic background information about these children. The names, ages, home addresses, and social histories given by the children or their families during psychological assessments often differed from information recorded on social services intake assessment forms. Inability to recollect, fear of stigmatization, or reluctancy to divulge information accounted for these discrepencies.

The three girls described here show similarities in their experiences and behaviors. Whether a victim of child abuse or a runaway, all demonstrated emotional and behavioral challenges in their immediate social and peer relationships. They each received intense counselling to bring them back to normal functioning. The therapeutic interventions mainly entailed regaining their trust, self-respect, and self-esteem. Attempts were also made to bring back their hopes and dreams. The children attended individual sessions until they were ready to join groups. For some, individual sessions continued once they had joined a group. Creative arts therapies interventions were an important part of the multidisciplinary approach of providing psychological, social and economic rehabilitation for these children.

The Sesame approach to drama and movement therapy

One of the therapeutic modalities used in this context was drama and movement therapy based on the Sesame approach pioneered and developed by Marian Lindkvist (Pearson 1996). This innovative approach was found to be successful with this group of children, whose capacity for free, open and joyful expression had become distorted, inhibited and interrupted by abuse and abandonment.

The Sesame approach to drama and movement therapy involves working obliquely, based on the knowledge that most of us reveal the nature of our difficulties through metaphor and symbol. Exploring drama and movement in a safe and structured environment enables people to find ways of expressing their needs, fears, anxieties and frustrations spontaneously and naturally. The Sesame approach uses holistic drama and movement interventions to promote healing and change through an indirect rather than direct approach. As described by Pearson (1996), it is based on three distinct theories: the psychology of Carl Jung, Rudolf Laban's Art of Movement, and Peter Slade's Child Drama.

The focus on opportunities for movement in a Sesame session is informed by the work of Rudolph Laban. Laban worked in the early 20th century as a dancer and choreographer, and developed a language of movement observation and analysis in order to find the connections between motion and emotion. For some people, using movement creatively helps them express that which may not be known to them primarily through talking. Together, client and therapist can explore what emerges through movement, dance and their own body language – using clients' movement as the symbols and images of what needs to be expressed.

The influence of the research work of Peter Slade on how children play spontaneously can be found within the art form of Sesame session work. His central contribution was observing that children spontaneously enact scenes from their imagination when left to themselves to play freely and dramatically. The transformation that Slade noticed in children when they were absorbed in forms of play which engaged their whole selves, physically and emotionally, has its counterpart in Sesame work with people of all ages and abilities. This link between the Sesame experience and Slade's research emphasizes that through drama and movement people can recapture experiences of past states of being in which enjoyment was possible (Pearson pp.94–103).

Each session follows a consistent structure, including a warm-up, main event, and grounding activity. The Sesame toolkit includes enactment, spontaneous dramatic play, and non-verbal expressions using movement and music. Verbal feedback is also encouraged to emphasize the importance of expressive language. The therapeutic process engaged in by the client and the facilitator is based in a non-threatening and creative space. The client is never judged by the quality of her contribution, as the work is not geared towards performance but towards process. All the work during a session is done within the art form, with no attempt at interpretation of personal material (Pearson 1996).

All these qualities of the Sesame approach make the process accessible to children who undertake the therapeutic journey of exploring and expressing a variety of emotions. During the process, they find ways of communicating their inner feelings in a non-judgmental atmosphere created by the playful and spontaneous structure.

Case studies
Rani

Rani is a nine-year-old girl who ran away from her village at the age of six and ended up on the city streets. She claimed that her mother was dead and that her father had remarried and worked in a city far from her village. She was left with her stepmother and stepbrothers. Rani did not go to school like her brothers, and did all the household chores. One of her chores was to make snacks and serve alcohol to her stepmother's male friends. They would often try to touch and fondle her, which Rani did not like. Her refusal to comply was met with severe physical punishment. She remembers overhearing her stepmother making arrangements to send her away as she was considered a burden on the family.

Rani asked her stepbrothers to help her look for her father in the city. They offered to help her run away at night. She remembers drinking milk her brothers gave her and falling asleep. When she woke up, she was on a railway platform, had a terrible pain in her abdomen, and bled during urination. She felt strange and angry at her brothers for abandoning her. She decided to go to the city and look for her father on her own. She got on the first train that arrived, without any ticket. She was caught, handed over to the police, and then to social services, who put her in a shelter home.

In the shelter home the housemothers did not know what to do with Rani's aggression. She would pick fights and hardly sleep at night. She would punch her abdomen whenever she menstruated and refused to bond with her peers. The psychologist who conducted her regular follow-ups referred her to drama therapy to give her an opportunity to work through her feelings. The rationale was that through drama therapy, Rani might be able to discover and express aspects of herself that might not emerge in her everyday life. Of necessity, the home tried to contain the violent rage that many children felt as a result of how they were treated, rather than letting them express it in the course of daily life (Pearson 1996). Drama therapy sessions would provide the opportunity for much-needed emotional expression.

When Rani first came to the sessions, attempts to engage in conversations with her were unsuccessful, despite her curiosity about the materials that were available. To encourage interaction in ensuing sessions, materials to stimulate sensory play, objects and puppets for storymaking and dramatic play, and dolls to explore and express family dynamics, were made accessible (Cattanach 1992). Rani would come in, look around, make eye contact, and somehow manage to smile. She would then sit in silence, look at the objects, flip through the storybooks, or play with the assorted textured and colored fabrics. The session would end with cleaning up and a reminder about the next session. This pattern repeated itself for about four sessions. During one such silent playing session, Rani reached for the objects representing human figures, a house, trees, and vehicles, and placed them in front of her. She sat in front of them for a while and made repeated eye contact with the therapist. Picking up from this non-verbal cue, the therapist made the first move and started to play house.

Rani's eyes followed the activity in silence and then she slowly reached for paper and a crayon. She drew a little girl in black with a big red blob surrounding the image. Then she took her crayons and began to hit the girl over and over again until the paper tore. She was visibly upset. She stood up and curled up on the therapist's lap. As Rani was supported in silence, she said, "Now I know why there was blood coming out from me… if I ever see them, I am going to kill them."

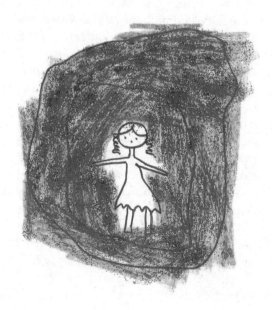

Figure 20.1 Rani's drawing

The power of non-verbal expression through a creative medium is clearly demonstrated in this session. Rani had been almost non-verbal during earlier sessions. Her images, however, "spoke" volumes. Up until Rani made this drawing, she had never understood that she had been sexually abused by her stepbrothers. She seemed to be unaware of what she was drawing as she drew it, but the unconscious surfaced spontaneously during the process of her creating the image. Her artistic process, along with the corresponding dramatization by the therapist, using familiar objects, helped to provide information concerning the actual incident and allowed repressed feelings to resurface where they could be addressed effectively (Kelley 1984).

After this revelation about the source of her aggression, the team decided that Rani should continue attending drama therapy sessions in order to heal, as well as to learn to ask for support from the adults around her. In subsequent sessions, Rani started to play more with the objects in the therapy room. In a ritualistic manner she would arrange and rearrange them, as if trying to recreate different scenarios from her past. She would role-play scenes from her past, such as serving alcohol to her stepmother's friends, often using animated voices. At times she would be overwhelmed, bang the stepmother doll and destroy the scenery. Once the outburst subsided, she would come and sit close to the therapist and ask for a story to be read. Her favorite story was the Indian version of Cinderella. Over time, Rani memorized the story and would recite certains section with animated vocal expressions. She would let out mournful cries when Cinderella was being mistreated. Her moment of total emotional freedom was when the fairy godmother granted wishes, and they came true.

This pattern of reading and dramatization continued until puppets were brought into the session to increase Rani's repertoire of expression. She was excited to see and handle the new props, manipulating them in different ways and using her body as well as her voice. She had a flood of ideas and asked to make her own personal fairy godmother. She said that the fairy godmother would grant her wishes, and in her imaginary world she saw those wishes coming true, especially being reunited with her father.

Rani began to verbalize more freely during this time, and it was crucial to allow her unconscious images and dramatic scenarios to become conscious through verbal connections and acknowledgement in order to achieve therapeutic change (Dokter 1990). Once she was able to understand, identify and name her abuse she suddenly found the words to express how she really felt, and they replaced her anger outbursts. She no longer suffered in silence but had the space and the medium to free her repressed images and give them a name. By verbalizing her needs, her wishes, her fears, and her anger, Rani seemed to make connections with her angry inner child. The fairy godmother was the rescuer that she used metaphorically to re-parent her hurt inner child. With her new-found words Rani seemed to want to be heard, not only by the therapist but by herself too. Finding her inner and outer voices was a therapeutic change which Rani embraced with new-found inner peace.

This inner peace was reflected in her relationships with the housemothers and her peers. During this stage, the housemothers began to notice positive emotional changes in Rani. She began making friends and asking for more support from the housemothers during some of her sleepless nights. She also started to cooperate with authorities to track down her father, still waiting for her wish to come true. The frequency of her individual sessions decreased and she joined a larger group.

Sadia

Sadia is ten years old, and has been looking for her biological family since she was seven. She has no idea which part of the country she is from. All she remembers is that her village is surrounded by large mountains and is always cold. Her parents would go out in the morning and come back late with firewood and water. From her descriptions it is assumed that Sadia is from Nepal, which neighbors India to the north.

Sadia remembered going to the village fair with her family. While she was taking a ride on the giant wheel with her parents, an accident happened and her only recollection was of waking up in the hospital. Her parents had perished in the accident and she was sent to stay with her uncle and aunt. From then on she was brought up by a nursemaid (caretaker or nanny). One night, the nursemaid ran away with Sadia. All she recalls is travelling for many days by bus and train. They finally stopped in a large city where she couldn't recognize the language that people were speaking.

They lived in a house with other girls of her age, and with a woman who said was her aunt. One day the nursemaid left, saying that she was going to work, but she never returned. During this time Sadia was taught the local language, to dance, to put on make-up, and at times was left alone with strange men who would do strange things to her which she never understood.

During a police raid one evening, Sadia was taken away with the other girls and handed over to the shelter home by social services. It was much later that she realized that she had been in a brothel in Kolkata and that the woman was not really her aunt. Sadia never saw the nursemaid again, and realized why she never came back to get her. Since then she has been trying to get back to her native home.

Sadia was different from many of the girls in the shelter home. She was cheerful, sociable, and very creative. She would occasionally suffer from bouts of depression and would behave in an unusual manner. If a parent came to visit another girl, Sadia would urge them to take her home with them. She would become aggressive and would have to be put in isolation. Her behavior would return to "normal" after a couple of days and she would be back to her cheerful self.

On one ocasion Sadia hid in the back seat of a parent's car and had to be returned to the shelter once she was discovered. The shelter authorities were thinking of sending her away to a more secure facility, as they could not handle her behavior. The resident psychologist referred her to drama therapy sessions, hoping these would help Sadia to explain why she was constantly trying to run away. As the situation required constant monitoring, it was decided that she would be kept under close supervision and be given the opportunity to attend intensive sessions every day for a week.

As soon as Sadia realized that the therapist had access to the outside world and was not a housemother, she begged to be taken away. She became inconsolable and it took much explaining and reassurance to pacify her. During the next session, the moment Sadia came in, she hugged the therapist. She seemed to be feeling fragile as her body was trembling and she was on the verge of tears. The therapist hugged her back and began to rock from side to side, humming a lullaby. Sadia slowly began to relax and stayed like that for the whole session. In subsequent sessions, the rocking and the humming became a ritual, with Sadia requesting certain tunes she remembered from her childhood. She would start humming a tune and the therapist would join in.

Gradually the hugging time decreased, until an initial hug at the beginning of a session would be enough for her. Sadia would ask to listen to stories about families or princesses and little girls being rescued and returned home. She would often draw pictures of being rescued. Telling made-up stories while drawing and playing imaginative games was therapeutic and allowed her to communicate her feelings, perceptions and wishes (Lawton and Edwards 1997). During role-playing she would alternate between being the rescuer and being rescued. The therapist took an active role in this exchange. Sadia would overly dramatize the rescue scenes, her dialogues and situations often influenced by Indian movies. Sometimes she would be rescued by being smuggled in the trunk of a car. She used chairs, cardboard boxes, fabrics and dress-up clothes to make the experience as authentic as possible. She would take on the powerful role of the rescuer while the therapist portrayed a vulnerable and defenseless character who was in mortal danger.

By engaging in experiential drama therapy sessions, Sadia slowly began to regain control of her confidence and of her past, as reflected in her improving social and emotional functioning. Sadia's depressive episodes decreased and she no longer tried to run away. Her individual sessions ceased and she joined a group, where she was able to explore other social roles. Seeing her remarkable progress, the social services decided to look for a foster home for Sadia until they could find a way to work with the Nepali authorities to return her to her biological family.

Baby

Eleven-year-old Baby was brought to the shelter home by her biological mother. Baby joined a group on peer relationships. Almost all the girls in the group agreed that the relationship between a mother and a child was pure and good. Baby did not want to share any thoughts and was very quiet. Baby was told by the therapist that there would always be a space for her in the group whenever she was ready to participate. After the end of the next session she came to the therapist and said, "All mothers are not good, at least, not mine," and she left the room.

Two weeks later, the house mother reported that sexually explicit books were found in Baby's possession during one of their surprise check-ups. As a consequence of her actions, all her extracurricular privileges were taken away. That night she was caught by the night guard, trying to run away from the shelter home. She was placed in a watch room. Her mother was informed about her actions, and Baby was warned that if she did not change her ways, she would be expelled from the shelter home.

To give Baby a chance to explain her actions without any pressure, she was referred to drama therapy sessions for a set number of sessions, as a meeting with her mother was scheduled in four weeks' time. The therapist used a time-limited task-based method of play therapy with this client (Cattanach 1994). This intervention can be used effectively to help a client solve a specific, well defined task or problem in a limited period of time. In Baby's case the task was to find out why she had attempted to run away and why she had pornographic books in her possession. The number of sessions, and goals, outcomes, and boundaries were agreed upon by the psychologist, the client and the therapist.

After an initial introduction, various postcard images representing family dynamics, human figures, and social situations were introduced. Baby was invited to choose images that she could relate to. After choosing them she was asked to sort them into "images that made her happy and images that made her sad". During this process Baby was very quiet. The only verbal contribution that ocurred was the therapist reflecting on her happy and sad choices. Baby only nodded. As the session came to an end, Baby asked if she could have a box of drawing materials to take with her.

In the following session Baby came a little early and was very tearful. She started by saying that living with her mother was like a punishment. She did not want to be expelled from the shelter or return to her mother's house. She began sharing her drawings which she had brought with her. The first drawing (Figure 20.2) showed a family scene. The caption read "Dad and us". She explained that she and her sister were both very happy with their parents.

Baby described how slowly she began to experience changes in her family. Her father's business was not doing well and he started drinking and gambling for quick money. Her mother's jewelry was sold to repay his gambling debts, and there was constant tension in the household. Her mother had to take up a job in the local hospital to support the family. It was during this time that Baby's father suddenly left home and never came back. In Figure 20.3 she and her sister are shown crying and, the caption reads, "We are hungry – Daddy please come back".

She explained that she had no idea when her mother started to bring strange men home. She noticed that the material situation in the house began to

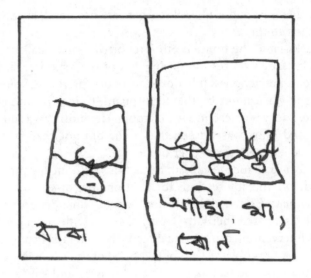

Figure 20.2 Baby's drawing: "Dad and us"

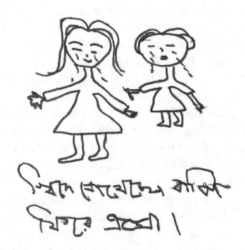

Figure 20.3 Baby's drawing: "We are hungry – Daddy please come back"

improve. They were wearing new clothes and going out to eat in restaurants. When Baby questioned her mother, she was told that these men were her father's friends and that they were helping them out. Baby left it at that until one day she accidentally saw her mother taking a stranger into her bedroom.

Her next drawing (Figure 20.4) showed her mother with a man in the bedroom, with herself and her sister crying outside. The caption read "New papa – no way".

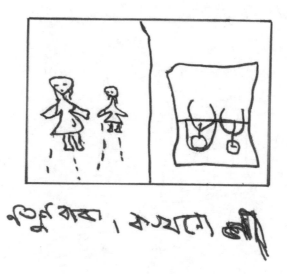

Figure 20.4 Baby's drawing: "New papa – no way"

Upon confrontation, Baby's mother admitted that these men were paying her for sexual favors. Baby felt betrayed and angry, and guilty that she had found out that her mother had become a prostitute. She also found out that her mother had lost her job at the hospital and could not get another one. Things got out of control when the men who came to the house began getting over-friendly with Baby and her sister. Baby's mother sent her sister to live with their grandparents, and Baby was sent to the shelter home. The next drawing (Figure 20.5) shows her mother bringing her to the shelter home and the caption reads "It's a lie, this is not Granny's place".

Baby continued to say that her mother had remarried and wanted to bring the girls home. Baby was not ready to go home, and stated that she would prefer to become a street girl than to go and stay with her mother and "that man". These developments caused Baby much anxiety. She had wanted to look at the sexually explicit materials to understand her mother's lifestyle. During the final session, with the resident psychologist attending, Baby was able to articulate her discomfort with the idea of returning home and the reasons behind her defiant actions at the shelter home. After careful re-examination of the situation, a solution was agreed upon. Baby would have a family session with her mother and the psychologist to discuss the option of returning home. Once at home, her progress would be monitored, and if there were any major concerns about the domestic situation, Baby would be allowed to return to the shelter.

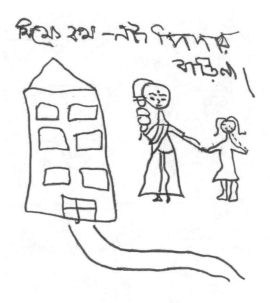

Figure 20.5 Baby's drawing: "It's a lie, this is not Granny's place"

Conclusions

As seen in these case studies, the Sesame approach to drama and movement therapy was found to be very successful in dealing with the trauma faced by Rani, Sadia and Baby. The sessions provided a space that allowed the children to use a variety of modalities to explore and express their emotions and to heal. Some of the children did not even realize what had happened to them. Engaging in therapeutic activities unlocked repressed memories and helped them to gain control over their pasts. The non-threatening approach provided an opportunity for the children to reclaim their lost childhood in a playful and spontaneous, yet structured, environment. They learned to develop healthy and trusting relationships with the adults in the shelter home through positive interactions. Based on the positive outcomes of the sessions and the responses of Rani, Sadia and Baby, it is hoped that more children in the city of Kolkata will be able to experience the magical space called Sesame.

Notes

Owing to the nature of the client group, real names have been changed and artwork has been modified to respect confidentiality, as well as to adhere to the Data Protection Act of the Indian juvenile justice system.

The authors would like to thank the children and staff of ABWF, and the editor and publisher of this book for giving them the opportunity to share their work with a larger audience.

References

Cattanach, A. (1992) *Play Therapy with Abused Children.* London: Jessica Kingsley Publishers.

Cattanach, A. (1994) *Play Therapy. Where the Sky Meets the Underworld.* London: Jessica Kingsley Publishers.

Child Relief and You (2005a) *Child Rights.* Accessed 24 August 2005 at www.cry.org

Child Relief and You (2005b) *Projects/Partnerships: Statistics.* Accessed 24 August 2005 at www.cry.org.

Dokter, D. (1990) 'Symbol and metaphor.' In P. Jones (1996) *Drama as Therapy, Theatre as Living.* London: Routledge.

Kelley, S. J. (1984) 'The use of art therapy with the sexually abused child.' *Journal of Psychosocial Nursing and Mental Health Services 22,* 12, 12–18.

Lawton, S. and Edwards, S. (1997) 'The use of stories to help children who have been abused.' In K.N. Dwivedi (ed.) *The Therapeutic Use of Stories.* London: Routledge.

Ministry of Indian Human Resources (2002) *The Indian Child: A Profile.* New Delhi: Government of India.

Pearson, J. (1996) (ed.) *Discovering the self through Drama and Movement – The Sesame Approach.* London: Jessica Kingsley Publishers.

UNICEF (2005) *Calcutta City-Level Programme of Action for Street and Working Children.* Accessed 24 August 2005 at www.childfriendlycities.org/resources/examples/india.html

US Library of Congress (1995) 'India: A Country Study.' Accessed 24 August 2005 at http://countrystudies.us/india/83.html

CHAPTER 21

A Safe Distance

An Intermodal Approach to Creating a Country Retreat for City Girls who have been Abused

Julie Lacy, Reina Michaelson and Carla van Laar

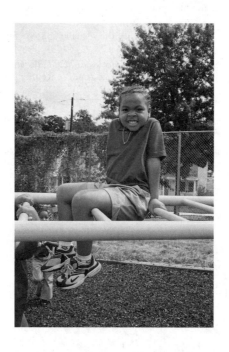

This chapter presents an intermodal approach of working with 10–18-year-old urban girls, within the setting of a country retreat. The girls have either been abused or are at risk of abuse, and some have learning disabilities. The retreat is a house set in ten acres of bushland, 160kms from Melbourne, Australia. The aim of the retreat is to provide a space where the girls can heal from traumatic life experiences and build self-esteem, resilience, and trust in others. It offers a safe environment where the girls can be themselves, and provides recreational, creative, and therapeutic activities. The modalities used include visual arts, narrative, play, drama therapy, playback theatre,

and psychodrama. The experiences of three girls during the retreat illustrate therapeutic principles and processes. While the voices of the girls are their own, names and identifying details have been changed. Therapist voices are also present to explain therapist insights and process.

Introduction

As practitioners we have arrived at a place of shared understanding by travelling different roads. In this chapter we author some sections in the first person, and co-author other sections collaboratively. Rather than "case studies", we present stories about our work with the girls.

Our literary style choice reflects our creative therapeutic practice. By using the first person voice we acknowledge and utilize the subjectivity of the therapist in forming authentic therapeutic relationships. From this perspective, authors are not conceived of as detached scientific observers of situations, but rather acknowledged as subjective, present and active co-participants in therapeutic encounters (Grainger 1999; Hyland Moon 2002; McNiff 1998). We have chosen a storying style in order to reflect the inherently arts-based nature of our work. Hyland Moon describes her style choice as "creative non-fiction, rather than clinical case histories" (p.15). Grainger argues that in researching and presenting the arts therapies, "art should be used to interpret art" (p.128). McNiff calls for discourses in arts therapies literature that more accurately reflect the creative processes and products utilized by arts therapists working creatively with clients. This is exemplified by our use of italics for dialogue, which mirrors dramatic interplay as a core element in our work.

As a facilitation and caregiving team, we share core values, the most central of which is "keeping children safe". Based on shared knowledge, we value thinking, talking, art-making, storytelling, playing, and acting as they relate to safety, self and body image, relationships, bullying, and emotional, physical and sexual abuse.

When utilizing education, visual arts, narrative, play, drama and role we continuously balance our interventions and responses along continuums of distance and closeness, as well as safety and challenge. This balancing involves planned and spontaneous decisions that are informed by our educational, caregiving, artistic and therapeutic sensibilities. This chapter highlights the creation of safety and distance, both physical and metaphorical, and how these translate into therapeutic interventions for the girls.

Background to the retreat and authors' approaches
Julie Lacy

As a psychodrama psychotherapist I use role theory and role dynamics as the underlying philosophy for retreat activities. Drama, play and role are shared elements in the fields of psychodrama, drama therapy and playback theatre.

While these modalities are distinctly different (Bannister 1997, 2003; Chesner 1995; Jennings 1990; Salas 1993), the combining of theory and practice from each can produce wonderfully creative and therapeutic processes for group participants (Blatner 2000).

Role theory relates to the body of knowledge associated with the interactive functioning of human beings (Clayton 1994). Roles encompass consistent patterns of thoughts, beliefs, feelings, behaviours, and interactions that can be developed and modified (Remer 2000). Role dynamics describes a methodology used to investigate, examine, negotiate, develop, change and create roles as they exist in relation to and/or in response to the self, other people, or objects (Blatner and Blatner 2000). Roles are "the actual and tangible forms which the self takes" (Moreno 1964, p.153).

The purpose of using drama, play, and role at the retreat is to offer experiences that enable the girls to express themselves through roles that enhance their safety and well-being and to develop their role repertoire – the range of roles from which they can express and relate. Role training is my method of choice to work with this group.

> Role training aims to bring about the development of specific, limited aspects of human functioning… it does not focus on a total personality reorganisation which is a major intent in a classical psychodrama session. (Clayton 1994, p.142)

Given that we are not engaging the girls in continuous regular retreats, it is essential that their therapeutic process be contained within the time boundaries of the weekend. Role training as opposed to classic psychodrama (where typically they would be revealing personal material in more depth) provides a safe and manageable process for the girls.

It is important, then, in this context, to distinguish my role as a role trainer from that of a psychodrama psychotherapist, and it is important that, as facilitators, we express ourselves through many roles such as supportive advocate, trusted co-creator, creative facilitator, caring teacher, excited motivator, safe boundary maker, interested listener, and inspiring leader. We also need to be spontaneous and develop new roles, should they emerge while relating to the girls.

Spontaneity is defined in psychodrama as an adequate response to a new situation or a new response to an old situation (Fox 1987). My aim is to enable the girls' spontaneity by providing safe activities using dramatic or role distancing (Blatner and Blatner 2000; Jennings 1990). The distance serves as a boundary between the girls and people, objects, or other parts of themselves, and provides safety for the girls as they engage and express. The intended therapeutic effect is to develop spontaneity by expanding their role system. This contributes to the development of their creativity, self-esteem, resilience, and appropriate interpersonal functioning.

Reina Michaelson

In 1995 I founded the Child Sexual Abuse Prevention Program (CSAPP) with the intention of reducing the prevalence and impact of child sexual abuse in Australia. Research available at that time increasingly acknowledged sexual abuse of children as a major social problem (Goldman and Goldman 1987). Furthermore, research indicated that there was a paucity of child sexual abuse prevention initiatives available in Australia, despite the potential effectiveness of education-based programs.

CSAPP provides a variety of workshops that seek to inform and empower children and young people ages 10 to 18. Topics include healthy body image, assertiveness, self-esteem, resilience, positive relationships, and bullying prevention. CSAPP's school-based "Staying Safe With People" program provides young people with information and skills that they can use to identify, avoid, or safely respond to unsafe or potentially abusive situations. All workshops are interactive and use a variety of teaching and therapeutic modalities, including didactic methods, theatre performance, visual arts, music, games, drama and action methods (Bannister 2003; Williams 1989). The workshops are implemented in schools by a team of experienced facilitators. Schools may request that the program be implemented as a preventative approach to personal safety, or to address a particular problem, such as a recent disclosure by a student.

The CSAPP retreat was created in response to the needs of children, as identified through CSAPP's school program, for a safe and rejuvenating environment that could encourage nurturing and supportive relationships with peers and adults (Michaelson 2001). Children who have participated in CSAPP's school-based program and who have been identified by their teachers as requiring further support are referred to the retreat. Retreats are typically run over a weekend or up to five days during school holidays. Up to eight children and six adults can attend a retreat program. Some children may attend the retreat once, while others may attend the retreat numerous times throughout the year, depending on their availability. The regular facilitators include a psychologist with expertise in child sexual abuse, a creative arts therapist, and a psychodrama psychotherapist. Other specialist facilitators may also attend, such as a self-defence instructor, storyteller, and bush gardener. Staff members from the participating school may also attend the retreat, such as the school psychologist, welfare coordinator, or classroom teacher.

Safety is a crucial element of the retreat program, and is achieved at a number of levels. The first is having the retreat physically located at a safe distance from the girls' everyday life – removed enough that they feel safe to explore issues that cause them discomfort, fear or pain, but close enough that they can return home if they need or want to. Another important factor is being surrounded by trusted adults with whom they feel safe or have an established relationship (Ambridge 2001).

Safety is also achieved by the adoption of "safety rules". These include general safety rules, such as the safe use of electrical appliances, fire safety and personal safety, as well as interpersonal safety rules. Disclosures of traumatic and/or abusive experiences in group settings are avoided by introducing an interpersonal safety rule. If a child has experienced unsafe touching of private parts it is safest if they share it privately with an adult they trust rather than with the whole group. We would say, for example, "You may feel like telling the whole group about your experience, especially if we are talking about the topic. However, after sharing such a personal experience with the whole group, you may wake up tomorrow morning and wish you hadn't told *everyone*. So, in order to help you feel safe, if you have a personal experience to do with unsafe touching of private parts that you wish to share with someone, it is safest to talk privately about that experience with an adult you trust in the group, rather than share it with the whole group." These safety rules are articulated and agreed upon by the girls at the beginning of the retreat. All adults model safe boundaries and appropriate touching, both with the children and with each other. For example, "Giving hugs can be good for saying hello or good-bye, or when someone is upset, but not all the time." It is important for girls who have had their personal boundaries violated and who have difficulty forming appropriate boundaries with others to experience this appropriate adult modelling.

Other principles from the "Staying Safe With People" program are interwoven in all retreat activities. Topics such as safe and unsafe touching, recognising early warning signs, the "No–Go–Tell" rule (if someone is making you feel unsafe, say no, run away and tell someone you trust, and keep telling until someone helps you), building a personal safety network, talking to someone you trust, persistence in telling, and remembering that the offender is always responsible in cases of abuse, are ever-present themes throughout the retreat experience.

Another important factor in the development of a safe environment is being prepared for, and responding appropriately to, disclosures of abuse. Girls who disclose are given the opportunity to share their experiences and feelings privately with one or more adults providing support. For example, "I'm glad you told me this. It can be difficult to share such experiences with others. You have been very brave, and I will work with you and help you to stay safe from now on." If a report to Protective Services is required, or ongoing counselling is necessary, this is sensitively explained (Palmer 2001).

Carla van Laar

My experience working in the field of creative arts therapy and my practice as a visual artist informs how I engage with the girls during the retreats. My philosophical approach is built on the arts, play, and narrative. The arts are integral to human experience. More than merely metaphor or rehearsal, the arts are ways of communicating, exploring, understanding, choosing, destroying, creating, transforming, knowing, and being (Bannister 2003; Hyland Moon 2002; McNiff 1998). When people are supported and secure, they can play within the arts, experimenting and taking reasonable risks. People safely experience ways of knowing, acting, and being that are transferable to many situations, through the therapeutic distance offered by creative play within the arts (Cattanach 1997). People can author their own life stories through their actions and inter-actions (Freeman, Epston and Lobovits 1997; White and Epston 1990).

I am aware that the girls have been referred to the retreat because they have been, or are at risk of being, emotionally, physically, and/or sexually abused. This general awareness persists until individuals choose to disclose more. Things that children should ideally take for granted, such as having a stable and caring home life, knowing what is appropriate behaviour, having strong social networks, or feeling safe, cannot be assumed in this context. In planning and facilitating activities I aim to create opportunities for the girls to feel safe, and to experience themselves as creative, valuable, active and contributing individuals in the world. My role as a therapist is to encourage, support, witness and cele-brate the girls as they bravely engage in these opportunities.

The retreat in action

After the two-hour drive watching the scenery change from city roads and power poles to dirt tracks and gum trees, we all piled out of the dusty van. Rain was drizzling but spirits were far from dampened. Even before the van was unloaded, the girls went straight to the dormitory bedroom, chose their beds for the night, and were settling in. Many hugs of greeting were exchanged between girls from different schools who hadn't seen each other since the last retreat. Within half-an-hour everyone was seated at the table (which was covered with a familiar patchwork tablecloth that the girls had created at a previous retreat), eating pizza and salad with the potbelly wood-burning stove blazing, and catching up on news. Hilde (12) accidentally spilled her juice on the tablecloth. Her reaction gave voice to the unspoken pain that the girls brought with them:

Hilde: *If anybody is going to spill something, spill it on my patch, because mine is the only one with a stain on it. Nobody else's has got a stain on it.*

Session One: "Totems" with Carla

After lunch I gathered the girls in the lounge for the first activity. Before I had figured out how to introduce the idea, I was offered the perfect lead.

Mia: *Is it something scary?*

Carla: *No – it's the opposite of scary! What would that be?*

The girls responded — *"brave"*, *"courageous"*, *"unfearful"*, and, with prompting, *"safe"*. Hilde demonstrated how difficult it was for her to feel safe by snuggling up on a dining chair before falling on the floor.

> **Hilde:**   *You're all nice and cosy…and then suddenly, someone rips the chair out from under you!*

As a group, we acknowledged that having the chair pulled out from under you would definitely make us feel unsafe, and used this opportunity to agree on how to behave towards each other during the retreat: with respect for safety and privacy.

The opening activity invited the girls to make totems about safety. This offered an opportunity to explore and create a protected environment for the rest of the weekend. We started by going for a walk through the grounds of the retreat, finding out how far it extended, and physicalizing the concept of safe boundaries by discovering the exact perimeters of the property. We walked through the long grass, discussing how to keep safe from snakes by making lots of noise, and how to keep safe from being lost by always staying together. We collected natural materials such as rocks, sticks, and grasses. Everyone was invited to find a place out-of-doors, close to the house, and to each use what she had found to create a totem as a guardian of the house for the weekend. Some of the girls worked together, and some worked individually.

They became engrossed in their constructions, some talking about meaning, others working silently. Zoe (17) and Mia (14) made an altar on a tree stump. They explained the significance of the different elements they had used.

> **Zoe and Mia:** *Flowers for welcoming and love. Pretty, when you see flowers you are happy because they're beautiful. Straw for calmness and gentle because they're so frail. A stick for strength. Rocks for togetherness, we'll all be here for each other, solid. An altar for remembrance, like a temple, it's yours only.*

In contrast, Hilde chose to revisit a grave she had made the year before for three dead mice. She told us about it.

> **Hilde:**   *I dug them up* [the dead mice] *and put them all back together again. It doesn't sound very pleasant but it was. The flowers represent the mice's souls blossoming in heaven. The dry grass represents the retreat, the outback. The green sticks represent the mice's lifelines. Did you notice that when I told you about the third mouse that died it was raining, but after I explained it all* [the totem] *the sun came out. I wonder why that was?*

In choosing to offer totems as a starting point, I made use of solid external objects, with the intention of providing aesthetic distance through which the girls could engage in an active meditation on the theme of safety. The different ways they engaged in this activity and expressed themselves within it enabled us, as facilitators, to have an understanding of where each girl "was at" at the beginning of the retreat. In particular, I was struck by Zoe and Mia's "altar", which seemed like a perfect formula for safety. Reina and I later reflected that it was like laying the foundations for a safe environment so that more difficult aspects of the girls' experiences could be creatively explored. We also reflected that Hilde's fascination with attending to the graves of three long-dead mice was in keeping with her frequent comments about death and dying.

Session Two: "Animal Planet" with Julie

The second activity the girls engaged in was drama-based. "Animal Planet" uses animal roles as a means of creating distance to explore reparative relating and role training in staying safe. Children who have been abused may have difficulties with maintaining appropriate physical and emotional boundaries (Bannister 1991, 1997, 2003). Animal Planet allows for the giving and receiving of safe physical touching including shaking hands, patting backs, and the occasional hug. This relating enables the girls to find safe ways to connect, interact, and give and receive care.

The girls made themselves comfortable on the lounge floor, closed their eyes and prepared for a journey to Animal Planet. They imagined themselves as their favourite animal and were asked to make a safe habitat for themselves. I prompted them to come out and play with the other animals, using their animal sounds and movements to communicate with each other. I asked half of them to pretend that they were wounded animals. The others were invited to find a way to care for the wounded ones. Hilde, in role as a lion, went to Zoe, who was in role as a wounded tiger, and pretended to scratch her across the face. Hilde then tried to care for another animal and tripped, yelling *"Ouch!"* It appeared to be difficult for her to be in the carer role and more natural for her to be wounded and attacking. When the roles of wounded and caring animals were reversed, Zoe moved immediately to Hilde to care for her, and Hilde was able to receive her empathic attention.

Carla entered Animal Planet in role as a threatening animal. In response, Hilde followed the animal to attack it. Mia, in role as a kangaroo, jumped away. The animals were given the power of language so they could discuss what to do about the threatening animal.

Zoe:	*How do we get rid of it?*
Hilde:	*You attack it.*
Zoe:	*Maybe we should go up to it and see how it reacts. Maybe it's shy or territorial, or just scared and acting tough to hide its fear. If we are friendly and welcoming, it might see that we are not threatening.*

Mia:	*I think we should step back in case it tries to attack us. We could run off if it attacks, or all of us could surround it and let it know it's on our territory. It can come in if it's not going to act dangerously.*
Hilde:	*We could give him* [the animal had become a "him" now] *a warning first. If he's not going to agree to what we are trying to do, we should attack it ourselves.*
Zoe:	*We should have a welcoming approach. If it doesn't work we can use self-defence and say "back off".*

Zoe was empathetic to the animal's feelings, and willing to be "trusting accepter", while also wary as "cautious planner". Hilde became "destructive attacker". She was keen to take control of the situation, but her suggestions to attack would have meant putting herself at risk, given the animal was much bigger and stronger than she. Mia's response as "careful organiser" reflected a safer and more boundaried approach. I asked the "animals" to look closely at the face of the threatening animal to help them decide whether they were safe having it near them.

Hilde:	*It looks angry and disturbed.*
Zoe:	*It needs to be helped.*
Hilde:	*It's evil.*
Mia:	*I'm scared of it, but the other part of me wants to help it.*
Hilde:	*It's not scary but I'm worried it's going to hurt the other animals like the cats and dogs. I'm not scared of it because I'm a lion!*

Hilde saw a disturbed inner state in the threatening animal and a propensity to attack. Zoe interpreted that it needed help. These observations could be compared to assessments of an abuser. Mia, despite her fear, wanted to help the animal. We are reminded that children in abusive situations can experience conflicted role responses, causing extreme confusion, especially when the abuser is someone the child loves or trusts (Ambridge 2001).

Pam, the school counsellor, now entered Animal Planet in role as Queen of the Animals to role-model a safe approach. She chose to be an albatross because they always steer people in ships to safe places.

Pam:	*I'm not seeing kind eyes. I'm seeing cold eyes and a hard mouth. I'm steering you all to a safe place now. Come with me.* [The animals happily followed her as she swept her wings up high and enfolded them in her giant wingspan. She turned to the threatening animal.] *I'm now banishing you from Animal Planet forever!*

I told the animals they were free to play safely again, which they did. Hilde ran to the couch, which the threatening animal had moved, and pushed it back to where it had been, thus re-establishing the safe boundary. We completed the session with everyone de-roling and sharing.

> **Zoe:** *I liked the way we worked together and shared care and respect towards each other.*
>
> **Hilde:** *The really mean animal treated me like I wasn't worth anything.*
>
> **Carla:** *That's a good way to tell if you are unsafe.*
>
> **Hilde:** *Its like you've been stabbed when people say, "You're nothing." You shouldn't even be in this world. Sometimes they don't even have to say anything. It's body language.*

Again, Hilde returned to her ever-present theme of non-existence. In previous retreats Hilde had found it difficult to play with the others, often sitting by herself and crying. In this sharing she was able to shed the distance of the animal role and speak about her own feelings. By expressing herself from the role of "worthless nothing" she was developing the progressive role of "courageous truth speaker".

Session Three: "Talent Show"

There are always unplanned, unfacilitated, but very significant moments during retreats. After dinner in front of the fire, we – Julie and Carla – had one such moment with Zoe. She confided that she had been crying six out of seven days a week, that she was feeling isolated and emotionally at the end of her tether, and that she wanted to move out of her home and care for herself. We discussed these things at length and in detail. We talked about how brave, strong and beautiful Zoe is, and also about people she can trust and turn to when she needs to talk. Through the act of talking and being heard, Zoe told us, she felt a lot better already.

When the conversation was finished we all gathered in the lounge room for the "Talent Show", a traditional feature of each retreat, which provides an opportunity for the celebration of the girls' strengths and talents. A red velvet curtain was hung as a backdrop, creating a sense of theatre. Traditionally, each girl performs an act for the group, such as dancing, singing, reciting poetry, or stand-up comedy. The atmosphere was celebratory and encouraging. Zoe opted to take a leadership role as "MC". She introduced the other girls' acts with encouragement and appreciation for their uniqueness, talents and courage. Her ability to make others feel good about themselves reflected the earlier conversation and illustrated her attempts to treat others in the way she wants to be treated.

At the end of the performances the girls were invited to visit the "Magical Toy Room", a toy-filled room painted with rainbows, trees, and waterfalls, to choose a toy to take home. We explained that each toy is a keepsake from this happy time, and serves as a tangible connection with their talents, strengths, and personal courage. Some girls have taken their toys with them to help them feel secure in exceptionally challenging situations, such as testifying in court.

Session Four: "Magic Shop" with Julie

The final session of the day was "Fantastic Magic Shop" an adaptation of the traditional warm-up activity, Magic Shop (Blatner 1997; Starr 1977). In this context we used it as a grand finale to the evening, co-facilitated by Carla as the shopkeeper in role as "beautiful Fairy Godmother", spinning a pink parasol. The shop became a therapeutic container in which the girls could spontaneously create what they needed through the distancing of fantasy (Bannister 2003). My role was "curious, supportive director", while Reina's was "excited, appreciative witness". The Fairy Godmother's task was to trade something the girls no longer wanted or needed for something they did want or need. I supported the girls to step up and start negotiating with the Fairy Godmother. Unwanted items were stored in an imaginary "safe" under the shop counter, and the new items were dramatically mimed and presented to the girls.

> **Zoe:** I'd like to get rid of some of my tears. I cry six days out of seven. If I could get rid of three-quarters of that it would be good. Everyone needs to cry every now and then so I'll keep a quarter for regular, normal times to cry...

Zoe used an imaginary vacuum-cleaner to draw out her river of tears, and used the reverse cycle to deposit them into the Fairy Godmother's upturned parasol.

> **Fairy Godmother:** Would you like me to use some of these tears to water the daffodils?
>
> **Zoe:** Yes, please, and then put the rest in the safe... I also need a fresh start.
>
> **Fairy Godmother:** Would you like one fresh from the fridge or the oven?
>
> **Zoe:** A vanilla fresh start with sprinkles on top. Plus some extra happiness. I really need one ASAP. In a colorful sparkly take-away bag made of satin with daffodils.

After building a solid foundation through her totem, expressing the caring part of herself in Animal Planet, and chatting privately about her problems by the fire, Zoe chose to use the distance of the Magic Shop to reveal her vulnerability, with the whole group as the audience. The group witnessed her in the role of "truthful self-nurturer" as she expressed her needs to those she trusted.

Having witnessed Zoe's exchange, Mia confidently stepped up to the shop.

Mia:	*Can I trade in all my anger? Can I give you my life's worth of anger?*
Julie:	*Do you want to give her all your anger?*
Mia:	*I think I'll keep a bit for myself, but I don't want to be angry all the time anymore. I'll keep some just to protect myself.*

In expressing her request for something new, Mia spontaneously engaged in the creation of her own internal "fantastic" safe place.

Mia:	*I would like my own secret garden so that no-one can bother me when I need time out and so nobody can come into it.*
Fairy Godmother:	*What kind of garden would you like?*
Mia:	*Like the Garden of Eden. No walls. No people. But with animals like Pegasus, plus a waterfall, with two trees and a hammock. Blue sky, no clouds, sun, fruit, but no forbidden fruit, and where the animals are playing with each other.*
Fairy Godmother:	*How would you like to have this garden?*
Mia:	*I'll have it compressed and put it in my heart so no one knows that I have it.*

Mia's expression of safety through her totem, and her warm-up in Animal Planet, appear to have enabled her to develop her spontaneity. By creating a safe garden into which she could retreat, and by placing it in her heart, she created the role of "protective self-carer". Her request that there be no forbidden fruit and no people seemed to free her from "scared carer" of others to "loving carer" of self.

Hilde stepped up to the shop.

Hilde:	*I don't know what I want to get rid of. Oh yeah – my cough. And my back pain. The pain is in my whole back. It's white, dead pain. Deadly pain. I'll just rip it out of my back. I'm just weird.*

Eighteen months earlier, at a similar retreat during Magic Shop, Hilde had asked for a new body because she felt her body was dead. In the interim she had spoken of wanting to kill herself. Throughout the retreat she suffered from a chronic cough and made frequent complaints about various bodily ailments, a common sign of embodiment of the trauma of sexual abuse (Bannister 2003). Hilde coughed into the parasol, then reached over her shoulder, wrenched the "pain" out of her back, and deposited both into the safe.

Hilde: *I don't know what to get [she spent some minutes deciding]... a unicorn. A white unicorn. Life size. Big enough for me to ride on. It would give me fun.*

Fairy Godmother: *Can you think of the name of the unicorn? The unicorn will come when its name is called.*

Hilde: *I can't think of a name.* [She spent more minutes trying.]

Fairy Godmother: *What does the unicorn look like?*

Hilde: *It's white with blue eyes... a pink horn... loves to eat salad and chips... Its name... is... Reina!*

Reina became the unicorn and Hilde rode on her back around the room, with the rest of us waving and calling up to her as she flew past us. When Reina put her down she was crying and laughing at once.

Hilde: *I'm just too happy! I'm too happy!* [She gradually stopped laughing and smiled through her tears.] *I really am alive!!*

I am aware that one of the medieval myths surrounding the unicorn is that it symbolises purity and innocence. I saw Hilde's choice as a beautiful act of claiming back her childhood. By naming the unicorn Reina, Hilde allowed herself to acknowledge and receive Reina's care, as her emerging role of "happy, alive child" was born.

All the girls' unwanted pain was left under the table in the "safe" overnight, and the next morning Carla brought the "safe" outside to the campfire. The girls, one by one, opened it and ceremoniously threw their pain into the flames.

Session Five: "Choose your own Adventure" with Carla

For Sunday morning we planned a breakfast barbeque and "choose your own adventure" outing to a local park, with the intention of giving the girls the opportunity to have experiences outside of the contained space of the retreat. The adventure outing is a regular event, and a common feature of these excursions is the inclusion of a portable CD player, with the girls' own choice of music providing a soundtrack for our wacky adventures. As we boarded the minibus, I spontaneously adopted the role of a kooky flight attendant named "Cabina Crew". Ms Crew explained the safety features of the craft, including the option of bells, whistles, flare guns, and our team of rescue helicopters if we were to land in crocodile-infested waters. Ms Crew then invited the girls to think about their adventure.

Cabina Crew: *It's your choice what we do when we get there... Some ideas might be something you have done before that you enjoy or something new.*

Mia:	*Can we play games?*
Zoe:	*Can it be Chick Footy?*
All:	*Yeah! Wow! Let's!*

"Chick Footy" is a game invented at a previous retreat. It involves turning up the volume of the girls' favourite pop songs, kicking the football to each other, running, wrestling, yelling, screaming, cheering, and generally being noisy and taking up public space!

On disembarking from our "craft" after "landing", Julie started cooking breakfast and it was my job to have a Chick Footy adventure with the girls. We discovered that the football had been left at home! As Cabina Crew, I officially sent an SOS message to Reina via my mobile phone, and loudly announced that there was no need to panic because our backup team was bringing the football to the park. This meant we had to fill time and try to keep warm on the bitterly cold morning. Zoe offered to lead us in some stretching exercises. Hilde sat to the side, shivering and complaining. I walked over to her and took her hands, gently pulling her to a standing position, propelling her forward with my hands on her hips.

Cabina	
Crew:	*Where are we going, Hildeena Crew? It's up to you. Come on everybody, all aboard, Hildeena is taking us on an adventure.*

The other girls obligingly joined the "train". Hilde started at a slow shuffle around the outskirts of the park, then, declaring it was boring, headed for the adventure playground and proceeded to dazzle us with a marvellous exhibition of her physical prowess, leading us through tunnels, around sharp corners, under low-lying obstacles, jumping from platforms with dizzying precision to the flying fox – all of which we had to follow! When Reina arrived with the football we were warmed up for a good game of Chick Footy.

In Australia the game of football is a very male sport, with women generally taking spectator roles. Chick Footy is definitely not a spectator sport! I found the sights and sounds of the girls claiming their rights to be seen and heard and actively enjoying their physicality very moving, not least because of my awareness of the traumas they have been through. Playing Chick Footy seemed to embody the exact opposite of Hilde's comment from the previous day, "you shouldn't even be in this world".

On our way back, after breakfast, Hilde happily adopted the role of fellow crew member Hildeena Crew, reminding passengers of safety requirements, helping to cross-check cabin doors, and navigating us back to the house.

Session Six: Assessing the Retreat – "Playback Moments"

In order to provide enjoyable and rewarding experiences that are relevant to the girls' needs, an evaluation is conducted at the end of each retreat. Different formats are used, including anonymous written feedback, or a playback theatre session (Salas 1993). The evaluation seeks to discover what aspects of the retreat the girls found most and least enjoyable, rewarding, useful and challenging.

We chose playback theatre. Playback is a theatre form where audience members tell personal stories that are real events from their lives and watch them immediately "played back" by actors and musicians. The performers may be brought in as a professional team, or they may be a part of the group. The storyteller is known as the "teller" and the facilitator of the playback theatre performance is called the "conductor". There are specific techniques or forms that the performers use to convey short moments, and a range of improvisatory styles to illustrate and interpret longer stories. This very flexible model is used throughout the world in a broad range of contexts, from clinical, to community, to corporate. It has been adapted for the retreat program to maximize teller and performer participation in a safe and playful manner, and to minimize concern for theatre aesthetic.

Sitting around the campfire, the girls reflected on challenging and important moments from the weekend. Julie conducted each girl in role as the "teller" to express their moments. Reina and the other girls were the audience. Carla role-modelled acting in every story moment, and was joined by two different girls from the audience who became actors in each story. As conductor, Julie directed the actors to sculpt with their bodies a "frozen moment" or "photograph" to show the story moment. The teller was invited to comment on how she felt after witnessing her moment played back.

Julie interpreted the girls' story moments, using role descriptions as a component of the evaluation. We contrasted the girls' commentaries about their most challenging moments with their responses to their most rewarding moments. We thus observed the girls' transition. They began the retreat in a "place" where they were relating through roles that isolate and inhibit. They travelled to a "new place" by exploring, discovering, developing and strengthening progressive, functional roles (Clayton 1994). Expressing themselves in these roles enabled them to experience connection and spontaneity. In practical terms, for the girls in their everyday lives, connection promotes their ability to form mutually respectful and caring relationships, while spontaneity enables them to adapt and respond creatively to challenges in their lives. This is best illustrated by their own voices, which we present with the closing thoughts.

Closing thoughts

Zoe: *I found it hard to push out the negative stuff from home and school and to focus on the good things happening. I was worried how my behaviour would affect other people.*

Zoe:	*I had a deep and meaningful conversation with Carla and Julie. I felt important and cared for and good about myself. I felt like dancing! It was really good.*

Zoe's story moments reveal her retreat journey from "depressed daughter", "isolated student", and "anxious acceptance seeker" to "truthful revealer", "trusting teller", "nurtured self-appreciator" and "joyful dancer".

Mia:	*Trying to remember who everybody is. I felt embarrassed that I should have known who you* [Julie and others] *were.*
Mia:	*Being here with all my friends and getting to know people even more.*

Mia's retreat story changes from casting herself as "forgetful, embarrassed retreat member" to being "comfortable retreat member", "accepted friend", and "happy socialiser".

Hilde:	*When I had to see the mice that had died, again, I was angry that nature had ruined their home, so I made a decision that I would fix it up and create a new mouse home. I buried the mice next to each other and made the new home nice and solid.*
Hilde:	*My most important moment was meeting everyone and spending time with my lovely friend Zoe and with Reina. I was very, very happy.* [The actors played back the moment.] *It's making me happy just looking at the photo of happiness!*

Hilde's retreat journey shows her being "angry mouse carer", "decisive creator", and "determined re-constructor", and seeing herself as "happy socialiser", "loving friend" and "happy self-appreciator".

Creating safety and distance for ourselves
Julie

A shared emotional debrief in the bus en-route home with Carla, a bath and lighting a candle to honour the courage of the girls and writing in my journal was how I created some distance for myself immediately after the retreat. The following day I dealt with the moments that had a profound impact on me in my personal therapy and supervision session, using psychodramatic methods. The effects of these processes both sustain a safe distance and deepen and enrich the privileged journey of working with these beautiful girls.

Reina

Enjoyable and fulfilling as the retreats are, they are also quite exhausting! In celebration of a wonderful retreat, I rewarded myself with a scented bubblebath, flickering candles and soft music. I reminded myself of the joy that is found in witnessing others transform pain and grief into joy and strength... And then I fell asleep!

Carla

My personal time to create safety and distance for myself comes when I go for a jog in the park, do yoga, and when I write or paint. After this retreat I was running in the winter sun around a local inner city park, when these words came to me:

Dear Zoe,
Thank you
for leaving your river of tears
in the vase
with the daffodils

It seems that they have been
magically transformed
by the colour
of the flowers

Because today, when I was jogging
I felt an amazing sensation
a buoyancy
an energy
carrying me onward

A golden river in full stream
flowing through
my heart and
washing away my doubts and fears

It was your tears
that you don't need so many of

Thank you
for leaving some
for me.

EPILOGUE: E-MAIL FROM ZOE TO CARLA TWO WEEKS AFTER THE RETREAT

Zoe: *Hey Carla, great to hear back from you… Yes the tears have lessened immensely!! How have things been for you?*

Note
Julie Lacy, Reina Michaelson and Carla van Laar have worked as a team in the Child Sexual Abuse Prevention Program (CSAPP) since 2000. Together they have recently co-designed and facilitate "Chill Skills", an anxiety prevention program for adolescents, with Anxiety Disorders Association of Victoria (ADAVIC).

References
Ambridge, M. (2001) 'Monsters and angels: how can child victims achieve resolution?' In S. Richardson and H. Bacon (eds) *Creative Responses to Child Sexual Abuse: Challenges and Dilemmas.* London: Jessica Kingsley Publishers.

Bannister, A. (1991) 'Learning to live again: psychodramatic techniques with sexually abused young people.' In P. Holmes and M. Karp (eds) *Psychodrama: Inspiration and Technique.* London: Routledge.

Bannister, A. (1997) *The Healing Drama: Psychodrama and Dramatherapy with Abused Children.* London: Free Association Books.

Bannister, A. (2003) *Creative Therapies with Traumatised Children.* London: Jessica Kingsley Publishers.

Blatner, A. (1997) *Acting-In: Practical Applications of Psychodramatic Methods.* (3rd edition). New York: Springer.

Blatner, A. & A. (2000) *Foundations of Psychodrama: History, Theory and Practice.* (4th edition.) New York: Springer.

Cattanach, A. (1997) *Children's Stories in Play Therapy.* London: Jessica Kingsley Publishers.

Chesner, A. (1995) *Dramatherapy for People with Learning Disabilities: A World of Difference.* London: Jessica Kingsley Publishers.

Clayton, M. (1994) 'Role theory and its application in clinical practice.' In P. Holmes, M. Karp, and M. Watson (eds) *Psychodrama since Moreno: Innovations in Theory and Practice.* London and New York: Routledge.

Fox, J. (1987) (ed.) *The Essential Moreno: Writings on Psychodrama, Group Method and Spontaneity.* New York: Springer.

Freeman, J. Epston, D. and Lobovits, D. (1997) *Playful Approaches to Serious Problems.* New York: Norton.

Goldman, R.J. and Goldman, J.D.G. (1987) 'The prevalence and nature of child sexual abuse in Australia.' *Australian Journal of Sex, Marriage and Family 9,* 94–106.

Grainger, R. (1999) *Researching the Arts Therapies: A Drama Therapist's Perspective.* London: Jessica Kingsley Publishers.

Hyland Moon, C. (2002) *Studio Art Therapy.* London: Jessica Kingsley Publishers.

Jennings, S. (1990) *Dramatherapy with Families, Groups and Individuals: Waiting in the Wings.* London: Jessica Kingsley Publishers.

McNiff, S. (1998) *Art-based Research.* London: Jessica Kingsley Publishers.

Michaelson, R. C. (2001) 'Development, Evaluation and Revision of the Child Sexual Abuse Prevention Program.' Unpublished manuscript.Victoria University of Technology, Victoria, Australia.

Moreno, J. L. (1964) *Psychodrama.* Vol.1. (3rd edition.) New York: Beacon House Inc.

Palmer, T. (2001) 'Pre-trial therapy for children who have been sexually abused'. In S. Richardson and H. Bacon (eds) *Creative Responses to Child Sexual Abuse: Challenges and Dilemmas.* London: Jessica Kingsley Publishers.

Remer, R. (2000) 'Secondary victims of trauma: Producing secondary survivors.' In P.F. Kellermann and M.K. Hudgins (eds) *Psychodrama with Trauma Survivors: Acting out Your Pain.* London: Jessica Kingsley Publishers.

Salas, J. (1993) *Improvising Real Life: Personal Story in Playback Theatre.* Iowa: Kendall/Hunt Publishing Company.

Starr, A. (1977) *Rehearsal for Living: Psychodrama.* Chicago: Nelson Hall.

White, W. and Epston, D. (1990) *Narrative Means to Therapeutic Ends.* New York: Norton.

Williams, A. (1989) *The Passionate Technique: Strategic Psychodrama with Individuals, Families and Groups.* London: Routledge.

The Contributors

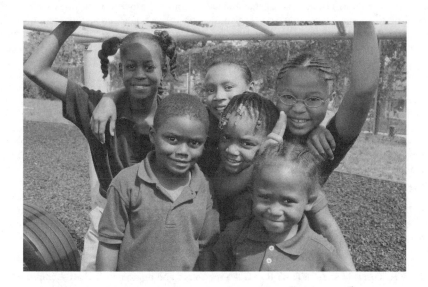

Vanessa Camilleri, MA, MT-BC (editor) is a third generation educator and has always been an advocate for underprivileged children. She is a classically trained pianist, which has allowed her the freedom of exploring improvization and personal expression through music. She received her B.A. in Psychology and Education from Vassar College in Poughkeepsie, New York, and her M.A. in Music Therapy from New York University. She has started two music therapy programs in inner city charter schools in New York City and Washington, DC, where she has focused on prevention through the development of social skills that enable children to succeed in their classrooms and in life. She has supervised undergraduate and graduate-level students of music therapy, published several journal articles and book chapters, and has presented at regional and national conferences. She has worked at several summer camps and after-school programs for at-risk youth, using drum circles and therapeutic activities to facilitate community building. She has held several administrative positions (discipline committee, student support team, middle states accreditation) and served on various school improvement and expansion committees. She is currently exploring the importance of social emotional learning in schools, and firmly believes that if children are socially and emotionally well, they will succeed academically and personally. She lives in Washington, DC with her husband, Steve.

Diane Austin, DA, ACMT is the Director of the Center for Music Psychotherapy at Turtle Bay Music School in New York City, where she offers a two-year certificate program in music psychotherapy, focusing on the voice. Dr Austin has maintained a private practice in music psychotherapy for 17 years, supervises music therapists, and has been a member of the Music Therapy faculty at New York University for 13 years. She is the co-founder and was the director of the music therapy program for adolescents in foster care at the Turtle Bay Music School, has lectured and taught internationally on the use of the voice in in-depth music psychotherapy, and her work has been published in many journals and books. She recently completed her doctoral dissertation, which illuminates her own method of in-depth music psychotherapy.

Mark Bottos, MCAT, DTR resides in Doylestown, PA and is a dance/movement therapist with over 17 years' experience of working with individuals with developmental disabilities and within the autistic spectrum. He is the Assistant Director of the Kardon Institute for Arts Therapy in Philadelphia where he coordinates several programs and supervises creative arts therapists and interns. Mark has co-facilitated rhythm-and-motion workshops with Flossie Ierardi, music therapist, for university-level music students and music educators. He is the President of the Pennsylvania chapter of the American Dance Therapy Association. In addition to his clinical and administrative work, he facilitates movement/dance improvisations and instruction in Latin and ballroom dances for adults and youth.

Tian Dayton, PhD is the author of *The Living Stage: A Step by Step Guide to Psychodrama, Sociometry and Experiential Group Therapy* (2005, Deerfield Beach, Fl: Health Communications) and of the bestsellers *Forgiving and Moving On* (1994, Deerfield Beach, Fl.: Health Communications) and *Trauma and Addiction* (2000, Deerfield Beach, Fl.: Health Communications) as well as twelve other titles. Dr Dayton spent eight years at New York University as a faculty member of the drama therapy department. She is a fellow of the American Society of Psychodrama, Sociometry and Group Psychotherapy (ASGPP), winner of their scholar's award, executive editor of the psychodrama academic journal, and sits on the professional standards committee. She is a certified Montessori teacher through 12 years of age. She is currently the Director of the New York Psychodrama Training Institute at Caron, New York, and in private practice in New York City. Dr Dayton has a Masters in Educational Psychology, a Ph.D in clinical psychology, and is a board certified trainer in psychodrama, sociometry and group psychotherapy. For further information log on to tiandayton.com.

Ashley R. Dorr, MA, LCAT, ATR-BC is a registered and board certified art therapist who is working in New York City at The Door, a Center of Alternatives. She has worked there since 2001 as an art therapist and senior counselor for a school suspension program with junior high and high-school students. She is also a professional facilitator for Free Arts, NYC where she facilitates groups with families. She has run art therapy groups for children around issues of trauma in relation to 9/11, and in relation to refugee experiences. In August 2005 she traveled to Sri Lanka, where she provided art therapy to children orphaned by ethnic war, poverty, and the tsunami.

Craig Haen, MA, RDT, CGP is a drama therapist who resides in New York. He is the Clinical Director of Adolescent Services for Kids in Crisis and serves on the advisory board of Creative Alternatives of New York. He is the co-editor, with Anna Marie Weber, of *Clinical Applications of Drama Therapy in Child and Adolescent Treatment* (2005, New York: Brunner/Routledge). He has been fortunate to work with children from the inner city in shelters, community centers, hospitals, residential facilities and schools.

Maria Hodermarska, MA, RDT, CASAC, LCAT is Clinical Adjunct Assistant Professor for the New York University graduate program in Drama Therapy and Gallatin School of Individualized Studies. She works as a consultant in community-based mental health programs throughout New York City providing supervision and direct care in the areas of substance abuse treatment and drama therapy.

Flossie Ierardi, MA, MT-BC, LPC is a music therapist residing in the Philadelphia area. She is the Clinical Coordinator for the Hahnemann Creative Arts in Therapy Program at Drexel University, where she teaches clinical musical improvisation. Flossie studied music therapy at Temple University, following undergraduate and graduate studies in percussion performance. She is also a clinical practitioner with Kardon Institute for Arts Therapy, where she served as community connections director. Flossie has co-facilitated numerous drumming and movement workshops with Mark Bottos, dance/movement therapist, at Immaculata University for under-graduate music students, and in the Circles of Healing series. She also facilitates drum circles for people of all abilities in community and institutional settings. Her clinical experience includes adult psychiatry, geriatrics, at-risk youth, children with autism, and children and adults with developmental disabilities.

Susan Kierr, MA, ADTR, NCC is a dance/movement therapist who has been working in schools and hospitals in New Orleans, Louisiana, for the past twenty years. Before that, she worked in Boston, Massachusetts, where she pioneered the use of dance/movement therapy (DMT) with people suffering from chronic pain and physical disabilities. Her publications include 'Therapy for patients with spinal cord injuries', an article in the *American Journal of Dance Therapy*, Vol. 4, No. 1, documenting the use of DMT with people who are paralyzed. She coauthored *The Overeaters*, (Susan Kierr Wise and Jonathan Wise, MD, 1985), a book describing overeating and applying the use of DMT to treatment, with the theoretical framework of Eric Erikson's stages of development. In *When Words are not Enough*, (ed. F. Levy 1995), Susan's chapter, 'Treating anxiety; four case examples', illustrates the use of DMT therapy with people who have anxiety disorders. Susan is currently on the board of the American Dance Therapy Association, conducts workshops internationally, and offers supervision to other dance/movemen therapists.

Juliane Kowski, MA, MT-BC, LCAT was born and raised in East Germany and earned her B.A. at a German teaching institute. She obtained a second and third B.A. at the Music University in Berlin, and worked as a performer and vocal teacher of contemporary music and jazz. She obtained an M.A. degree in Music Therapy at New York University and completed her post-graduate AMT training with Benedikte Scheiby. She has worked for the Association for Help for Developmental Disabilities, with emotionally disturbed children at the Cumberlandt Family and Health and Support Center in Brooklyn, NY, with school-age children affected by 9/11 through the New York City Music Therapy Relief Project, with children and families suffering from trauma, grief and loss at the Lutheran Medical Center in Brooklyn, NY, and has established a private practice. She is married and has two sons. The family recently moved from New York to Jackson Hole, Wyoming, where she is working with the local public school system and is estab-lishing a private practice.

Julie Lacy, MA, AdDipArt, DipP'drama and GrpAnalysis, BA, DipT is a psychodrama psychotherapist, educator, actor and screenwriter. A teacher since 1980, and a graduate of the National Theatre Drama School (Australia) in 1985, Julie trained in the UK at the London Centre of Psychodrama and Group Psychotherapy and was the founding artistic director of London Playback Theatre (1991). She has worked as a therapist and arts-based psycho-ed facil-itator since 1992 in prisons, schools, community mental health, and private practice, in the UK, Hong Kong, and Darwin and Melbourne, Australia. She resides in Melbourne, where she prac-tices as a freelance therapist, facilitator, lecturer and screenwriter. Julie currently facilitates in Deakin University's Arts Lab program in the School of Nursing, La Trobe University's Master of Art Therapy program in the School of Public Health, and teaches in the School of Education at Victoria University. She is also writing and directing a documentary film about volunteers mentoring young people in the juvenile justice and child protection systems.

Janet K. Long, MA, LMFT, ART-BC has an art psychotherapy private practice in Oakland and Carmel in California, treating children, adolescents and adults. A licensed marriage and family therapist, she is also a practitioner of the Trager approach to psychophysical integration. She is an adjunct professor at the California College of the Arts in Oakland and at the University of California, Berkeley Extension. She has been practicing art therapy for 34 years in hospitals, schools, clinics, and agencies. She was the recipient of the Northern California Art Therapy Association's (NCATA) Distinguished Person Award in Education 1990, the Helen Landgarten

Award for Clinical Excellence in Art Therapy 1994, the U.C. Berkeley Extension Award for Excellence in Instruction 1998, the 2002 American Art Therapy Association Award for Service to Children, and the 2005 Honorary Life Membership Award by NCATA. She has published widely in the field of art therapy, and is a practicing artist who has exhibited her paintings, photographs and mixed-media sculptures in Europe and the United States.

Dorothy (Dali) McGuire, MAAT, LCPC is an art therapist and licensed clinical professional counselor at the Community Counseling Centers of Chicago (C4) where she currently coordinates individual, group and family art therapy services for the child and adolescent programs at C4. As a member of C4's art therapy team and under the direction of Joanne Ramseyer, ATR, LCPC, she also provides art therapy to adults with chronic psychiatric disorders and has co-curated several exhibits of client art work in the community over the past ten years. Ms McGuire is an alumna of Smith College and the School of the Art Institute of Chicago (SAIC) and has lectured and presented on art therapy topics including trauma and violence at SAIC, Northwestern University and Concordia College in Illinois.

Reina Michaelson, BA, GradDipEdPsych, PhD has a Bachelor of Arts from La Trobe University (1992), a Graduate Diploma in Education Psychology from Monash University (1993) and a Ph.D in Psychology from Victoria University (2001). In 1995 Reina established the first Australian school-based Child Sexual Abuse Prevention Program (CSAPP Inc.), and was the Young Australian of the Year (for Community Service) in 1997. CSAPP received the Australian Violence Prevention Award in 1998, and the National Child Abuse Prevention Award for Innovation in 2001. Reina's Ph.D, documenting and evaluating the development of CSAPP, was awarded the Vice Chancellor's Medal for Excellence in Research (2001). Reina has also established a retreat for abused and traumatized children. She has assisted a number of developing countries to develop their own prevention programs, including Malaysia and Vietnam. In addition to her work as Executive Director of CSAPP, Reina works as an international consultant with UNICEF.

Mary K. O'Brien, PhD has over 19 years of experience in the field of public health, with particular emphasis on violence prevention, program evaluation and health communications. Dr O'Brien is the founder and Executive Director of a non-profit organization called "A Better Philadelphia," whose mission is to address the root cultural causes of violence in the Delaware Valley region. She currently serves as a board member of Women Organized Against Rape and has served as a member on the board of directors for the National Clearinghouse for the Defense of Battered Women and for Women Against Abuse. She is involved with the Philadelphia Health Department's Division of Early Childhood, Youth and Women's Health in addressing issues of domestic violence in Asian communities in Philadelphia, and is a member of the policy team for the Philadelphia Women and Youth Death Review Team.

Linda Odell, MA has 16 years of experience with at-risk and troubled youth. For 10 years she worked as a classroom teacher for emotionally disturbed youth and transition coordinator for a residential treatment provider, developing curricula and programming for juvenile offenders throughout Colorado. Ms. Odell served as a guidance counselor in Costa Rica, developing service-learning programs with international middle-school students. She is currently employed by the City of Alexandria, developing youth programs for the 18th District Court Service Unit. Ms Odell holds a Master of Arts degree in special education from University of Northern Colorado, and has completed postgraduate studies in Language and Literacy with University of Colorado's Bueno Center for Multicultural Education. Ms Odell is co-creator and co-manager of the SOHO program and mentor to a SOHO graduate, Tiffany.

Suzannah Scott-Moncrieff, MA, MT-BC, LCAT is a graduate of New York University's Music Therapy program. She is currently employed as a music therapist at the Tomorrow's Children's Institute in New Jersey, where she specializes in using music therapy to meet the special needs of children with brain tumours, and their siblings.

Priyadarshini Senroy, MA, DMT, CCC is a drama and movement therapist residing in Toronto, Canada. She works with children with special needs and mental health issues. She is also on the board of the Creative Arts in Counseling Chapter of the Canadian Counseling Association. She has taught at various training programs in India, Thailand and Singapore. She has international experience in facilitating workshops in the UK, USA, and Canada. She has presented her multicultural work using drama and movement therapy at conferences and has contributed to newsletters and journals all over the world.

Sonali Senroy, BA is a counselor and therapeutic storyteller residing in Kolkata, India. She works with at-risk children, women and adults in her private practice. She has taught at various training programs in India, Thailand and Singapore. She has international experience in facilitating workshops in the UK, USA, and Canada. She has presented her multicultural work using drama and movement therapy at conferences and has contributed to newsletters and journals all over the world.

Laura Soble, MA, LMFT, REAT is a licensed marriage and family therapist and registered expressive arts therapist, and has an arts-based private psychotherapy practice in Oakland, California, specializing in children, adolescents and adults. She provides consultation and supervision on integrating the arts into the therapy process, and has presented widely at conferences, agencies and schools. Drawing on her background as a theatre director and musician, she employs a multimodal approach to using the arts and sandplay in therapy. She has created prevention programs for young people, blending the arts, therapy and education with focuses including violence prevention, nicotine dependence, and anger management. She has had articles published in the *Arts in Psychotherapy Journal*, and the *Journal of Sandplay Therapy*.

Dan Summer, ATR-BC is an art therapist in New York City. He is currently working with chemically dependent adults at Woodhull Medical center in Brooklyn NY. He graduated with a Masters Degree in Creative Arts Therapy from Hofstra University. He worked as a consultant for September Space, a program devoted to helping individuals process grief, loss, and trauma after 9/11. He worked as a consultant with Women against Violence, where he facilitated educational workshops on domestic violence and abusive relationships. He has worked with several after-school programs facilitating individual and group therapy for inner city youth, providing a safe environment, addressing conflict resolution, social deficits, and low self-esteem.

Carla van Laar, MCAT is a visual artist, therapist, author and educator. She lives in Melbourne with her family. An exhibiting and community artist since 1990, Carla graduated from the Master of Creative Arts Therapy program at the Royal Melbourne Institute of Technology (RMIT) in 2001. She now teaches in this program, and is also a doctoral researcher within the School of Education at RMIT. In 2001, whilst working within the juvenile justice system, Carla established Melbourne's first volunteer mentoring program for young people in custody. In addition to her ongoing work with CSAPP and ADAVIC, Carla is a staff member of the therapeutic team working with adolescents who have offended sexually, in the Male Adolescent Program for Positive Sexuality (MAPPS) in the Adolescent Forensic Health Services (AFHS) department at the Royal Children's Hospital (RCH), Melbourne. Carla's first book, *Bereaved Mother's Heart* (Bendigo, VIC: St Luke's Innovative Resources) explores the use of visual and text-based arts in living with grief and trauma, and will be published in 2006.

Subject Index

poems 159–60, 162, 183, 184, 219–20,
    298
    see also songwriting
poetry therapy 67, 182–3, 184
pollution, in inner cities 30
positive expectations, as a protective factor
    54
positive regard, in dance and movement
    therapy 237
positive transference 116
post-traumatic stress disorder 47–8, 60,
    123, 202
poverty
    and behavioral problems 44
    and delinquency 42–3
    and education 28–9, 44, 45
    effects 220
    and health 30
    and home environments 23–4
    predictors 23
    as a risk factor 19, 22–4
    statistics 16, 23, 28
    see also low-waged employment; welfare
        dependency
power
    in drama therapy 225
    and Whiteness 216
preschool education, as a protective factor
    53
pretend play, in play therapy 108, 111,
    112, 114
printmaking, in art therapy 176–7
problem-solving, in art therapy 123
problem-solving skills, as a protective
    factor 53–4
Project Yield 193
    see also Focus Youth Photography
        Project
prostitution, risk factors 36
psycho-opera *see* operatic play
psychodramatic therapy
    benefits 198–9
    empty chair 207, 208–9, 210
    journaling 206–8, 210
    locograms 203–4
    masks 204, 209–210
    memory sharing 205
    picture sociometry 203
    sculpting the self 209

song sharing 204–5
    theoretical background 283–4
    see also role training
psychodynamic play therapy *see* play
    therapy
psychological hardiness *see* resilience
psychological make-up
    as a protective factor 53–4
    as a risk factor 18–19
psychosocial adjustment 43–4
PTSD *see* post-traumatic stress disorder
purpose, in emotional literacy 201

racism
    coping skills 172
    as a risk factor 21–2
    see also minority ethnic groups
rage *see* aggression; anger
rapport, development of 234
reality rehearsal, in analytical music
    therapy 107, 112
relationships, development of 81–3, 261
repetitive play, in traumatized children
    106
residential care in India 269–70
    see also adolescents, in foster/residential
        care; drama and movement
        therapy
resilience 50, 181, 205
resistance 96, 116, 122, 133–4
risk factors 17–20
    see also environmental stressors; societal
        stressors
risk taking, in art therapy 123–4
rituals 101–2, 233–4, 236
role-definition 70–71
role models 62, 82, 90, 221
role play
    in drama therapy 185–6
    in play therapy 108, 111, 112, 113
role theory 218, 284
role training 284, 289–91
room remodeling, in art therapy 155–6,
    157
rules, for therapy 84, 87, 98, 99, 166–7,
    233–4, 286

Safe Expressions program
    art therapy 262–3

Author Index

Vanessa Camilleri begins this remarkable and unique volume by describing the complex context that creates the fabric of life for inner city, at-risk youth. This fragile fabric brings the need for arts therapies approaches with at-risk children into sharp focus. Pervasive societal, environmental, and domestic stressors easily shred this fabric, damaging lives and societies. The transformative nature of the creative arts therapies approaches engagingly described in this volume can moderate these effects to generate positive behavioral and emotional outcomes that affect individuals and communities.

Camilleri brings together an impressive, international group of creative arts therapists to describe work with children-at-risk from Chicago to Calcutta. This book is rich, original, timely, and inspiring. *Healing the Inner City Child: Creative Arts Therapies with At-risk Youth* is a must for all who care about the welfare of children. Its many resources include compelling accounts of arts therapies interventions, and goals and processes common to all creative arts therapies approaches. It should serve as an inspiration to creative arts therapists in training and in professional practice, and as a vital resource to school and community organizers who value the health and resilience of children.

Robyn Flaum Cruz, PhD, ADTR
Associate Professor, Lesley University Division of Expressive Therapies
Editor-in-Chief, The Arts in Psychotherapy